T0298363

TOXIC SEXUAL POLITICS

Toxic Sexual Politics

Toxicology, Environmental Poisons,
and Queer Feminist Futures

Melina Packer

NEW YORK UNIVERSITY PRESS
New York

NEW YORK UNIVERSITY PRESS
New York
www.nyupress.org

Please contact the Library of Congress for Cataloging-in-Publication data.

ISBN: 9781479828616 (hardback)
ISBN: 9781479828623 (paperback)
ISBN: 9781479828647 (library ebook)
ISBN: 9781479828630 (consumer ebook)

New York University Press books are printed on acid-free paper, and their binding materials are chosen for strength and durability. We strive to use environmentally responsible suppliers and materials to the greatest extent possible in publishing our books.

Manufactured in the United States of America

10 9 8 7 6 5 4 3 2 1

Also available as an ebook

To the anthropologist,

for the biochemist,

who together made me.

Their unsavory rages, their massacres and rapes, their atrocious rituals of militarized masculinity sprang not only from the economic lust for spices, silver and gold, but also from the implacable rage of paranoia.
—Anne McClintock

CONTENTS

LIST OF FIGURES AND TABLES

A Different Kind of Family History

Each of my paternal grandparents fled Eastern Europe shortly after the Bolshevik Revolution of 1917, arriving in New York City as children, along with thousands of other Jewish refugees. Had they not left when they did, they would have succumbed to either Stalin's purges or Hitler's gas chambers. Instead, as new immigrants in the United States, they enjoyed the opportunity to create a middle-class family with four children, living comfortably into their nineties. Along with fond memories of my grandmother's soup and my grandfather's humor, I recall their stories of survival shared around the dinner table.

Ironically, it was my maternal grandparents—who suffered neither anti-Semitism nor refugeehood—whose lives ended abruptly and prematurely. In the late 1960s, they moved to the San Joaquin Valley of California, settling into a small house nestled between vast grape vineyards and peach orchards. The seemingly pastoral landscape surrounding their home was sprayed heavily and frequently with pesticides. My mother remembers her parents routinely wiping toxic residues off their car windshield, in order to see out of it, with their bare hands. My grandfather, pictured in approximately 1976, blissfully unaware of the toxicity surrounding him, was trained as a chemist. He taught in public schools and became an active member in California high school science teachers' organizations toward the end of his career. Teaching chemistry, he believed and imparted what the agricultural-chemical corporations advertised regarding their products' safety, efficacy, and exigency.

I was only two years old when cancer took them away, and I can recall no memories of our chemically aborted relationship. As an adult, I learned that the "slow violence" of toxic environmental pollution is a direct descendant of the rapid brutality of fascism:[1] the same chemical

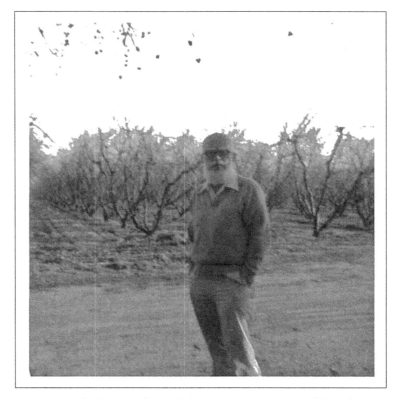

Figure 0.1: Author's maternal grandfather, circa 1976. Courtesy of the author.

weaponry that scientists developed for the world wars was repurposed as agricultural pesticide in the postwar years.[2]

It was not until my early thirties, while working on my PhD, that I interviewed one of my two maternal aunts seeking to learn more about her parents'—my grandparents'—sudden diagnoses. I preface this book with excerpts from our conversation because this personal history shapes my political, and physiological, position.

> AUNT: They moved to a fifty-five-and-older kind of community. It was real nice and they had their own little house. It was nice. So that's where they were when they got sick. . . . First she got it. And then he got it. Her first operation was on his birthday in August [1982], and he went in the hospital on her birthday in October [1982]! And then they—well, he passed away that December [1982] and she passed

away the following September [1983]. About nine months apart. . . .
When we would go to see my dad, [my mom] would say: [*whispers
emphatically*] *"Is he really going to die? Is he really going to die?"* And
I had to be the one to say, "Yeah, we have to be here for him."

MELINA: It seems like it happened so quickly.

A: It did.

M: Do you remember how it came on? Or when they noticed something was wrong? Did they attribute it to something?

A: They came up to see us in December [1981], and she was having
these really horrible stomach aches. And she said [*gestures with her
hands around her abdomen*]: "It's like, I feel like I'm having a baby. It's
all cramping."

And I said, "Well, did you go to the doctor?"

And she said, "Yeah, I went and I had a pap smear and all that and
everything was okay."

[*Sighs exasperatedly*] Like they checked, right? That was the summer that we . . . came and saw you guys [on the East Coast]. And I
can still remember calling, from your house, and that's when they
discovered she had the ovarian cancer. So then we drove home [back
to California]. . . . And then, his back started bothering him. He
started having real bad back pains, back here [*gestures toward her
midback*]. . . . He had esophageal cancer that had metastasized. . . .
They tried radiation and my dad wouldn't do it, after he had a couple
[treatments], he got too sick. And then they did chemo, and after a
while he just couldn't handle that. . . . He just said, "I've had a good
life, I don't understand all the pain. I'm done."

M: I'm sure this is hard for you to talk about, so we don't have to dwell
on this, but with the cancers, there's some suspicion that it was not
congenital, that it was exposure—

A: Oh, definitely! Oh, it's not in our genes [*pauses deliberately for emphasis*]. It was *environmental* [her emphasis]. You were never there, I
don't think, where they lived. . . . It was a little town, it's a bigger town
now, but then it only had 3,000 people. They lived on a grape vine-
yard and a peach orchard . . . and [the growers] used pesticides. And
my dad would just brush them off the car like that [*gestures with her
forearm, swiping across a surface vigorously and impatiently*] and they
[*speaks slowly and emphatically*] *drank their water out of a well.* . . .

I would come home for vacation, like Easter or whatever, and I can still remember my mom going, "Remember that nice Mr. S that lived right down there?"

I'd say, "Yeah."

"He's got cancer!"

Next time I come home, "Oh you know his wife has it now!"

None of 'em—because you see pesticides were just starting to get the bad name. And those were the bad pesticides. And they were breathing it in, and they were walking—we'd walk out into the vineyards and get grapes and we'd wash 'em off but, you know, we were all ignorant. So, given the fact there is no [family] history of it, [the oncologist] said, "This is a case of environmental pollution."

M: Did they make those connections when they saw all their neighbors getting sick, and then they got sick—did they talk about it in that way?

A: [*Shakes her head*] No. And nobody really did then. And it—I mean, I don't—I just think—like with the water, I mean, they were drinking this polluted, polluted water, because of all the pesticides on both [crops]. And no, it didn't—I mean, later they realized, you know when the news was coming out, if you lived in the San Joaquin Valley in these certain areas. Bakersfield is one of the very worst. And a lot of the young men are sterile. They can't even have kids. I mean, it's so affected their bodies. Yeah. So I'm a believer that it was brought on that way. And if you think about it, your mom hasn't had any issues, [the middle sister] hasn't had any issues, I haven't had any issues. If it were genetic by now one of us would have had some little somethin'. But we haven't. . . . It's not a genetic—I mean, you might have a predisposition, cellwise, if you get polluted, but it wasn't something in the family history.

M: How old were you all?

A: I was thirty-six.

M: And your parents were . . . ?

A: Sixty-six. Sixty-six. And that's pretty young.

M: Was there anger too, especially knowing it was environmental?

A: We were all upset. But I guess for me I just had to go into the mode of, "I've gotta be there, I've gotta help, I've gotta—I don't have the time to scream and yell and get mad."

After listening to my aunt's story, I realized something that in retrospect is rather obvious: people who are dying of cancer, and those caring for them, typically do not have the time, energy, or emotional capacity to respond politically. This particular kind of violence—toxic exposure—is so visceral, so intimately and deeply debilitating, if not deadly, that perhaps it is no wonder agrochemical corporations continue to produce and deploy pesticides with practical impunity, despite all the evidence pointing to these chemicals' culpability. They are literally killing the opposition.

Several months later, I asked my other aunt to add her perspective on the tragedy. She too remembered how almost everyone who lived in that area died of cancer. Moreover, she recalled the valley's migrant farm workers who had "terrible health problems"—infants born with severe deformities, spontaneous abortions and miscarriages, infertility, and so on. In her memory, she and her sisters did briefly consider filing a lawsuit, but "none of us had any money" and worried the chemical corporations would drag their case out for decades—"[suing] was impossible back then." She mused further: "That whole area of former vineyards and orchards is now covered with suburban housing. I doubt that the people who live there now know the cancer history of that [place]." After a pause, she continued, "I think [we sisters] were . . . dumbfounded and deeply saddened by our mother's inability to make sense of it all. She was literally blindsided! Of course, she had already been given a terminal sentence when our father was diagnosed. After her first surgery, they gave her one to three years, and she barely made it over a year. Our father was of course blindsided and confused too. Both had been so healthy all their lives and they thought they were moving to a safe place out in the country."

To what extent do my two sets of grandparents' different, but related, toxic environmental exposures become my biological and sociological predisposition to these linked threats? I have a family history of cancer, among other health issues, but not in the strictly physical way the biomedical establishment would have me understand. Family medical history is always already social, racial, political, and environmental. Genetics, by contrast, seem almost inconsequential.

I wonder, too, how my grandfather might have taught chemistry differently, if at all, or whether my grandparents would have chosen to teach in California's Central Valley had they been educated then in the political economic histories of pesticide deployment that I know now. What larger and broader social forces, for that matter, constitute the *preconditions* for chemical warfare, ethnic cleansing, chemical pest control (as it were), and the supposedly neutral science of poisons?

Toxic Sexual Politics brings attention to toxicology's role in making the political *this* personal, or, conversely, how the science of poisons obscures such relations. I hope my work helps transform toxicological training such that persecuted peoples and their allies, acting on behalf of life-threatened biodiversity around the planet, can more meaningfully promise: never again—to anyone.

Introduction

Finding the Man in the Science

All dimensions of state power, and not merely some overtly "patriarchal" aspect, figure in the gendering of the state. The state can be masculinist without intentionally or overtly pursuing the "interests" of men precisely because the multiple dimensions of socially constructed masculinity have historically shaped the multiple modes of power circulating through the domain called the state—this is what it means to talk about masculinist power rather than the power of men.
—Wendy Brown[1]

Masculinist Science Feminizing Frogs

My favorite meme about so-called gay frogs—feared to be feminized by toxic chemicals—is captioned "You have to be male or female!" Directly beneath this exclamation is a cartoon drawing of a clinic-blue, gloved human hand holding a green frog, whose legs dangle passively under their suspended body. The frog appears to be calmly responding, or at least thinking, "bro relax I am literally just attractive." Underneath this image and text is a scene from the gay cowboy movie *Brokeback Mountain*, showing Heath Ledger's character, Ennis, hugging Jake Gyllenhaal's character, Jack, from behind. I wish I knew whom to credit for this clever visual, but memes defy proprietary authorship by design.[2]

Mediatized panic over the specter of gay frogs, including queer mockery of this panic, has a more traceable history. Beginning in the 1990s, scientists began sounding the alarm over synthetic substances called endocrine-disrupting chemicals, which interfere with naturally

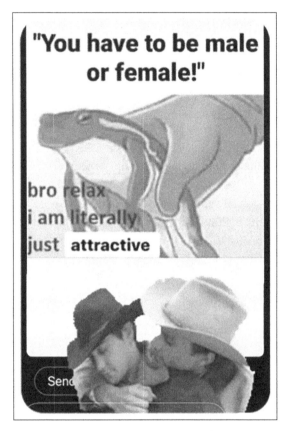

Figure 1.1: One of many memes about gay frogs.

occurring hormones and thus interfere with all kinds of bodily functions and organ development, including but not limited to reproductive organs. While these environmental health scientists meant well, and hormone-interfering chemicals do appear to cause serious health issues, including cancer and diabetes, the science and advocacy around these chemicals almost exclusively focused on their reportedly feminizing effects, in terms of reproductive organs as well as what's understood as sexual behavior.[3] One 2008 documentary lamented the "disappearing male," for instance, and a 2021 book by epidemiologist Shanna Swan,[4] publicly endorsed by famed environmental activist Erin Brockovich, despaired over the threats that "plummeting sperm counts" and "shrinking penises" posed to humanity.[5]

Frogs, meanwhile, have been a model organism for laboratory science for as long as laboratory science has existed.[6] And frogs make sense to study in the context of toxic environmental exposures because they spend so much of their lives in the water, where so much chemical pollution circulates. Scientists studying the effects of endocrine-disrupting chemicals on frogs widely reported that individual frogs exposed to these chemicals displayed same-sex sexual behavior, exhibited both female- and male-marked phenotypes, and as tadpoles changed sex during development, resulting in what researchers and journalists variously called "gay," "intersex," or "transgender" frogs (with "sad sex lives" to boot).[7] Queerness was thus characterized as a *bad* outcome of toxic exposure, and media outlets—both mainstream and fringe—were quick to jump directly from frog to human bodies and behaviors.[8]

Framing same-sex sexual behavior, transness, or intersex conditions as both unnatural and undesirable has a long and ugly history that continues to rear its ugly head, as demonstrated by recent and proliferating statewide bans on gender-affirming care and sexuality education.[9] But labeling frogs as harmed by toxicants because toxicants "make them gay" is not only socially wrong, it's also biologically wrong. Frogs, among many other animal species, engage in same-sex sexual behaviors in the wild all the time.[10] And tadpoles, it turns out, change sex all the time, irrespective of chemical exposure.[11] Intersex frogs, meanwhile, can still successfully mate to produce offspring.[12] Scientists overwhelmingly assumed that intersex frogs and male-male frog sex—nobody seemed concerned about female-female frog sex—demonstrated evidence of chemical harm because that's what biological sciences like toxicology have taught them. I hope my work helps correct this scientific and popular miseducation, for the sake of stamping out stigma as well as injustice. Toxic environmental pollution, as environmental researchers and activists have amply documented, is indeed demonstrably harmful, while its demonstrable harms are vastly and unevenly deployed. The challenge I offer, and rise to, is how to organize effective political action against the poisoners without stigmatizing the poisoned. Throughout this book I push people to ask not simply *what* makes a poison but rather *who*?

Chemical Agents

The American Chemistry Council is the oldest trade organization in the United States. The group was founded in 1872 as the Manufacturing Chemists Association, and its members later renamed it the Chemical Manufacturers Association before opting for yet another rebrand circa 2000 as the American Chemistry Council.[13] The rhetorical transition—from manufacturing chemists to chemical manufacturers to no mention of manufacturing whatsoever—is telling. I venture a guess that this lobbying organization's new moniker, American Chemistry Council, was intentionally chosen to closely resemble that of its scholarly counterpart, the American Chemical Society. My research suggests that the distinction between chemical trade and chemical science (never mind chemical policy) is not so neatly delineated in any case.[14]

Alongside the US Federal Reserve, the American Chemistry Council has tracked domestic, industrial chemical production since 1919. Exact volumes are hard to pin down, however, as prior to 1972, chemical production—which was significant, given the world wars—was subsumed under the more general categories of "manufacturing, mining, and agriculture."[15] One might turn to the US Environmental Protection Agency's Chemical Data Reporting (CDR) system, established in 1986, but this gauge is extremely limited.[16] CDR relies on chemical manufacturers to report their own production data, and they only are required to report on toxicants produced in excess of 25,000 pounds annually. (There is an exception for the subset of toxicants specifically regulated by the Toxic Substances and Control Act [TSCA] of 1976, *which excludes pharmaceuticals and pesticides*, as well as food and cosmetics;[17] TSCA toxicants must be reported if their annual production volume exceeds 2,500 pounds. What a relief.) Additionally, this federally mandated reporting of *some* toxicants does not include chemical production stemming from processing or use—only manufacturing. Needless to say, additional chemicals are produced during processing and use. Even with its sizable limitations, not all of which are listed here, CDR statistics are staggering: this mere fraction of US toxicant production volume totaled 7.1 trillion pounds in 2020 alone (figure 1.2).[18] In terms of the number of different synthetic chemicals actively circulating, estimates range from 9,000 (if one asks the chemical industry) to 85,000

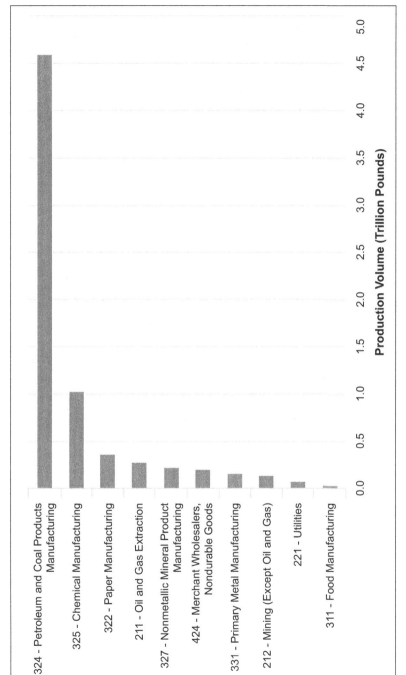

Figure 1.2: (Partial) Production Volume of the Top Ten US Chemical Manufacturing Sectors in 2020. US Environmental Protection Agency 2022.

(if one asks environmental health scientists).[19] While total toxicant tonnage remains evasive by volume, the American Chemistry Council is eager to boast of its industry's production totals by dollar, valued at $614.2 billion in 2022. The United States is currently the world's second-largest industrial chemical producer, after only the People's Republic of China, responsible for approximately 11 percent of global toxicant production.[20] Notably, in contrast to Environmental Protection Agency data, American Chemistry Council data include chemicals produced via processing and use.

Even if precise numbers were attainable, I argue throughout this book that strictly quantitative measures cannot capture the expanse of chemical exposure. Chemicals are slippery, diffuse, gaseous, volatile. As medical anthropologist Vincanne Adams writes of the ubiquitous pesticide glyphosate, better known as Roundup, such synthetic substances have an "ability to shape-shift into a biological-then-chemical-then-biological thing," to say nothing of "the human constituencies, institutions, and politics that have played important roles" in manufacture, deployment, and ingestion.[21] When does the measuring of DDT begin or end (to name another one of tens of thousands of toxicants) given how its chemical structure changes as it is metabolized and remetabolized by various organisms, or given how it persists in the environment, and in our bodies, long after production ceases?[22] There seems to remain not a single synthetic-chemical-free space on this planet, and there will never be such a space well into the (un)foreseeable future, as some metabolites of radioactive toxicants possess "half-lives"—the length of time it takes for half of its constitutive elements to decay—in the millions of years.[23] These somewhat inconceivable, and often visually imperceptible, metric tons of toxicants are strongly associated with all manner of physical and mental health ills, ailing all manner of organisms (and their future offspring), including asthma, Alzheimer's, cancers, cardiovascular failures, diabetes, depression, miscarriage, multiple sclerosis, sterility, and silicosis, among numerous other diagnoses. Increasing evidence points to a plethora of mysterious new infirmities not yet named, temporarily (?) grouped under the general headings Multiple Chemical Sensitivity (MCS) or Toxic-Induced Loss of Tolerance (TILT).[24] More-than-human animals and plants are likewise adversely affected at alarming numbers the world over; even microbes and bacteria cannot seem to escape the effects of toxic exposures.[25] Our thoroughly—and unevenly—chemically saturated condition led some scholars to pronounce this world "permanently polluted" in 2018.[26] Incidentally, the Oxford word of the year for 2018 was, you guessed it, *toxic*.[27] How did we get into this toxic mess?

Before shedding some light on the enabling preconditions for permanent pollution, it's worth pausing for a moment to define *toxic*, at least for the purposes of this project. Oxford chooses its word of the year based on the following criteria: "A word or expression that is judged to reflect the ethos, mood, or preoccupations of the passing year, and have lasting potential as a term of cultural significance."[28] Oxford linguists define toxic as "poisonous," and further note that this mid-seventeenth-century English word began as the ancient Greek *toxikon pharmakon*, referring to plant- or animal-derived toxins that hunters and warriors, presumably, smeared on the tips of their arrows—one of the earliest forms of chemical weaponry, it would seem.[29] Notably, *toxikon* is the ancient Greek word for bow, not for poison. *Pharmakon* is ancient Greek for poison, and yet medieval Latin borrowed the Greek *toxikon* for its *toxicus*, meaning poisoned. The English word *toxic*, or poisonous, emerged from this Latin derivative. Given how toxic chemicals have been and continue to be violently deployed, it is perhaps fitting that today's *toxic* stems from the poisoner's bow rather than the poison itself.

Without dwelling too long on Oxford's singular decision regarding the 2018 word of the year, I want to reiterate that Oxford chooses this word to reflect the year's "ethos, mood, or preoccupations." The top two word collocates, or words "habitually used alongside" toxic in 2018 were (first) chemical and (second) masculinity.[30] My training in feminist science studies tells me this pairing of collocates is no coincidence. Indeed, I use toxic to refer not only to the poisonous properties of synthetic chemicals themselves but also to the masculinist prerogative, as political scientist Wendy Brown might term it, to invent and disseminate such poisons. It would be overly simplistic to suggest that all chemicals are always toxic, but I submit that it is equally sloppy to suggest, as prominent toxicologists have since the inception of their discipline, that synthetic chemicals are generally safe, even harmless. *Toxic Sexual Politics* argues that founding toxicologists' interested decisions about whether and to what extent a synthetic chemical is toxic are uncertain at best, sexist and white supremacist at worst. Put another way, toxic exposures are not produced by toxicants alone.

Social studies of science and environmental justice scholarship generally present two main causes of our permanently polluted world: corporate greed and structural racism.[31] I started the research that morphed into this book, way back when as a fledgling PhD candidate, because I believed the reasons for today's ubiquitous and unevenly distributed toxic environmental pollution were not fully explained by such "deceit and denial" accounts,[32] meaning those that blame corrupt chemical manufacturers and revolving door regulators (the latter referring to former chemical industry employees who become chemical regulatory agency bureaucrats, and vice versa). Reams of evidence point to corporate culpability around numerous toxic disasters, and I have no reason to disbelieve the meticulous documentation of the many, reputable researchers who thoroughly demonstrate the industry malfeasance and regulatory failures behind toxic exposures.[33]

What I found unsatisfying about many of these accounts, however, was the contrasting of "sound science" against "sounds like science," to quote epidemiologist David Michaels's turn of phrase.[34] Critical race theory and feminist science studies, relevant elements of which I will share in these pages, taught me that "sound science," too, is political through and through. Even the excellent interventions from environmental justice (EJ) literature,[35] which places greater emphasis on the second overarching cause of permanent pollution—structural racism— tends not to question the validity of the basic science of poisons itself, toxicology.[36]

The US environmental justice movement emerged out of the racial, sexual, and economic justice movements of the 1960s and '70s.[37] Poor people and people of color recognized that they were being unjustly exposed to more toxicants than their wealthier and white counterparts and organized to bring polluting industries and enabling regulators to account for these uneven exposures.[38] While I am fully in support of environmental justice, I join other EJ-supportive science studies scholars in cautioning EJ activists against leveraging toxicological findings for their campaigns, even when scientific studies corroborate polluted communities' lived experiences of illness.[39] I advise against using toxicology for environmental justice because my research reveals both how uncertain and how interested (as opposed to disinterested) the science of toxicology is.[40] In other words, today's toxicology rests on an incredibly unstable foundation both methodologically and politically. This scientific discipline was initially designed for and by people enthusiastic about toxicant use—by those drawing the poisoned bows, not those pierced by the poisonous arrows.

Toxicology: The Basic Science of Poisons

Founded in 1961, the US Society of Toxicology seems to have arrived on the global toxicant stage rather belatedly, in light of the reality that chemical manufacturers (or was it manufacturing chemists?) synthesized some of the first industrial toxicants, phosgene and mustard gas—both chemical weapons, nonincidentally—in 1865, nearly one hundred years prior.[41] Surely a basic science of poisons was well in demand well before 1961. As I will detail in chapters 1 and 2, the founding fathers of the US-based scientific discipline of toxicology were not overwhelmingly concerned with tens of thousands of new toxicants' potential hazards, but were rather more enamored with synthetic chemicals' potential for better living, to borrow DuPont Corporation's tagline of the time ("better living . . . through chemistry").[42] I submit that the midcentury US scientists who contrived of modern toxicology, which they self-titled "the basic science of poisons," devised this simultaneously basic and applied discipline in order to *make toxicants safe*, and thus assure their continued production and limited regulation.[43]

I am not arguing that US toxicology's founding fathers were simply industry shills—though, importantly, early toxicological experiments were almost exclusively funded by the US Department of Defense.[44] As mentioned, I myself have always found the deceit and denial thesis to be missing something—surely blaming bad apple scientists is too simplistic. Instead, my argument is a critical race feminist intervention: I argue that US toxicology emerged out of a specifically white supremacist and masculinist epistemic entitlement, engaging in a sort of chemical gaslighting, if you will.[45] The scientific elites who codified toxicology, several of whom readers will meet in chapters 1 and 2, occupied particular gender-, race-, and class-privileged social locations, positions which empowered them to *grant themselves the authority* to define what makes a toxicant safe (and measurable), what chemical risks are acceptable (and to whom), and how much of an exposure is tolerable (where, for whom, and for what). I further argue that toxicology's inherent biases undermine the usefulness of toxicological findings for environmental justice struggles, despite toxicologists' best intentions, by focusing on the environmental toxicology and ecotoxicology of endocrine-disrupting chemicals (EDCs), which is the sub-field fretting about feminized frogs.[46]

I do not mean to sound flippant; EDCs are a class of toxicants that have become ubiquitous throughout our environments, being constitutive components of such commonplace objects as plastic bottles, receipt paper, or body lotion, among many other items. EDCs are particularly alarming to scientists and other environmental health advocates because they have been shown to interfere with our bodies' hormonal processes via the endocrine system. Hormonal disturbances, in turn, can adversely affect fundamental aspects of physiological development and function, leading to a range of serious health issues, including different cancers and cardiovascular and metabolic failures.[47] Moreover, because EDCs either mimic or override bodies' naturally occurring hormone signals and hormone receptors, these particular toxicants may be more harmful at lower doses than at higher doses, upending the core tenet of toxicology: "the dose makes the poison" (an apparent contradiction I elaborate on in chapter 2). My work does not question the urgency of attending to EDC contamination, but rather how EDC toxicology inadvertently—or by design—reviles the poisoned more than the poisoner.

Critical Race and Feminist Theory

In proposing that EDC toxicology is inherently masculinist and white supremacist, I am not name-calling individual EDC scientists. Rather, I am drawing from the intellectual and activist traditions of critical race feminism, which help explain how *institutions* can be racist and (hetero)sexist, not merely individuals.[48] Ideologies such as racism and sexism are structural and structuring, meaning that supposedly neutral entities like the law, or science, are in fact built in ways that preserve the advantages of dominant members of society and developed in ways that privilege the worldview of the dominant culture. Legal scholar Kimberlé Crenshaw's highly influential intersectionality theory, for example, stems from how US discrimination law allowed for only white women's experience of gender discrimination and only African American men's experience of race discrimination, thus cornering African American women into "a location that resists telling" and erasing African American women's intersectional experiences of discrimination[49]—which are sometimes similar to white women's and sometimes similar to African American men's, but are oftentimes only experienced by African American women as uniquely (not additively) *both* gender *and* race discrimination.[50] Intersectionality has since been applied well beyond the black-white or woman-man binary, as Crenshaw's concept helps illuminate the multiple, contingent facets of all people's complex social identities in different times and places.[51]

Similar to critical race theory, though more focused on sex and gender, feminist theory describes how supposedly neutral institutions are inherently patriarchal. Political scientist Wendy Brown, whose pivotal "Finding the Man in the State" article inspired my title for this introductory chapter, demonstrates how the modern state can be masculinist "without intentionally or overtly pursuing the 'interests' of men."[52] Brown argues that modern state structures assume and build on preexisting patriarchal social orders such as the private sphere (coded female) versus the public sphere (coded male). Even when women are granted civil rights then, they are merely expected to conform to an existing system that was derived by and for elite men.[53] The standardized nine-to-five workday (brought about by working-class agitation, ironically[54]) effectively, if simply, illustrates what Brown means by "the Man in the State": a nine-to-five workday makes sense only for socially and economically privileged men who are so fortunate as to have wives or domestic servants at home, caring for children and preparing meals, among other forms of reproductive labor.[55]

Women, thanks to generations of activism, are no longer as explicitly excluded from pursuing careers in public, and it's important to note that historically, poor women of all ethnicities could hardly have hoped to avoid working for a living.[56] In any case, the nine-to-five workday continues to disadvantage women who work such hours outside the home yet remain primarily responsible for childcare and other domestic arts inside the home.[57] In short, critical race and feminist theory show how the past's more rampant forms of white supremacy and patriarchy persist structurally and implicitly (of course, explicit racism and sexism hasn't gone away). EDC toxicology is no exception—or, to paraphrase Brown, science can be masculinist without overtly pursuing the interests of men.

For example, recent efforts by science and policy elites to include fence-line communities—meaning those who are disproportionately more burdened by toxic environmental exposures—in epidemiological studies do not deign to question the toxicological precepts of those studies.[58] As political scientist Sarah Wiebe notes from her research alongside Indigenous (Aaamjiwnaang) EJ movements in what's called the Chemical Valley in Canada, "When citizens are brought 'into' a conversation about health and, in this case, about the recognition of reproductive health concerns, a paradox of engagement becomes apparent: citizens are expected to adopt the terms of dialogue or debate, which may not necessarily provide a context for empowerment and the recognition of particular claims."[59] Toxicology does not generate neutral data and, moreover, does not accommodate all the evidence that exceeds quantitative categories.[60]

Postcolonial and Feminist Science and Technology Studies

Postcolonial and feminist science and technology studies (STS) show how today's dominant form of biological science, which is widely perceived as purely factual and objective, emerged from the historical, sociocultural, and economic contexts of European imperialism, the transatlantic slave trade, and Christian patriarchy, and thus bears the imprints of those violent formative years.[61] Even such seemingly neutral categories as "species"—important to this book because of toxicology's decisions about which animals may be used as substitutes for humans when testing toxicants—are steeped in racist and sexist ideologies. Critical historians of science have brilliantly, and disturbingly, shown how European and Euro-American taxonomies of so-called human races and animal species were devised in tandem, meaning that fictions of racial hierarchies remain inseparable from species taxonomies.[62] European naturalists and explorers (who are often framed as innocently joining missionary, merchant, and militaristic vessels to the New World[63]) considered people, or "primitives," in the parlance of that time, from Africa and Asia to be lesser forms of human, less advanced specimens on a Darwinian evolutionary scale.[64] Black people in particular were seen as the "missing link" between apes and humans, and this racist "chain of being" is still invoked today, insidiously reappearing in everything from contemporary genetics and anthropology to animal welfare and wildlife management.[65] Dominant science's hierarchies of species, whether from hairy monkey to white man, or invertebrate to vertebrate, have become so integrated into the realm of common sense, so internalized and normalized in contemporary culture, that the systematic killing of *millions* of animals per year for scientific research barely registers for either the general public or highly trained specialists, as I discuss in chapter 5.[66]

Importantly for my ensuing analysis of EDCs in particular, which affect hormones and hence reproductive and sexual development, postcolonial and feminist STS demonstrate how sex and gender are always already racialized as well. Elite Europeans constructed enduring ideals of white, Victorian femininity against the constitutive difference of women of African descent especially—conflating sex categories with gender in the process. Dominant ideologies about proper feminine behavior and normal female anatomy were based on a specifically white ideal, which, in turn, was positioned explicitly against and as superior to the hypersexualized and animalized Black female Other.[67] (This co-constitution of race, sex, and gender certainly complicates Crenshaw's intersectionality thesis, but I digress.[68])

Heterosexuality is racialized too.[69] Because Western European and Euro-American notions of ideal-type masculinity and femininity, including a binary system for sex, gender, and sexuality, were shaped in constitutive opposition to the varying cultures of sex, gender, and sexuality observed in those societies deemed primitive, the heterosexual norm is also the white norm.[70] Such white supremacist conceptions of sex, gender, and sexuality are why EDC toxicology's assumptions about normal sex and sexual behaviors, deliberated in chapter 4, support my overarching argument that EDC toxicology is inherently white supremacist and heteropatriarchal, even when its practitioners do not identify as such. Again, to paraphrase Wendy Brown, this is what it means to talk about masculinist science rather than the science of men.[71]

Western European and Euro-American scientific knowledge production, what I refer to as *dominant science,* is shaped by what its powerful practitioners want to believe and want others to know, steeped in specific historical and cultural contexts. Founding US toxicologist Louis J. Casarett, for instance, colorfully described several conniving women of "Ancient Rome" and the European Medieval and Renaissance periods, repeatedly presenting "the distaff set,"[72] as he categorized the female of the human species, as murderous sorceresses. Casarett juxtaposed these irrational if clever ladies against rational, enlightened men, most famously Paracelsus (c. 1493–1541), who swoop into the historical record, cleaning up lady poisoners' and primitives' acts of nonscientific poisoning, a choreography I describe in greater detail in chapter 3.[73]

Postcolonial and feminist STS also highlights other(ed) forms of scientific knowledge production that predate and persist through colonial encounters, many of which do not subscribe to dominant science's Cartesian framework, or one that conceptualizes the mind as separate from, and superior to, the body.[74] Several different, marginalized traditions view the cosmos and its inhabitants (material and spiritual) as interdependent and porous,[75] in stark contrast to dominant toxicology's approach, which presumes that a toxicant designed to kill insects or rodents or fungi can somehow remain safe for what are termed nontarget organisms and ecosystems.[76] (Note that my critical race feminist analysis of US toxicology does not throw the toxicological-findings baby out with the toxicology-methods bathwater; more on this distinction to come.) Cultural geographer Max Liboiron insists moreover that pollution *is* colonialism: twentieth and now twenty-first century US and Canadian scientists who determined so-called tolerable levels of pollution presumed that the land and water was theirs to pollute in the first place.[77] They (we) are polluting stolen territories, without Native and First Nations peoples' permission, with pollutants that emerge from (settler) colonial scientific and economic structures, which, in turn, determine what is an acceptable, measurable, amount of pollution. These are not innocent, apolitical definitions and measurements, however quantitative or mathematical they might appear.[78] Thus even an EDC toxicologist who measures the adverse effects of chemical contaminants today in an effort to *reduce* contamination can be participating in a colonial knowledge system.

Critical Environmental History

In addition to the environment's uses and abuses, what constitutes the environment more broadly is inextricable from sexual and racial hierarchies. US notions of wilderness, shaped during the conservation and preservation movements that presaged late twentieth-century environmentalism, are intimately intertwined with white supremacist and masculinist ideologies. Famed conservation figures like John Muir, Gifford Pinchot, and Theodore Roosevelt were ardent eugenicists who believed Native Americans were lesser forms of human who should be removed from their ancestral homelands because they were incapable of properly stewarding (read: controlling) the natural landscape.[79] And yet even as powerful white men relegated men of color, especially Black and Indigenous men, to the realm of the primitive or savage, they simultaneously fetishized and envied what they imagined to be these othered men's hypersexuality and animality, given how they positioned Black and Indigenous peoples as closer to Nature (and further from Culture). For all its widely touted benefits, Western civilization, including the rapidly industrializing and urbanizing US frontier, was seen as feminizing. Fearful that their manhood and social power was slipping, elite white men (alongside their elite white women allies) enthusiastically embraced environmental causes *as* eugenics, advocating for the preservation of wild spaces and segregated national parks to enable rugged, outdoor recreation that would guarantee the continued virility of able-bodied, heterosexual white men, who would thus germinate future generations of this allegedly superior human race.[80]

We shall see how these eugenic notions of racial and environmental purity and (white) male virility persist into contemporary environmentalism vis-à-vis EDC contamination, as anti-toxics advocates and scientists alike mobilize tired tropes of lowered intelligence and declining sperm due to chemical exposures.[81] Sociologist Scott Frickel's study of genetic toxicologists, markedly, found that the scientists "who led the movement to establish genetic toxicology had far more enduring loyalties to human genetics and its promise to cure genetic disease than to toxicology and the emerging field of environmental health. They also harbored stronger commitments to the politics and social activism of an older, and largely discredited, eugenics movement than to a new wave of environmentalism. . . . Chemical mutagens threatened the long-term integrity of the human gene pool as well as the environmental health of living individuals and communities."[82] Addressing the flip side of this feared feminization coin, *Toxic Sexual Politics* also analyzes performances of (hyper)masculinity in modern-day "weed scientists," who overwhelmingly rely on toxic substances, power tools, and militarized metaphors to "control noxious weeds," as I describe in chapter 3. Overall, I rely on critical environmental historians to argue that Euro-American, Christian, and (settler) colonial ideologies—wherein White Man is entitled to dominion over Nature, Woman, Nonwhite Human, and Animal, while His Culture is superior to a feminized and racialized Nature—taint even the most well-intentioned toxicology and anti-toxics advocacy.[83]

Queer Ecologies and Critical Disability Studies

Finally, the scholarly activist fields of queer ecologies and critical disability studies also enrich this feminist study of EDC toxicology. These scholars and activists urge researchers to recognize that the so-called normal or natural physiologies and behaviors that EDC scientists rely on to mark postexposure physiologies and behaviors as *ab*normal or *un*natural are likewise based on heterosexist, racist, and ableist ideologies.[84] EDC research overwhelmingly assumes that same-sex sexual behavior, in amphibians, birds, and so on, is an *adverse* outcome of EDC exposure, despite the widespread prevalence of same-sex sexual behavior across a multitude of species.[85] This scientific literature also characterizes frog "sex-reversal," for example, as harmful and unnatural, when in fact wild frogs frequently develop both female- and male-sexed phenotypes irrespective of exposure to EDCs.[86] What is more, EDC research tends to conclude that physical intersex characteristics in frogs, such as individuals with eggs cells in their testes, threaten species survival when in reality these frogs (labeled intersex) can still mate and reproduce successfully.[87] Queer ecology, however, is not simply about naturalizing same-sex sexual behaviors and intersexed physiologies, but also about "asking different questions" and asking questions differently.[88] Whereas environmental-health-leaning toxicology has tended to ask "How are toxicants making organisms abnormal?," an EDC toxicology informed by queer ecology and feminist biology might ask instead "What human and chemical agents have historically and are currently altering this organism's environment (broadly defined), and what can we learn about the capaciousness of eco-biological processes from the myriad of different ways that different organisms adapt and interact?" Sociologist Myra Hird suggests, for instance, that the work is not so much about queering nature as it is about reconceiving how the world is "naturally queer."[89]

Scientist feminists point out that concerns about adverse cognitive and developmental outcomes of EDC exposure[90]—"threatening our fertility, intelligence, and survival"[91] to borrow the subtitle of one of the earliest scientific advocacy publications—are disturbingly resonant with eugenicist anxieties about the devolution of the so-called white race (in the event that good stock fail to restore their vitality in wild outdoor spaces with vigorous activities or interbreed with people of color, poor people, so-called feeble-minded people, or people with bodies labeled deformed).[92] Again, these criticisms are not meant to suggest that EDC researchers are card-carrying eugenicists. My concern, rather, is that the framing of well-intentioned research on the adverse outcomes of EDC exposure inadvertently reproduces the very same eugenicist logics that generate environmental injustices in the first place, in the sense that marginalized people are disproportionately more exposed to toxic chemicals because they are fundamentally disregarded as lesser and hence disposable humans, while the spaces where they live, learn, work, play, pray, and eat are rendered pollutable.[93]

Environmental toxicologists and ecotoxicologists counter, however, that physiological functions *are* harmed by endocrine-disrupting chemicals, as evidenced by piles of ecological, biological, experiential, and medical studies.[94] The environmental health researchers I interviewed were also quick to point out the political economic asymmetries of synthetical chemical production and deployment, as compared to academic and governmental research (putting aside for the moment how these categories—industry, academy, government—overlap and intersect).[95] As one state-level environmental health regulator freely admitted to me, "The laws in which we operate are limited; they're implemented in a way that's friendly to [chemical manufacturers]."[96] And an environmental toxicologist working for a national nonprofit declared that "the whole way the system is set up is backwards; we're chasing something that's already happened, it's like trying to get a cat back in the bag. Places are already contaminated, people are invested. . . . [Chemical] risk assessment was set up for the time [1970s–1980s], but now we know it's underestimating risk, and industry thinks it's overestimating."[97] Because the chemical industry already holds an enormous financial advantage over government officials and hence environmental regulations, anti-toxics advocates find it politically (and environmentally) dangerous to downplay the adverse effects of EDC exposure in any way, shape, or form.

Toward Critical Toxicity Studies

The challenge for critical feminists and EDC toxicologists, including of course those who identify as both, is to communicate the urgency of reducing toxic pollution—by *both* better regulating chemicals *and* reining in corporate power—without resorting to eugenicist and masculinist tropes of deformity, low intelligence, queerness, or weakness.[98] As disability justice activist Eli Clare asks, "How do we witness, name, and resist the injustices that reshape and damage all kinds of bodies—plant and animal, organic and inorganic, human and more-than-human? And alongside our resistance how do we make peace with the reshaped and damaged bodies themselves, cultivate love and respect for them?"[99] Importantly, critical feminist STS interventions are not simply about politically correct language. As mentioned, decades of EDC research on frogs in particular has been built on the homophobic and ableist assumptions that same-sex sexual behavior is abnormal, that frog sex changes are unnatural, and that intersex frogs cannot produce offspring.[100] The violent histories that EDC research unwittingly recites by deploying such terms as "demasculinization" and "chemical castration" is a form of violence in and of itself.[101] By assuming and perpetuating the white supremacist and heteropatriarchal ideologies that queer, transgender, intersex, neurodivergent, and disabled bodies are somehow aberrant (read: abhorrent), the work of prominent EDC researchers and anti-toxics advocates reinforces social stigma as well as judicial, material, and biomedical inequity.[102] Social science scholars and activists have well-documented the unjust ways that people who are marked as queer, trans, disabled, nonwhite, and foreign struggle disproportionately more to receive the medical care they need, safely access transportation and public restrooms, survive bullying and other forms of violence in schools and sports, and so on.[103] Put another way, feminist critique of EDC research and advocacy is not simply about problematic language or social stigma on a conceptual level, it's about how scientific theories can be complicit in prejudicial mistreatment on an undeniably material, visceral level—and sometimes fatally so.[104]

Feminist STS scholars and EDC toxicologists alike (again, not that these groups are mutually exclusive) want healthy, happy families and ecosystems, however these may be defined. Environmental humanities and queer ecologies scholar Nicole Seymour reminds us that "skepticism of natural categories can coexist with sincere investment in the natural world."[105] The main difference between the approach of critical feminist STS versus EDC toxicology seems to be the attention paid to unchecked chemical corporate power, which demonstrably threatens the livability of all life. EDC toxicologists tend to sweat the small stuff—molecular biology, cellular mechanisms of action, subtle genetic shifts occurring over generations—whereas critical feminist STS tends to scale up to the structural stuff—legacies of imperialism, corporate and transnational capitalism, white supremacy and heteropatriarchy.[106] In an attempt to venture beyond the feminist critiques canvassed above, while conducting the research for this book I spent considerable time in the weeds, literally and figuratively, with EDC (or EDC-adjacent, as in the case of weed science) toxicologists across the political economic spectrum: from industrial chemical manufacturers and industry-funded practitioners to government regulators and advocacy-oriented researchers. My queer feminist methods are described in greater detail in the appendix.

Before turning to this book's organization, allow me to concede at the outset that a major shortcoming of *Toxic Sexual Politics* is its US focus. China regularly surpasses the United States in terms of annual production of industrial chemicals, rendering the geographic focus of my analysis somewhat misplaced. Readers might argue that the end of US toxicant empire is already upon us, especially given more and more mainstreamed environmental health social movements. The most ubiquitous pesticide on earth, for example, glyphosate (more commonly known by its US brand name, Roundup), has come under increased scrutiny for its carcinogenicity and endocrine-disrupting effects in North America, Western Europe, Australasia, and Southeast Asia. Several states and countries have enacted legislation to ban the substance, prompting US-based advocates to speculate that a federal ban may be imminent.[107] However, according to agricultural economics researchers, "China has enough glyphosate capacity to satisfy the global demand even if all other glyphosate manufacturers cease production."[108] I contend, nevertheless, that the specifically US roots of contemporary, transnational practices of toxicology merit critical feminist scrutiny. While the United States' stint as global toxicant hegemon may indeed be waning, the norms of toxicological knowledge production that were fabricated by US-based toxicologists in the heyday of US empire—roughly the mid-twentieth century—have been widely exported and normalized worldwide, buoyed by the authoritative force of a supposedly politically neutral, culture-free Science.[109] Thus, at the risk of committing some of the same Euro-American-centric analytical crimes for which I indict dominant toxicology, I submit that unsettling the core concepts and origin stories of the scientific field of US toxicology is an essential initial move for destabilizing its explanatory and regulatory power on a global scale.

Book Organization and Overview

I did not expect to write a queer ecofeminist historiography of toxicology in the United States, and where I end the book—laboratory animal liberation!—was even less expected. I can explain. *Toxic Sexual Politics* is loosely divided into two parts: chapters 1 through 3 constitute the first part, chapters 4 and 5 the second. In chapter 1, I pivot from scientist feminist Donna Haraway's critique of the "god trick," or how dominant science purports to "[see] everything from nowhere."[110] Drawing from my close analyses of scientific texts and ethnographic research in toxicology classrooms and conferences, I show that when it comes to chemical exposures, environmental toxicology performs something more like a *devil* trick, wherein toxicants *appear* from nowhere. US toxicologists are not trained in, and oftentimes actively discouraged from, connecting the chemical substances under study to the sociopolitical preconditions for these same toxicants' massive production and uneven deployment. In other words, the devil trick works to conceal not so much the social location of the scientist (as in the god trick), but rather the social location of the toxicant.

My textual and ethnographic data show that this depoliticization of toxic pollution and toxicological practice extends from undergraduate- and graduate-level US toxicology programs and toxicology textbooks, where the devil trick is arguably the most blatant, to environmental health advocacy in both research and regulatory spaces, where the devil trick may be the most treacherous. While recognizing that textbooks do not represent all of toxicological practice, I contend that the messages revealed in such outward-facing training tools are representative of the disciplinary norms and scientific rigor that leading toxicologists wish to establish and propagate, and hence a rich source of qualitative data for a critical feminist STS analysis such as this one. Furthermore, as scientist feminist Celia Roberts finds in her study of endocrinology textbooks, "It is difficult, to say the least, not to be seduced by the level of certainty and clarity that is offered in these [textbook] descriptions of biological systems."[111]

Refusing to be seduced by the certainty that leading toxicologists offer in their textbook descriptions of toxicants is my task in chapter 2, where I suggest that the founding fathers of US toxicology cloak themselves with the *magical authority* to know toxicants (including what makes them supposedly safe), even as they fully admit that toxicological experiments require an unavoidably uncertain mixture of prediction, extrapolation, and interpretation. Toxicology is "both a science and an art,"[112] textbook authors assure readers; or, as one of my interviewees memorably summarized, "Toxicology is like forecasting the weather."[113] Thus, for chapter 2 I focus on toxicological methods, which derive from the central tenet "the dose makes the poison," a mantra attributed to the late medieval alchemist, physician, and theologian Paracelsus (1493-1541). I analyze the dominant US toxicology textbook, *Casarett & Doull's Toxicology: The Basic Science of Poisons*, alongside other scientific publications on toxicology, to reveal toxicologists' unarticulated anxieties regarding what dominant science *can* know about toxicants. Toxicology consists of predictions and probabilities calculated from exposure experiments conducted on animals (predominantly rodents), typically focusing on one chemical at a time, in controlled laboratory conditions—the gold standard being a two-year rodent study.[114] Rather than admit that such methods are inadequate to the task of protecting human and environmental health from tens of thousands of newly synthesized chemical substances, early US toxicologists authoritatively presented their emerging discipline as the best possible and most rational response to toxic uncertainties, convening a highly curated congregation of early European Enlightenment historical characters to solidify their shaky science, including especially Paracelsus. I further suggest that the charm of historical apothecaries like Paracelsus allows modern toxicologists to naturalize, if not romanticize, the apparent enigmas of industrial pollutants.

Anti-toxics environmental advocacy groups, too, increasingly turn to dominant science to confer greater legitimacy to their campaigns against toxicant hazards, even if they recognize scientific findings to be a "double-edged sword" when it comes to environmental justice (EJ) demands.[115] Despite its unstable foundations and uncertain practices then, toxicology is leveraged by both industry-leaning and public-health-leaning groups as the superior, authoritative form of knowledge about toxic environmental exposures. Thus, drawing parallels between dominant science's historical legacies of marginalizing other ways of knowing, and contemporary society's privileging of toxicology's knowledge claims above all others, I argue in chapter 2 that toxicology's *magical authority* is a reinforcing symptom of the white supremacist and masculinist entitlement that undergirds this uncertain science.[116]

Chapter 3 breaks away from the books and ventures beyond indoor classrooms and conferences to encounters in the outdoor, experimental field site. Here, my queer eye turns to what is called weed science, or the study of pesticides' effects on agricultural commodity crops, primarily. I pivot to the toxicology-adjacent field of weed science for several reasons. First, many pesticides are also endocrine-disrupting chemicals, and second, pesticides are chief among those synthetic substances that toxicologists used to refer to as "economic poisons" because they were deemed economically necessary despite their hazards.[117] Third, many toxicants synthesized for use as chemical weaponry immediately before and during the world wars were directly repurposed, and rebranded, as industrial agricultural chemicals after World War II's end. Fourth, unlike industrial toxicants manufactured and deployed within indoor, factory settings, pesticides are sprayed outside, entirely uncontainable by factory walls, and thus constitute toxic environmental exposures in an even more diffuse way than the toxic exposures we might experience via plastics, carpeting, or lead paint, to name a few everyday examples.[118]

The devil trick and magical authority feature prominently in weed science's use of toxicology as well, but I found these concepts did not adequately explain, or prepare me for, my participant observation of a weed science conference in 2019. The hypermasculinity of this particular setting of toxicology was so overt and overwhelming (to me) that I felt compelled to conceptualize a third term: *toxicant masculinity*. Pesticide brand names, never mind the massive, systematic dissemination of these toxic substances—408,000 tons deployed for US agriculture and 4.12 million tons worldwide in 2018 alone[119]—struck me as almost comically masculinist. Some choice selections include Prowl (pendmethalin), Regiment (bispyribac-sodium), Stinger (clopyralid), Cadre (imazapic), Roundup (glyphosate), Mission (flazasulfuron), BattleStar (fomesafen), Gunslinger (picloram plus 2,4-D), and Macho 4.0 (imidacloprid). Chapter 3 offers close readings of (auto)ethnographic vignettes from the weed science conference I attended, half of which was held outdoors at state agricultural research stations. My field notes, including brief, informal interviews with conference attendees, are further supported by textual and visual data from other weed science publications and spaces, with the help of an interlocutor who works in this applied discipline. Without being naive about the global entrenchment of industrial agriculture and its undeniable dependency on synthetic chemicals, I end chapter 3 by suggesting that *toxicant masculinity* is generating its own demise; the more pesticides are deployed, the more weeds and weed scientists alike develop resistance.

The second part of the book, consisting of chapters 4 and 5, extends the critical feminist analyses laid out in the first part by dwelling in the daily particulars of one ecotoxicology laboratory. I asked this laboratory's principal investigator, as laboratory leaders are called, if I may closely observe and participate in his lab's weekly meetings because I knew the lab focuses on EDCs (based on lab members' publications), and because they proudly describe themselves as committed to environmental health *and* social justice on their website. Just as my weed scientist interlocutor in chapter 3 points a way toward a more ecofeminist (or at least less agro-masculinist) sort of agricultural production, toxicologists who explicitly align themselves with environmental and social justice hold promise for a more queer relationship with nature—queer in the sense of provocatively and productively countercultural and queer in the sense of the "effective ecological values," which Nicole Seymour describes as "caring not (just) about the individual, the family, or one's descendants, but about the Other species and persons to whom one has no immediate relations."[120]

Perhaps unsurprisingly, declaring one's commitments to environmental and social justice proves easier than putting said commitments into practice. Chapter 4 documents my attempts to play the role of scientist feminist interventionist as I observed this extraordinary group of EDC toxicologists consider the merits of a critical feminist approach to their scientific studies, per my prodding. I gently challenged my interlocutors to engage with intersectional feminist critiques of toxicology more deeply, while they generously taught me that toxicologists are not necessarily as positivist nor as disinterested as their outward-facing publications might imply. My main finding from this ethnographic experiment is glaringly obvious in hindsight: the cultural norms and economic pressures of dominant science are so overbearing, and yet also so insidious, that a couple semesters of engagement with critical feminism is not nearly enough to unlearn and uproot generations of (internalized) indoctrination regarding the proper performance and practice of dominant science: coolly clinical and quantitative. Building from feminist and critical disability scholars' analyses of care work, I end chapter 4 with an invitation to justice-committed toxicologists to expand on their existing care for one another—care work largely compelled by the challenges of navigating a particularly politically charged and implicitly patriarchal scientific field—and extend such acts of care in ways that refuse the tacit eugenicism and masculinism of mainstream toxicology. To quote Nicole Seymour once again, "The shirking of stable identities, epistemologies, and ontologies . . . might lend itself most effectively to empathetic, politicized advocacy for the non-human natural world . . . a specifically queer ecological ethic of care: a care not rooted in stable or essentialized identity categories, a care that is not just a means of solving human-specific problems, a care that does not operate out of expectation for recompense."[121]

In chapter 5, I turn my critical feminist STS lens from lab members' care for one another to their care for the exterior, natural world, inclusive of the more-than-human animals they are wholly enchanted by and yet deliberately expose to toxic substances, oftentimes killing them at the end of an exposure experiment. Here I use "enchantment" in reference to a different sort of spellbinding than that conjured by *magical authority*; in chapter 5, I mean enchantment in the sense that German philosophers Max Horkeimer and Theodor Adorno used the term, namely to critique the European Enlightenment philosophy of rationalizing, mechanizing, and utilizing nature (which Horkeimer and Adorno describe as "disenchantment," and which, in turn, leads to fascism, in their analysis).[122] The contemporary specialists in EDC toxicology I observed for twenty weeks, who publicly commit to supporting EJ movements, appear torn between their own (re)enchantments with nature, which motivate their worthy efforts to study and help reduce toxic pollution, and the disenchantment with nature that dominant scientific training demands, including the killing of innocent animals for the sake of an experiment.[123]

My analysis of lab meeting field notes and interview transcripts finds that these EDC toxicologists reconcile this tension via what I call *fishy exceptionalism*; fish are similar enough to humans that they can feel an affinity with them, and hence seek to improve their fish (and ultimately human) lives, yet also different enough from humans that they can feel less uncomfortable exposing fish (as opposed to mammals) to toxicants and subsequently ending their lives. Some fish arrive to the lab already dismembered, scraps donated from willing fisheries, and hence "reduced to their DNA and RNA" as one lab member put it.[124] Others are captured from the wild by the scientists themselves, only to meet their deaths in these same scientists' laboratory; still others are bred in the lab, often from captives taken from the wild, never to return.

Importantly, there is nothing unusually cruel about this lab's fishy practices; their experiments on fish are perfectly in line with a highly standardized, widely normalized operating procedure across dominant science, complete with approval from Institutional Animal Care and Use Committees (IACUC, the more-than-human counterpart to Institutional Review Boards for research with human subjects).[125] My observations of and conversations with this particular group of EDC toxicologists suggests that the lab's resistance to feminist critique (as canvassed in chapter 4) and deliberate choice to experiment on fish in particular, are avenues through which they might fulfill dominant science's demands for a pure, apolitical, ascendant truth.[126] Seeking a sort of *pure pollution*, a study of toxicants that avoids messy, political dramas—whether those of manufacturing chemists or animal liberationists—my toxicologist interlocutors find refuge in clean, sleek statistics and cool, slippery fish, neither of which require the kind of physical and emotional touch that diving into protracted, undeniably political battles with industrial polluters would necessitate.[127]

Overall, I hope *Toxic Sexual Politics* adequately shows that the toxicant does not preexist its making, and that the toxicant, too, is racialized and sexualized.[128] This book's concluding chapter is more of a speculative epilogue, where I trace the contours of a study of toxicants that is unflinchingly pessimistic,[129] in the words of scientist feminist Michelle Murphy, about today's permanently polluted world, and yet willfully optimistic about how we might better care for one another in what Murphy calls the chemical aftermath,[130] including holding perpetrators accountable. Reclaiming eugenicists' use of the term *drag*—as in "the drag of the race," or the fear that poor breeding will result in a lower quality gene pool—in the outro, I play with queer ecofeminist desires for a study of toxicants that explicitly, care-fully situates toxicants in their sociohistorical contexts, while simultaneously prefiguring a world where all bodies and identities—whether female, male, trans, intersex, disabled, queer, melanated, more-than-human, microbial, weedy, fungal, fishy, fat, young, old, sick, and so on—are fiercely, generously, handled with care.

1

The Devil Trick

There simply is no way to talk about human death or human societies when you are using a language designed to talk about weapons.

—Carol Cohn[1]

"Keeping Our War Fighters Healthy"

The Society of Toxicology conference I attended, where I was to copresent my first biomedical science conference poster, was located in one of those conveniently-near-the-airport-but-completely-inaccessible-by-public-transport sort of complexes. The conference center's opening atrium resembled an airplane hangar, where slim, rectangular boards on wheels sat in orderly rows, waiting for posters to be hung. The conference's more formal presentations with invited speakers took place in the next room—a squat, wide, dim rectangle without windows, under fluorescent lighting and dropped ceilings. Overall, the event felt to me like part academic meeting, part trade show, and part investor pitch, complete with chemical company swag and multiple iterations of "Thanks to our sponsors."

After some short yet obsequious opening remarks, during which a representative from the local Society of Toxicology branch repeatedly thanked an extensive roster of chemical industry sponsors for funding the day's proceedings, the first speaker took the stage and the conference presentations officially began. Our opening speaker hailed from the US Army's Division of Public Health. *Already I am learning things*, I thought to myself as I typed furious notes. *The US Army maintains a Division of Public Health?!* My bewilderment did not end there. The US Army toxicologist proceeded to share how the military applies the "latest innovations in toxicology" to determine the extent to which substances they use in manufacturing cause skin irritations. This bears repeating: the US military wants to know whether the processes and ingredients with which they produce munitions might irritate the skin of those producing them. The presiding toxicologist repeatedly insisted, "*Of course* we don't want to be poisoning the communities around us [through the toxicity of munitions factories], . . . *of course* we want to keep our war fighters healthy" (original emphasis). *War fighters? Does he mean soldiers? Is "war fighters" more diplomatic?*

Needless to say, examples abound of the US Army deliberately poisoning civilian and military communities alike, inclusive of their natural environments, such as the atomic bombs deployed in Hiroshima and Nagasaki, Japan, and at sites such as the Marshall Islands during World War II and into the so-called Cold War; Monsanto and Dow Chemical's toxic Agent Orange herbicide during the Vietnam War; the US invasion of Iraq; and massive, toxic defoliation campaigns in the name of the War on Drugs in Colombia, among numerous other examples.[2] Researching the skin irritating potential of products designed by the world's most powerful military seemed to me, at the risk of being glib, a prime example of getting lost in the wrong details.

As the speaker continued with his presentation, I became increasingly anxious and agitated. I began fidgeting in my toxic, plastic chair, looking around somewhat frantically at the other conference participants, hoping to share a commiserate glance with anyone else discomfited by the presentation. Many audience members seemed lost in their laptops, or else stared straight ahead, perhaps in rapt attention or with thoughts entirely elsewhere. Desperate for some sign of solidarity, I leaned over to whisper excitedly in a colleague's ear: "Is he talking about making sure weapons designed to kill people don't irritate the skin?!" My colleague was busy behind her laptop, working on other tasks and had not been listening. However, for my benefit she paused typing for a moment to tune in the speaker. She then quietly nodded in agreement, as if to say (I imagined, reassuring myself), "Yes, worrying about the skin irritating potential of ammunition seems rather misplaced."

Admittedly, I cannot be sure that the other audience members were not also questioning the presentation, but the impression I received, based on the room's overwhelmingly underwhelmed response, was that measuring the skin irritating potential of munitions that are ultimately meant to kill constituted a perfectly standard toxicology inquiry. How can this be? This chapter offers an explanation.

Let me be clear from the beginning that I do not wish to paint all toxicologists with the same brush. At the risk of amplifying already hegemonic narratives, I intentionally direct my critical feminist lens toward the most dominant voices, including authors contributing to the textbook *Casarett & Doull's Toxicology*, ranking members of the Society of Toxicology, and authors of toxicology literature reviews from various scientific journals.[3] Those social scientists and historians who have studied toxicology before me have movingly chronicled several of the public-health-aligned, even activist, efforts of many a professional toxicologist.[4] (Notably, even the reform-minded toxicologists concerned with chemical mutagenesis met with resistance from the Society of Toxicology in 1971.[5]) I encountered an encouraging number of reflexive toxicologists through the course of my ethnographic research as well, whom readers will meet in the chapters ahead. Such exceptions notwithstanding, textbook narratives are representative of a discipline, or rather, they are the representation that dominant members of the discipline want to broadcast. As sociologist C. Wright Mills noted, regarding the critical value of textbook analysis, "By virtue of the mechanism of sales and distribution, textbooks tend to embody a content agreed upon by the academic groups using them. . . . Since one test of their success is wide adoption, the very spread of the public for which they are written tends to ensure textbook tolerance of the commonplace. . . . the aim [of critical analysis] is to grasp typical perspectives and key concepts."[6]

Reading multiple editions (1975 to 2019) of the dominant US toxicology textbook, *Casarett & Doull's Toxicology: The Basic Science of Poisons*, through a critical feminist lens, I show how toxicologists are trained to separate toxicant industry from toxicant science, depoliticizing toxic exposures and their adverse outcomes in the process. In 1975, toxicology textbook authors presented industrial chemicals as risky but essentially beneficial and unequivocally necessary.[7] By 2019, the authors of *Casarett & Doull's Toxicology* minimize and relativize the twentieth and twenty-first centuries' plethora of toxic exposure catastrophes as "countless unforeseen events," while the toxicants involved in such disasters still remain only "potentially" harmful.[8] Rarely, if ever, are chemical corporations named, and more rarely still are specific synthetic chemicals affiliated with their specific manufacturers.

The Devil Trick

Donna Haraway uses the term "god trick" to describe the tendency of dominant science to assume a neutral "view from nowhere."[9] Relatedly, I suggest contemporary toxicology performs something more like a *devil trick*, wherein toxic substances *appear* from nowhere. (More extreme forms of the devil trick, one of which will emerge later in this chapter and at choice moments throughout this book, I came to refer to as *chemical gaslighting*.) Consider, for example, the opening lines of the most recent edition (the ninth, published in 2019) of *Casarett & Doull's Toxicology*: "Humans are smart but vulnerable. We need to be prepared for countless unforeseen events that could compromise our health and well-being. Toxicology arose as a way to understand, prevent, mitigate, and treat the potentially harmful consequences of many of the substances we are exposed to."[10]

Contemporary, leading practitioners position toxicology as a response to the "potentially harmful" substances that appear from nowhere and from no one in particular. Are these "countless events" really "unforeseen"? By whom? Are their consequences only "potentially harmful"? To whom? Who is the "we" passively exposed to substances here?[11] While toxicologists are not trained to ask these questions, environmental justice (EJ) activists and scholars are, and they have gathered an abundance of material and cultural evidence to provide important answers.[12] Yet the narrow, scientific scope of toxicology continues to be privileged above these more holistic knowledge claims. For example, in *Hardeman v. Monsanto* (2019), the second of three highly publicized toxic torts brought against the chemical manufacturer Monsanto (which had just recently been purchased by Bayer Corporation, in 2016), the US federal judge presiding explicitly forbid the plaintiff's bar—at the defense's insistence—from presenting ample evidence of Monsanto's role in ghostwriting scientific papers and subsequent government regulations on the toxicant under trial: glyphosate, or Roundup, the most ubiquitous herbicide on earth.[13] This case "bifurcation," as it came to be called, underscores how nonscientific evidence is considered subjective and thus overly partial. In order to be objective and impartial, in other words, the plaintiff's claim that Roundup caused their cancer must rest on the scientific evidence alone, which is presumed to be purely factual and hence neutral. If the jury found Monsanto/Bayer guilty based on the science, then a second part of the trial could proceed wherein the plaintiff's bar presented evidence of scientific corruption on the part of the corporation. The major irony—that the first part of the trial was to rely on the very same scientific evidence that the corporation had a significant hand in shaping—was not lost on the plaintiffs, nor the numerous environmental health advocates closely watching this and other Roundup trials.[14] As it turned out, Monsanto/Bayer lost the first, science-only part anyway, and soon after lost the second, science-corrupted part as well.

Toxicologists employed by the US Army and Monsanto are perhaps too easy (or too powerful?) for a critical feminist science and technology studies (STS) scholar like me to pick on. Not all US toxicologists are military apologists and industry sell-outs, as previous social studies of toxicology have documented and my own ethnographic research has corroborated.[15] However, as I argue throughout this book, contemporary endocrine-disrupting chemical (EDC) toxicology remains haunted by the ghosts of its founding fathers, whose masculinist and militarist ideologies shaped "the basic science of poisons" such that fundamental questions like "Who invented and profits from this synthetic chemical?" and "Why is it legally deployed?" are relegated dangerously outside the discipline.[16] When even public-health-aligned toxicologists remain uninformed of, or politely decline to confront, their discipline's historical emergence and embedded biases, then environmental justice futures become that much more elusive.

The conference's closing speaker illustrated this danger well. A PhD candidate gave the final presentation; she had been invited to speak after winning a Society of Toxicology prize for excellence in student research. From my perspective, her early career experiments provided a strange counterpart to the US Army toxicologist's opening presentation. Likewise focusing on munitions, but from a markedly different standpoint, this speaker presented her toxicological research on the effects of chemical weapons on children's developing brains, based, as most toxicological findings are, on rodent experiments. In her own succinct summary, she declared, "The goal of my PhD research is to develop a juvenile model for chemical warfare exposure."

It was nearing the end of a long day, and despite the speaker's clarity, initially I wondered whether I had heard her correctly. *First healthy "war fighters," and now "juvenile models for chemical warfare"?!* To be sure, this academic researcher was not defending the use of chemical weaponry on children. Rather, like many other environmental toxicologists today, this scientist was laboring to understand more precisely how synthetic chemicals harm rodents, specifically their neurological development in this case, in an effort to provide scientific evidence that might help prevent future atrocities of the sort. While approaching their military topics from widely divergent vantage points, these two toxicologists concerned with war-related exposures shared several commonalities. Both focused on the minutiae of complicated experimental processes, down to cellular mechanisms and microscopically precise measurements, emphasizing in turn the abstract, depoliticized calculations that distance both the toxicology and the toxicologist from the brutal, historical-material facts of chemical warfare.

Whether working for the US Army or the academy, then, my research evidenced that on the whole, toxicologists are not trained to ask how and why synthetic toxins came to be manufactured, by whom and for whom, not to mention how and why such chemicals came to be legally deployed, and against whom. Instead, toxicologists are trained to clinically demonstrate their scientific objectivity via numerical abstractions, based on Cartesian and colonial concepts of bodies and boundaries (as summarized in this book's introduction). Even though this academic toxicologist may be considered one of the good guys, so to speak, her public health-aligned presentation left me just as disheartened as the "keeping our war fighters healthy" session.

Overall, the toxicologists I observed, described in more detail in chapters 3 through 5, were experts in study design protocol and cellular mechanisms but just as skillfully (if unwittingly) elided structural and social mechanisms like political economy and patriarchy. Even those toxicologists working for anti-toxics advocacy groups, whom I observed and interviewed, saw toxicology itself as neutral. "Basic science is basic science,"[17] stressed one of my interviewees, an internationally renowned public health expert. All the political stuff, they reasoned, comes from outside the science, distorting an otherwise pure knowledge base. Another of my anti-toxics interviewees concurred: "Science is at the core. Science is the base [of our advocacy campaigns]. First you have to get the science right."[18] While many were also quick to point out that scientific data are not the only requisite component of chemical policy, they nonetheless firmly believed that sound science was free of politics, and that the political "interference," as two different interviewees termed it, enters much later.

What policy solutions may be derived from this supposedly impartial knowledge base? Who needs to know whether the manufacturing of munitions irritates the skin, and why? How did the toxic effects of chemical weapons on children's neurological development become an unremarkable scientific research question? My study of people who study toxicants suggests that toxicology cannot tell us what we need to know about toxic chemicals in order to protect people and other life from these hazardous substances. In an exception that perhaps proves the rule, one of my interviewees, then-director of a federal public health agency, seemed to agree: "I would like to see more common sense; a lot of times we're crunching numbers and dancing on the heads of pins . . . we tie ourselves up trying to do these precise calculations. . . . If a chemical is bioactive, it's bioactive."[19]

Another interviewee, a toxicologist who worked for an international organization against pesticides, was similarly unusual (among my interlocutors) in acknowledging that the entire, globalized system of industrial agriculture needed to be uprooted in order to effectively regulate pesticides: "The [toxicological] data is not enough . . . it's really naive [of researchers] to think that. . . . Just changing [chemical] risk assessment wouldn't be sufficient, we have to totally alter the way we do farming."[20]

Again, these interview quotes stood out to me precisely because they were outliers among the experts with whom I spoke, the toxicology textbooks and articles I read, and the toxicology courses and conferences I attended. Toxicology has always been a predictive and uncertain science, as I elaborate in chapter 2. For environmental justice's sake, I believe scholar-activists ought to pay particular attention to who makes these scientific predictions, how these scientific predictions are made, what worldviews these scientific predictions are predicated on, and which people and places tend to benefit or suffer because of such toxicological guesswork. Neither the god trick nor the devil trick will lead us out of the very toxicity such partial visions helped generate in the first place.

Chapters 4 and 5 chronicle my more collaborative research with environmental justice-aligned EDC toxicologists. In what remains of this chapter, I return to my concept of the devil trick, underscoring its presence in foundational toxicology textbooks and persistence in contemporary toxicological practices.

The Ultimate Authority

"Most trusted." "World's leading and most authoritative." "Landmark." "Gold-standard." "The ultimate authority in toxicology." These are but a few of the accolades the McGraw Hill publishing company boasts for their "all-in-one overview" textbook *Casarett & Doull's Toxicology: The Basic Science of Poisons.* Currently in its ninth edition, *Toxicology: The Basic Science of Poisons* was first published by Macmillan (now McGraw Hill) in 1975, initially edited by Louis J. Casarett, PhD (1927–1972), who unfortunately passed away before the text's publication, and the more recently deceased John Doull, MD, PhD (1922–2017). Their surnames, Casarett and Doull, have remained in the textbook's title ever since, despite the subsequent procession of expert editors carrying the torch. Contributors now total at seventy, with some of the original thirty-six authors continuously updating their chapters for each new edition—1980, 1986, 1991, 1996, 2001, 2008, 2013, 2019—and entirely new sections and authors being added to the two most recent. Notable additions include endocrine-disrupting chemicals (as a topic, beginning 1996) and the retired corporate vice president of worldwide regulatory sciences for Monsanto Corporation (as a contributor, also in 1996, coincidentally).

A certain Harold C. Hodge (1904–1990) wrote the foreword to the first, 1975 edition of *Toxicology: The Basic Science of Poisons.* Hodge was a prominent US toxicologist of the time, serving as the Society of Toxicology's first president in 1961, and the federally appointed head of the US Atomic Energy Commission's (AEC) Division of Pharmacology and Toxicology—the AEC is more commonly known as the Manhattan Project. By 1975, Hodge was a professor emeritus of pharmacology at the University of California, San Francisco. Over two decades later, investigative journalist Eileen Welsome brought to light some of Hodge's less favorable claims to fame in her Pulitzer Prize–winning exposé, *The Plutonium Files*,[21] which told of unethical experiments Hodge designed and implemented, injecting uninformed human subjects with uranium and plutonium in the name of scientific discovery and US empire.

A condensed version of Hodge's foreword appears in the second edition (1980) of *Casarett & Doull's Toxicology: The Basic Science of Poisons* (hereafter *Casarett & Doull's*), but is not included again in subsequent editions, or from 1986 on. I suspect that the disappearance of Hodge's foreword by 1986 has less to do with his unethical behavior, as *The Plutonium Files* would not be published for another thirteen years, than with mere publishing convention. By the third edition, two new editors and several new contributors had joined, rendering the updated textbook different enough from the original to warrant new frontmatter. Generally, dominant science has been slow to publicly confront or otherwise reckon with its harmful histories, and post–*Plutonium Files* editions of *Casarett & Doull's* make no mention of Hodge's disturbing decisions. In 1990, when Hodge passed away, the University of California memorialized him as "unarguably the dean of American toxicology. . . . loyal, affectionate, charming . . . the epitome of a scholar and a gentleman."[22] Perhaps in that Cold War moment of midcentury US history, Hodge's unethical experimentation on human subjects was neither uncommon nor censured, at least not among the science and policy elite. Welsome's research documents how the AEC knowingly approved of, and expressed gratitude for, Hodge's professional guidance. To my knowledge, the University of California, never mind the US government, has yet to publicly grapple with the amoral actions of their "unarguabl[e] dean of American toxicology."

Louis J. Casarett (1927–1972) was one of Hodge's PhD students, while John Doull had worked directly under E. M. K. Geiling, another of the most prominent toxicologists of the early twentieth century (whom Frederick R. Davis profiles in his history of toxicology vis-à-vis DDT, *Banned*).[23] Casarett was a graduate student of Hodge's at the University of Rochester, New York, in what would become that institution's first Department of Pharmacology. After joining the faculty at Rochester himself, Casarett eventually gained a tenured position at the new University of Hawai'i medical school. He met his future coeditor, John Doull, through the National Institute of Health's "Toxicology Study

Section," in which they were both members. While the textbook was initially Casarett's idea, his wife, Peggy Casarett, and Doull ended up taking on the majority of the editorial work because Casarett was diagnosed with brain cancer shortly after chapter drafts began arriving. (Doull's wife, Vera, did the work of indexing the book. While Peggy Casarett is listed as a contributor and thanked explicitly in the preface, referred to by her full name, Margaret, Vera remains unmentioned in the textbook.) In any case, Casarett's obituary confirms that "the emergence of *Casarett & Doull's Toxicology: The Basic Science of Poisons* in 1975 was a landmark event in toxicology and a fitting memorial to Lou Casarett's dedication to toxicologic education."[24]

Doull had the good fortune to live a much longer life than Casarett, building an illustrious career along the way. He completed his graduate work at the University of Chicago under E. M. K. Geiling, perhaps an even more prestigious pharmacologist-turned-toxicologist than Harold C. Hodge. Geiling is memorialized as the "Father of Toxicology," and I reuse such patriarchal language intentionally. Geiling oversaw the first "Tox Lab" in the country, established in 1941 with US military funding. According to science historian Frederick R. Davis, Geiling was a rather imposing principal investigator, micromanaging his staff's and students' personal lives to the point of discouraging marriage and hand-selecting Christmas gifts. Such blurring of professional and personal boundaries apparently "inspired . . . loyalty," though I cannot help but wonder who did (or would) *not* fit in to the Tox Lab family and why, as well as how such lab loyalty may have manifested itself in experimental designs, omissions, or conclusions.[25] I expand on the patriarchal underpinnings of contemporary toxicology laboratory culture in chapter 4. One of Geiling's many successful students, Doull eventually became President of the Society of Toxicology (1986–87) himself, decades after Hodge's inaugural post (1961–62), and served for multiple government agencies, including the National Institute of Health, the National Academy of Sciences, the Environmental Protection Agency, and White House Advisory Panels, appointed to the last by President George H. W. Bush in 1993.[26]

Both Casarett and Doull are credited as authors of the textbook's first edition (1975) preface; sometime shortly before publication, Doull alone added a brief paragraph of gratitude and *in memoriam* for Casarett. This "preface to the first edition" reappears in full in all subsequent editions, immediately before each subsequent editorial team's new preface. Casarett and Doull's 1975 preface emphasizes toxicology's breadth of applications and relevance, describing the science as fundamental to students and practitioners both well within and far outside the discipline—including "community health, agriculture, food technology, pharmacy, veterinary medicine, and related disciplines"—and justifying the textbook's organization "to facilitate its use by these different types of users." Unit I is "primarily mechanistically oriented," Unit II focuses on "the systemic site of action of toxins," Unit III adopts "a more conventional approach" wherein "toxic agents are grouped by chemical," while in Unit IV "an attempt has been made to illustrate the ramifications of toxicology into all areas of the health sciences and even beyond." This fourth and final unit is "intended to provide perspective for the nontoxicologist."[27]

In addition to coediting the entire textbook, Casarett wrote the opening two chapters, a history of toxicology and overview of core concepts, respectively. The content of these two introductory chapters remains almost verbatim up through the eighth edition (2013), despite being republished under different author names along the way. Casarett and his contemporaries presented twentieth century industrial toxins as risky but necessary features of the inevitable march of modern progress, the harms of which toxicologists are expertly trained to measure and mitigate. "Don't worry your pretty little head," their texts seem to say. Casarett writes, for example, "In the modern enlightenment of industrial practice, great expenditures are made to maintain a safe working environment. Despite this fact, the proliferation of new, potent, and complex chemicals and processes project the continuing spector [sic] of industrial and occupational overexposure. More alarmingly, the hazard of the plant and the potential danger of its effluent spill over into the general populace. Within the plant and in the community, the toxicologist has found a contributory role."[28]

Witness Casarett's immediately positive spin on the situation: "The modern enlightenment of industrial practice," within which "great expenditures are made to maintain a safe working environment." He at once assumes that industrialization is not only a good thing, but also an enlightened project, and moreover that working environments are safe and will continue to be under a toxicologist's watchful eye. The toxicologist's "contributory role," within this modern enlightenment of industrial practice, was quite literally to *set the terms of toxicity*, operating under the assumption—and this point is crucial—that such a thing as "safe use" of a synthetic chemical exists.[29] Casarett concludes his 1975 introductory chapter with the following summary:

> *A central element of toxicology is the delineation of the safe use of chemicals.* To use the term "poison" alone is inadequate as any effective chemical is a poison. . . . The toxicologist has as a major part of his discipline a contribution to make to the identification of "hazard," defined as the probability that injury will result from a chemical under specific conditions, and to establishment of limits of "safety," defined as the practical certainty that injury will not result from use of a substance under specified conditions of quantity and manner of use. These contributions may be made in many ways, most of which represent measures of "toxicity," defined as the capacity of a substance to produce injury.[30]

Notably, this founding toxicologist includes scare quotes around the terms *poison*, *hazard*, *safety*, and *toxicity*, acknowledging that these are not absolute, but rather constructed categories.[31] Given centuries of chemical disasters, concurrent with the "slow violence,"[32] as environmental humanities scholar Rob Nixon memorably terms it, of ubiquitous yet uneven toxic exposure, sensitive readers might note several assumptions laid bare by Casarett's definitions. First, and as mentioned, founding toxicologists assumed that synthetic chemicals may be used safely: "A central element of toxicology is the delineation of the safe use of chemicals." Second, disciplined toxicologists granted themselves the authoritative, masculinist prerogative to decide what constitutes "safe use" of a hazardous substance, based on mere probabilities: "The toxicologist has as a major part of his discipline a contribution to make to the identification of 'hazard,' defined as the probability that injury will result from a chemical under specific conditions." I elaborate on this masculinist prerogative, which I term *toxicant masculinity*, in chapter 3. Third, and relatedly, these scientific judgements that "establish limits of safety" for the public could be extrapolated "with practical certainty" from "specific conditions" staged in laboratory experiments. I call this "practical certainty" the *magical authority* of toxicology, discussed in more depth in chapter 2. Fourth, and likewise discussed in chapter 2, toxicity is considered measurable and knowable *enough*—trust the wizardly, "trained judgement" of the paternal, scientific expert.[33] Last but not least, and my focus for this chapter, toxicants are assumed to be inevitable (and generally desirable) for the "modern enlightenment of industrial practice." It is this presumed, unremarkable inevitability of synthetic chemicals that I characterize as the *devil trick*.

Out of context, founding toxicologists' assumptions are not necessarily bad. After all, by design, dominant science relies on hypotheses and explores unknowns, no matter the field. Science studies scholar Bruno Latour has indeed suggested that all scientific facts are "fabricated"; in any case, toxicology is not unique among sciences in relying on prediction and extrapolation.[34] However, as in Haraway's concept of the god trick, the devil trick erases the political economy and political ecology of toxicant manufacturing and deployment. What is more, the devil trick effaces toxicology's own rationalizing and enabling role in industrial chemical production.

Early toxicologists, for all their masculinist presumption and unethical experimentation, were at least more forthcoming about their political positions than contemporary textbook authors. For instance, our inaugural Society of Toxicology president Harold C. Hodge complained in his foreword to the first edition, in what I read as a direct attack on Rachel Carson's 1962 best-seller, *Silent Spring*, that: "The dangers of the indiscriminate overuse of pesticides have been so dramatized that some beneficial substances, irreplaceable at present, are banned rather than controlled."[35] Casarett also makes his allegiances clear, opining in the second chapter of the first edition, titled "Toxicological Evaluation," that "one could define a poison as any agent that is capable of . . . destroying life or seriously injuring function. As pointed out in Chapter 1, this is unsatisfactory because it includes virtually every known chemical . . . but it says nothing about the circumstances and conditions under which exposure to the agent occurs. The statement 'There are no harmless substances; there are only harmless ways of using substances' (Emil Mrak, member, Commission of Pesticides) correctly notes that a poison produces harm only within prescribed conditions of usage."[36] Having just explicitly and uncritically aligned himself with the interests of pesticide manufacturers, Casarett strongly implies that poisons don't kill people—people mishandling poisons kill people. Expert toxicologists, by extension, are necessary to educate pesticide users about these harmful substances' "prescribed conditions of usage," which, in a rather circular logic, toxicologists themselves have defined.

Remarkably, Casarett asserts that certain definitions of poisons are unsatisfactory because they "say nothing about the circumstances and conditions under which exposure . . . occurs"—and yet the entire discipline of toxicology avoids substantive discussion of the sociopolitical circumstances and conditions under which exposure occurs, context which could certainly help determine what makes a substance harmful, not to mention who makes a harmful substance. As I have written elsewhere, contemporary toxicology now offers the clinical framework "Adverse Outcome Pathways" (AOPs) rather than locate toxicants in political context. "The AOP abstractly begins when the toxicant touches the skin, is metabolized by the liver, or signals a DNA methylation. . . . In toxicological terms, the first "key event" in an AOP is the mechanistic delivery of the toxicant under study. Said delivery is cropped at the cellular level, not, say, at the level of the factory, farm, or household where toxicant exposure occurs, nor at the level of the government institution making toxicants legal."[37]

Casarett and his contemporaries insist that toxicants are only harmful if and when people are improperly trained in their use, thus insisting that toxicants not be banned. Instead, the general populace and government officials should defer to the expertise—or *magical authority*, see my next chapter—of toxicologists such as Casarett and Doull, who will diligently ensure that the modern enlightenment of industrial practice advances unimpeded.

As time wore on, powerful social institutions shaped modernity such that all industrialized and industrializing countries became increasingly dependent on "economic poisons"; industrial chemical production, meanwhile, skyrocketed (see the introduction), and the devil trick became more insidious. Allow me to offer a few more textbook examples before turning to the devil tricks of a contemporary US toxicological classroom.

In the fifth edition (1996) of *Casarett & Doull's*, reproductive toxicologist John A. Thomas echoes Casarett's 1975 sentiments regarding the "modern enlightenment of industrial practice," rephrasing this

generous description about twenty years later as "an industrial renaissance." Thomas writes, "The twentieth century has undergone an industrial renaissance, and through scientific and technical advances there
has been a significant extension in life expectancy and generally an enhanced quality of life. Concomitant with this industrial renaissance . . .
[the] production of synthetic organic chemicals has risen from less
than one billion pounds in 1920 . . . to over 200 billion pounds in the
late 1980s."[38] Note how the "concomitant" massive production of industrial chemicals is deidentified and despatialized. "Scientific and technical advances" of whom? Or rather, which corporations are producing
these 200 billion pounds of toxicants, which governments are enabling
such productions, and where (or against whom) is this tonnage deployed? Importantly, Thomas's chapter details, in distanced, clinical
fashion, several severe toxic effects of this triumphantly termed "industrial renaissance." The production of synthetic organic chemicals, as he
phrases it, is nevertheless foregrounded as inevitable, and desirable—
"generally an enhanced quality of life"—even within the context of serious, long-term toxic outcomes. As Thomas goes on to matter-of-factly
describe, "In the United States, male factory workers occupationally
exposed to 1,2-dibromo3-chloropropane (DBCP) became sterile. . . .
Factory workers in battery plants in Bulgaria, lead mine workers in the
state of Missouri, and workers in Sweden who handle organic solvents
(toluene, benzene, and xylene) suffer from low sperm counts, abnormal
sperm, and varying degrees of infertility."[39] Such apparently run-of-the-
mill worker sacrifice is presented as an acceptable, and indeed expectable, price paid for "generally an enhanced quality of life" (excluding
that of the factory worker, clearly). Meanwhile, the entities responsible
for and profiting from toxic exposures are left unnamed, unless being
commended for their efforts to delineate "harmless ways of using substances." Thomas, for example, swiftly brushes past "the thalidomide
incident" to emphasize instead some of the (rather weak) top-down
responses to this particular catastrophe.

In brief, thalidomide, a pharmaceutical sedative, was widely prescribed to pregnant women across Europe in the early twentieth century as a treatment for morning sickness, even though it had not been
adequately tested for toxic reproductive effects. Thousands of children whose mothers had ingested thalidomide were born with severly

malformed or entirely missing limbs, as well as more dangerous conditions like congenital heart disease, while thalidomide-induced miscarriage and death were alarmingly common (the neonate mortality rate is estimated at 40 percent).[40] In 1960, the German pharmaceutical company Chemie Grünenthal collaborated with the US-based William S. Merrell Company (later Richardson-Merrell, now part of Sanofi), to market and distribute thalidomide throughout the United States. Controversy remains as to whether Chemie Grünenthal and the Merrell Company knew at that time of the drug's teratogenic toxicity (meaning toxic to the fetus).[41]

Notably, then Food and Drug Administration (FDA) newcomer Dr. Frances Kelsey battled much corporate bullying for denying the thalidomide application—she later recalled her new boss had given her the assignment assuming it would be a rote approval.[42] Dr. Kelsey subsequently received a Presidential Medal of Honor from President John F. Kennedy for preventing the widespread sale and use of thalidomide in the United States. But Thomas omits such historio-political details in his 1996 *Casarett & Doull's* chapter on reproductive toxicity: "The impact of new chemicals (or drugs) on the reproductive system was tragically accentuated by the thalidomide incident in the 1960s. . . . This episode led to an increased awareness of the potential hazards of chemical and drug toxicity in the reproductive system and brought forth laws and guidelines world wide [sic]. . . . In 1985, the American Medical Association (AMA) Council on Scientific Affairs charged an advisory panel on Reproductive Hazards in the Work Place to consider over 100 chemicals with the intent to estimate their imminent hazards."[43]

"The intent to estimate" the "imminent hazards" of "over 100 chemicals" hardly makes a dent in the 200 billion pounds of industrial renaissance Thomas celebrated a mere few paragraphs earlier. In true devil trick fashion, Thomas's brief mention of this meager effort says nothing about who manufactured thalidomide or what systems approved its use (in the European context; and were it not for Dr. Kelsey, likely in the US context as well). "The impact of new chemicals" is not denied, but neither is it explained. "Chemical and drug toxicity" simply *is*, while toxicologists work industriously to increase awareness and sharpen their measuring tools. Let us jump ahead to the eighth edition (2013), wherein textbook contributor Michael A. Gallo demonstrates a rather extreme twist on the devil trick, descending into what I call *chemical gaslighting*.

Toxicological Potential

Louis J. Casarett did not live to see his textbook in print, and his introductory chapters have been minimally updated by new contributors beginning with the second edition (1980). Gallo joined the team of authors (replacing Casarett on chapter 1) beginning with the fourth edition (1991), but up through the eighth edition (2013) much of Casarett's original first chapter text remains, altered here and there with some politically correct edits, such as changing "early man" to "early humans" and omitting the term "primitives."[44] (See my chapter 3 for a critical feminist rereading of these specific sections.) Echoing his predecessors' "modern enlightenment of industrial practice" (Casarett in 1975) and "industrial renaissance" (Thomas in 1996), Gallo writes triumphantly in 2013 of synthetic chemicals' "toxicological potential" following the dawn of an "industrial and political revolution." He writes, "The 19th century dawned in a climate of industrial and political revolution. Organic chemistry was in its infancy in 1800, but by 1825 phosgene ($COCl_2$) and mustard gas (bis[β-chloroethyl]sulfide) had been synthesized. . . . By 1880 over 10,000 organic compounds had been synthesized . . . and petroleum and coal gasification by-products were used in trade. Determination of the toxicological potential of these newly created chemicals became the underpinning of the science of toxicology as it is practiced today."[45]

Once again, the inescapable presence of industrial chemicals is cast as both inevitable and desirable, despite inherent dangers and damaged workers, while the corporations synthesizing such "newly created chemicals" (not to mention the people and places suffering from toxic exposures) remain largely unidentified. In 2013, as in 1975, US toxicologists surely could not ignore, as Casarett phrased it, how, "alarmingly, the hazard of the plant and the potential danger of its effluent spill over into the general populace."[46] Even Hodge, the prestigious US toxicologist who injected uninformed human subjects with radioactive chemicals, acknowledged the hazards of industrial-chemical-saturated societies. In his 1975 foreword to the textbook's first edition, Hodge declared, "The pioneer industrial physician Alice Hamilton found primitive methods of manufacture in the 'dangerous trades' that engendered widespread poisonings of workmen as they earned their livelihood. . . . World War I brought new agents of chemical warfare—chlorine and mustard gas— that maimed and killed. Who could have foreseen that the slowly mounting concern over poisonings, which initially called forth almost trivial attempts to control and prevent injuries, would provide the impetus for efforts that grew in breadth and intensity until from their confluence sprang a new science, toxicology?"[47] Hodge clearly credits toxicological scientists (whom at the turn of the twentieth century were primarily trained as biochemists and pharmacologists, a subset of which branched off to form the new discipline of toxicology; more on this lineage in my chapter 2) for providing the *real* answers to widespread poisonings—as opposed to the "trivial attempts" of social movement leaders and early environmental health advocates like Alice Hamilton.

Echoing his forefathers Hodge and Casarett, Gallo's chemical gaslighting goes even further, as he frames toxicology as the solution to pollution, rather than its rationalization: "The contributions and activities of toxicologists are diverse and widespread. . . . They are involved in the recognition, identification, and quantification of hazards resulting from occupational exposure to chemicals and the public health aspects of chemicals in air, water, other parts of the environment, foods, and drugs. . . . In doing so, they share . . . the responsibility for using this information to make reasonable predictions regarding the hazards of the material to people and the environment."[48] Here, sensitive readers will see yet another instance of the devil trick, as "hazards resulting from occupational exposure" and "chemicals in air, water, . . . foods, and drugs" simply exist, with no apparent source or cause. Gallo takes the devil trick a bit further than his predecessors, though arguably Hodge was not too far behind. For instance, while chemical manufacturers generally go unnamed in toxicology texts, Gallo makes a point to *commend* some of the largest corporations for their diligence, simultaneously insinuating, similarly to Hodge, that the engaged public's trivial attempts at banning beneficial substances or reducing workplace exposures are some combination of overreactive and unscientific (read: feminine and irrational). "The discipline [of toxicology]," he writes, "expands in response to legislation, which itself is a response to a real *or perceived tragedy*. . . . The major chemical manufacturers in the United States (Dow, Union Carbide, and DuPont) established internal toxicology research laboratories to help guide decisions on worker health and product safety."[49]

Perhaps in reference to such catastrophes as the thalidomide "incident," Gallo strongly implies that public and legislative responses to toxic exposures are just as likely to be merited as "dramatized"—as Hodge complained regarding DDT and Rachel Carson: "[Chemical regulation] itself is a response to a real or *perceived* tragedy."[50] Gallo, moreover, presents Dow, Union Carbide, and DuPont—all three of which have since merged to make one mega-corporation DowDuPont, which, in turn, recently rebranded as Corteva[51]—as wholly committed to "worker health and product safety." Suffice it to say that decades of activism and research demonstrate quite the opposite.[52] Tellingly, Gallo places major chemical manufacturers' toxicology research laboratories on equal footing with those of the US government (such as those in the Department of Health and Human Services or the Environmental Protection Agency [EPA]), as if the financial resources and research intentions—"worker health and product safety"—of privately and publicly funded toxicology laboratories are equivalent. One of my more industry-sympathetic toxicologist interviewees echoed this sentiment in 2019 when he complained to me, reflecting on his own experience, that working for the US EPA was "probably no different from [working for] a [chemical] manufacturer."[53] Toxicologists across the political spectrum tend to agree that the EPA is not as well-resourced as chemical manufacturers (in terms of funding, capacity, and personnel), even if they disagree on whether the EPA *should* be better equipped.[54]

Like the "unarguable dean of American toxicology" Harold C. Hodge, Michael A. Gallo, whom the Society of Toxicology honored in 2021 with their Founder's Award for Outstanding Leadership,[55] similarly depicts DDT, the main pesticide of Rachel Carson's searing critique, in an exclusively flattering light: "It was also during this time that DDT and the phenoxy herbicides were developed for increased food production and, in the case of DDT, control of insect-borne diseases."[56] Gallo's silence around DDT's adverse effects, or at least political controversies, is so deafening it is hard for a critical reader such as myself to conclude that such omissions were oversights. Gallo's positive spin on the Manhattan

Project, my final textual example for this chapter (discussed next) and easily one of the most galling instances of toxicological devil trickery, lends further credence to my claim that dominant toxicology is tacitly aligned with the economic interests of chemical manufacturers and militarist prerogatives of the Man in the State.

All's Fair in Science and War

The work of buttressing modern toxicology's uncertain predictions did not end with its founding fathers' magical historiographies (more closely analyzed in the next chapter). Contemporary toxicologists writing for the authoritative textbook *Casarett & Doull's* continuously labor to justify their inherently uncertain discipline, perhaps especially because of the field's codependency with chemical industry. Toxicologists' efforts to justify "economic poisons" often take the form of patriotic and epistemic duty—for country, and for science! The US federal government deemed the risks of nuclear warfare, including for example Hodge's violations (experimenting with uranium and plutonium on uninformed human subjects), necessary risks to take for the sake of US dominance. Casarett too, in his day, described toxicologists' varied contributions rather altruistically: "The bewildering array of economic poisons in use today is testimony to the diligence of chemists, agronomists, botanists, and entomologists concerned with control of biologic pests by toxic agents. The same poisons represent a challenge to those concerned with maintenance of ecologic balance, with conservation of the environment, and with protection of the health of man, all objectives to which the toxicologist may contribute."[57] In leading US toxicologists' eyes, modernity's "bewildering array" of synthetic toxins are a testament to scientific diligence, with toxicologists ready and willing to rise to the challenges presented by economic poisons.

Wartime justifications in particular, such as for nuclear and other chemical weapons, tend to extend beyond the official exit from the battlefield, such that the desperate measures of desperate times are not just rationalized but rather celebrated. Consider Gallo's way of introducing toxicology students to the Manhattan Project, which led directly to the United States dropping atomic bombs on Nagasaki and Hiroshima, Japan, in 1945, among many other toxic, collateral damages.[58] Gallo writes, "If one traces the history of the toxicology of metals over the past 45 years, the . . . story commences with the use of uranium for the 'bomb' . . . Indeed, *the Manhattan Project created a fertile environment* that . . . revolutionized modern biology, chemistry, therapeutics, and toxicology."[59] To cast the Manhattan Project as something that "created a fertile environment" is perhaps the epitome, or nadir, of what I am calling *chemical gaslighting*. The embodied experiences of people overexposed to industrial and military toxins, as well as the material evidence of ecologies deeply damaged by these toxic substances, are cleanly omitted.[60] Perhaps, in line with what political scientist Carol Cohn observed during her work with US defense intellectuals, "there simply is no way to talk about human death or human societies when you are using a language designed to talk about weapons." Whereas midcentury US toxicologists like Hodge and Casarett dismissed early environmental movements as unscientific and overreactive while positioning toxicologists as scientific patriots (the earliest of whom did indeed almost exclusively work for the US military), late twentieth and early twenty-first century toxicologists like Thomas and Gallo quickly skim over toxic public health disasters as unfortunate accidents—the cost of doing business, some might say. And well into the twenty-first century, an award-winning toxicologist like Gallo has completely revised indefensible atrocities, namely the US deployment of atomic bombs on Japanese civilians at the twilight of World War II, into revolutionary advances for modern science. Thuy Linh N. Tu notes the same disturbing tendencies among dermatologists contracted by the US military, who repeatedly remarked that the perplexing, debilitating skin diseases wrought by US chemical weaponry during the Vietnam War had nevertheless worked wonders for the field of dermatology.[61]

By the twenty-first century, industry- and nuclear-friendly toxicologists have taken the devil trick to new depths, beyond their twentieth century counterparts' casting of toxicants as inevitable, (begrudgingly) beneficial, and conspicuously unattached to any producers. For contemporary practitioners like Gallo, the devil trick descends into a chemical gaslighting—arguably the very antithesis of "the destroyer of worlds," as cocreator J. Robert Oppenheimer himself described the atomic bomb, would be none other than a "fertile environment."[62]

"Countless Unforeseen Events"

Although textbook examples of toxicology's devil tricks abound, I trust I have made my point clearly enough based on the selection of quotes above, spanning the oldest to the most recent edition of the authoritative US toxicology textbook *Casarett & Doull's*. Rereading these dominant toxicological narratives helped me understand what I perceived as dark ironies and misplaced anxieties at the Society of Toxicology conference I described at the opening of this chapter, where a toxicologist employed by the US military expressed genuine concern over the skin irritating potential of munitions manufacturing, while an award-winning PhD candidate in toxicology earnestly focused her research on juvenile models for chemical warfare exposure. Neither US Army scientists nor US university researchers are expected, as toxicologists, to historicize and contextualize the sociopolitical sources of toxic weaponry. Having learned and perhaps internalized the devil trick, toxicologists at various points along the political spectrum present toxicants as inevitable and apolitical, while the "contributory role" of their toxicological expertise is simply to determine "safe use" and "potential hazard."

Michael A. Gallo is admittedly an egregious example, 2021 Society of Toxicology award notwithstanding. Certainly not all US toxicologists are as sympathetic to Dow, Union Carbide, and DuPont nor as rosy-eyed about DDT and the Manhattan Project. While he exerted considerable influence over the discipline's identity and toxicologists' training, having written authoritative histories in the dominant US toxicology textbook for several decades, Gallo's contributions to *Casarett & Doull's* ended in 2013. With Gallo's departure, so left, at long last, Louis J. Casarett's original, 1975 foundation and framing. I can only imagine why the most recent, ninth edition, textbook's new contributors chose to completely rewrite the introductory, historical chapter. I would like to believe Philip Wexler and Antoinette N. Hayes read Gallo's (and, beneath several coats of chapter paint, Casarett's) questionably celebratory take on synthetic toxicant production and chemical warfare and decided they could not condone such one-sided, glaringly incomplete narratives in 2019.

Whatever their reasons, Wexler and Hayes's 2019 introductory chapter "The Evolving Journey of Toxicology: An Historical Glimpse" provides an appropriately somber and humble discussion of twentieth and twenty-first century toxicants, drawing, for instance, explicit connections between chemical warfare and pesticide development.[63] However, the devil trick is still omnipresent. Again, their opening sentences, quoted earlier in this chapter, state that "humans are smart but vulnerable. We need to be prepared for countless unforeseen events that could compromise our health and well-being. Toxicology arose as a way to understand, prevent, mitigate, and treat the potentially harmful consequences of many of the substances we are exposed to."[64]

As late as 2019, toxicologists are still not trained to ask where toxicants come from and who profits from their use and toxicology retains its innocently contributory role, having curiously arrived on the (post) exposure scene to understand, prevent, mitigate, and treat. The US discipline of toxicology, as I argue throughout this book, and as historians Linda Nash and Frederick R. Davis have documented,[65] was (and is) no innocent bystander to the "modern enlightenment of industrial progress," but rather plays a contributory role, to borrow Casarett's phrase, in rationalizing and normalizing toxic chemical exposures. And yet many contemporary environmental toxicologists in the United States, such as the PhD student I quoted in this chapter and my interlocutors in chapters 4 and 5, would not patronizingly insist that there are "harmless ways of using substances" as the likes of Casarett, Hodge, and Gallo do. Nevertheless, prominent US toxicologists' habit of both omitting sociohistorical context and presenting industrial chemicals as inevitable, desirable, and apolitical—the devil trick—has made such elisions and erasures not just normal but preferable.

While they might certainly have disagreed internally or withheld judgement, nobody at the Society of Toxicology conference I attended batted an eye at either the US Army toxicologist's or the PhD candidate's presentations on toxic weaponry, signaling tacit approval of these presenters' respective concerns for "keeping our war fighters healthy" and developing a "juvenile model for chemical warfare exposure" simultaneously.

Name That Environmental Health Hazard

Casarett & Doull's functioned more as an encyclopedic reference text in the toxicology courses I observed, as opposed to regularly assigned reading. However, this authoritative tome and its notable devil trickery seems to have left a lasting impression on toxicological training in the United States, and, arguably, has been exported globally as dominant science has in general. Both of the toxicology courses I witnessed (one as an auditor and one as an enrollee) offered selective and highly decontextualized history lessons to introduce their university-level students to the basic science of poisons, following the patterns laid out by the textbook. Incidentally, neither of the toxicology professors I observed were white men, a happenstance that speaks to my point, drawing from Wendy Brown's foundational work, that US toxicology can be masculinist without "intentionally or overtly pursuing the 'interests' of men."[66] Put another way, one does not have to be a white man toxicologist to internalize and reproduce *toxicant masculinity* (discussed in my chapter 3). One of my toxicology professors even opened the first lecture with many of the same conspicuously curated historical characters as the textbook, starring "the dose makes the poison" Paracelsus (c. 1493–1541), featured in my chapter 2, and Percivall Pott (1714–1788), one of Britain's first industrial hygienists, as they were called then. (Industrial hygiene is known today as occupational health.[67]) Reiterating Casarett's "harmless ways of using substances" logic, this particular toxicology instructor imparted Percival Pott's legacy by way of attributing the prevalence of scrotum cancer among chimney sweeps to their lack of proper hygiene—recall that the historical moment here is mid-eighteenth century London—as opposed to the systematic oppression of the emergent working class of a newly industrializing society, the economic asymmetries of which produced these workers' disproportionate exposures to carcinogenic chimney soot.[68] Making matters worse, in my view, the toxicology students (predominantly undergraduates, in this classroom) erupted in laughter at the professor's wry editorial: "I guess chimney sweeps didn't think to wash their hands before touching [their genitals]."

Percivall Pott himself, who helped establish the field of industrial hygiene, now occupational health, by documenting the strong correlations between chimney soot exposure and scrotum cancer, was considerably more sympathetic, if patronizingly so, to the plight of the eighteenth-century London chimney sweep. Writing in 1775, he lamented, "The fate of these people seems singularly hard; in their early infancy, they are most frequently treated with great brutality, and almost starved with

cold and hunger; they are thrust up narrow, and sometimes hot chim-
nies, where they are bruised, burned, and almost suffocated; and when
they get to puberty, become peculiarly liable to a most noisome, painful,
and fatal disease."[69]

I would like to believe that, if pressed, this university-level toxicology
professor would have acknowledged, as the discipline's celebrated Percival Pott did, that chimney sweeps ought not be blamed for their scrotum cancer diagnoses. After all, the very premise of occupational health,
and a core contribution of toxicology, is the laudable goal of worker
safety. However, especially as compared to my training in the critical
humanities and social sciences, toxicologists-in-training displayed a
striking lack of concern for or curiosity about any given toxicant's sociopolitical and historical context, a lack which toxicology's devil trick
only exacerbates, from my perspective. (What little historical context is
provided tends to be borderline fantastical, as described in my chapter 2,
or else grossly incomplete, as discussed throughout this chapter).

Based on my ethnographic research, upper-level toxicology courses'
dearth of sociopolitical context, a lack also apparent across multiple
editions of *Casarett & Doull's*, was perfectly normal(ized). Indeed, a
question about classism or racial capitalism would have likely thrown
the professor off track, interrupting the lecture and annoying the other
students. One afternoon, for instance, recalling an experience that had
been shared with me,[70] I somewhat impulsively called out "the police" as
an example of an environmental health hazard, stopping the toxicology
instructor mid-chalkboard. It was the first day of a graduate-level toxicology course I had enrolled in as a participant-observer, and to break
the ice the professor asked students to name examples of environmental health hazards, calling out popcorn-style. My interlocutors enthusiastically suggested: Arsenic! Benzene! Formaldehyde! Chlorpyrifos! I
waited a bit to see if anyone would offer an unconventional environmental health hazard before offering one myself: "The police!" The instructor
stopped writing on the board and everyone turned around in their seats
to peer at me, curiously. I had certainly outed myself as a social scientist.

A day or two later, I ran into one of these students on campus, an
advanced PhD in toxicology who also appeared to be the only Xican@
woman in the course. She laughed and winked at me knowingly, re-
marking on how confused the professor looked when I offered an

explanation as to why, and for whom, the police could be considered an environmental health hazard.[71] Months later in my fieldwork, more intimate conversations with graduate students revealed their latent critical thinking, but still I did not sense in them the same strong desires I felt for a science-in-context. My toxicologist colleagues neatly separated social concerns from scientific practices, as they have been trained.

Dominant science's tendency to remove—or revise—its own historical, cultural, and political context is of course the substance of much STS. I was thus rather discouraged when one anonymous STS reviewer dismissed my work in 2020 with the comment (and I paraphrase), "Of course toxicologists are bad historians—who cares?" I focus on toxicologists' interested historiographies because I believe the stories toxicologists tell about their discipline matter gravely. As many other STS scholars have elegantly demonstrated, discourse shapes science—what questions are asked, what scientists claim to know, where and how scientists look for answers, which answers are found, and who counts as a scientific expert.[72] As feminist physicist Evelyn Fox Keller writes, for instance, "The ways in which we talk about scientific objects are not simply determined by empirical evidence but rather actively influence the kind of evidence we seek (and hence are more likely to find)."[73] Scientific disciplines' own origin stories and historiographies likewise actively influence the kind of evidence sought and found. Furthermore, traditionally trained scientists maintain a disproportionate hold over public opinion and policy in the United States, deeply influencing the decision-making of politicians, regulators, judges, journalists, and lay residents, not to mention junior and aspiring scientists.[74]

Returning to the classroom, I also felt alien observing graduate students nod their heads in appreciation and listen attentively to guest speakers, most of whom were practicing toxicologists "thrilled" to share their biotech company's latest innovation in "drug delivery," to cite one visitor. During the question-and-answer period for such guest lectures, students would ask about the technicalities of a particular drug or device in development, rather than question biomedicine's turn to for-profit industry or inquire after the *social* conditions producing the specific disease being so expensively and entrepreneurially treated (e.g., type 2 diabetes[75]). Surprisingly, the strongest pushback any toxicologist

guest speaker received was regarding an inexpensive, somewhat frivo-
lous household cleaning product. (The student toxicologists-in-training
expressed rather pointed skepticism about the safety of wet wipes containing an anti-microbial chemical, one of the best-selling items manufactured by the corporation this speaker represented.)

This same invited visitor shared a story that well illustrates dominant
toxicology's distancing from sociopolitical context. Offered as a word
to the wise from a (paternal) professional to a (childlike) student, this
corporate-employed toxicologist solemnly shared a harrowing anecdote
about a chemical manufacturing firm in Japan—not hers—that recalled a
consumer product because several Japanese children died after exposure
to its synthetic chemical constituents that were mistakenly deemed safe by
company toxicologists. What disturbed me most about the speaker's delivery, never mind the content of the anecdote, was her emphasis of concern.
Rather than offer this as a cautionary tale about the limits of toxicology,
the story was framed as one of a sloppy toxicology laboratory that could
cost a toxicologist her job, not to mention wreck her conscience. To be
sure, the speaker felt horribly about the preventable deaths of innocent
children, but such tragedies did not lead her to openly question toxicological methods or regulatory processes of chemical risk assessment. Rather,
she stressed the importance of designing rigorous toxicological experiments, lest one contribute to toxicant-induced mortalities.

Was I the only person in the classroom, I wondered, questioning industry toxicologists' claims that their work "helps people live better"?
Did the guest speakers believe these altruistic claims themselves? Certainly there is an element of self-selection in any undertaking, including
my own. (Interestingly, it was one of my more industry-friendly interviewees who suggested to me that toxicologists self-select into careers,
recommending I read Nancy Neil, Torbjörn Malmfors, and Paul Slovic's
"Intuitive Toxicology: Expert and Lay Judgments of Chemical Risks,"
published in 1994.[76] I say more on this self-selection in the next chapter.)
Yet overall, my textual analyses and in vivo experiences demonstrate
that US toxicologists are not trained to understand, nor encouraged to
confront, the power asymmetries reproducing uneven toxic exposures.
Instead, and as ever, US toxicology plays the devil trick.

If environmental toxicologists—who know all too well how harmful industrial chemicals can be for human and more-than-human

ecologies—are neither educated about nor encouraged to locate toxicants in historical, social, and political context, then how indeed can toxicology be expected to "understand, prevent, mitigate, and treat" the "harmful consequences of many of the substances we are exposed to"? My collaborative, ethnographic work with environmental justice-aligned toxicologists, detailed in chapters 4 and 5, grapples more directly with this question. The next chapter analyzes how the *devil trick* spawned *magical authority* as founding US toxicologists displayed their masculinist prerogative, and white epistemic entitlement, to confidently categorize and claim control of toxicants.

2

Magical Authority

Mansplaining typically stems from an unwarranted sense of entitlement on the part of the mansplainer to occupy the conversational position of the *knower* by default: to be the one who dispenses information, offers corrections, and authoritatively issues explanations. . . . The concept of epistemic entitlement, which I'm introducing here, is obviously closely related to [philosopher Miranda Fricker's] idea of testimonial injustice. But these are distinct and complementary. Whereas testimonial injustice involves unfairly dismissing a less privileged speaker—typically, after she has attempted to make a contribution—epistemic entitlement involves peremptorily assuming greater authority to speak, on the part of a more privileged speaker. Understood in this way, we can see that epistemic entitlement is a common precursor to, and cause of, testimonial injustice.
—Kate Manne[1]

White empiricism is conceptually distinct from epistemic injustice because it describes a resistance not just to testimony but also to empirical fact.
—Chanda Prescod-Weinstein[2]

Glass Goblets and Tall Tales

Daniel Goldstein, former "Lead, Medical Sciences and Outreach and Distinguished Science Fellow" at the Monsanto Company, chose a picture of antique-looking apothecary bottles as the banner image for his LinkedIn and Twitter pages (see figure 2.1).[3] Having retired in 2018, after nearly twenty-five years of employment with this chemical corporation,

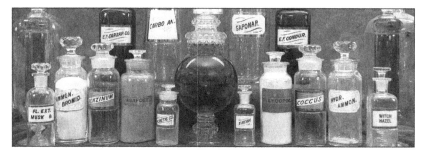

Figure 2.1: "Apothecary Historian and Collector." Goldstein 2020.

Dr. Goldstein now titles himself "Consultant in Medical, Industrial, and Environmental Toxicology; Apothecary Historian and Collector." Hence the antique-y bottles, I presume. Enveloping mysterious powders and potions, labeled with bespoke tags revealing equally mysterious (to the uninitiated) Latin names, these boldly colored and oddly shaped glass jars evoke quaint if eerie historical herbalists and apothecaries, or perhaps more wizardly concoctions for the Harry Potter generation.

Those who are more familiar with Goldstein as one of the expert witnesses for the defense in *Johnson v. Monsanto* (2016)—the first trial in which a civilian fatally diagnosed with non-Hodgkin's lymphoma won against the corporation for marketing its flagship and carcinogenic Roundup herbicide as safe—may be surprised by this industry toxicologist's affinity for the pharmacopoeia of yore.[4] Yet, as this chapter will elaborate, the founding fathers of US toxicology have aligned the discipline with a distinctly curated, one might even say fantastical, history of early science since toxicology's inception, enlisting primarily European phytomedicinal practitioners in their toxicological (tall) tales.[5]

The most frequently invoked is Paracelsus (c. 1493–1541), who is often misquoted for the core toxicology tenet "The dose makes the poison." In this chapter, I offer an explanation for why toxicologists repeatedly invoke Paracelsus, among their choice historical characters, and erroneously so. I also scrutinize toxicological methods in finer detail, underscoring the deep and enduring uncertainties that characterize this scientific discipline. I argue that early US toxicologists contrived a historiography that would buttress their shaky claims of knowing toxicants (in ways that were overwhelmingly beneficial to chemical manufacturers), curating a Euro-American, masculinist, and triumpha-list genealogy of toxicology that would lend rigor and stability to what can only be a highly predictive and uncertain science.

Endocrine-disrupting chemicals (EDCs) are especially illuminating for my argument because this class of toxicants appears, counterintui-tively to some, to be more harmful at lower doses, deeply unsettling tox-icology's core tenet of "the dose makes the poison" (which suggests that smaller doses are less harmful, if not harmless). Because they mimic nat-urally occurring hormones, even at low levels EDCs can wreak havoc on physiological functioning, particularly in critical developmental stages such as in utero, neonatal, or puberty, leading EDC researchers to insist rather that the *timing* makes the poison.[6] Despite "the timing makes the poison" findings of contemporary EDC research, dominant toxicol-ogy texts persist in emphasizing "the dose makes the poison" (alongside Paracelsus-as-progenitor), and thus extend the *magical authority* that chemical regulators and policymakers have historically accepted, and continue to act on, as rational, scientific truth. As this chapter's anal-yses will show, even when the uncertainty of toxicology experiments *is* acknowledged, toxicological evidence is still held to be superior to other(ed) forms of toxicant knowledge, namely the embodied experi-ences of those exposed.[7] US chemical regulation relies on toxicological findings to derive legal, material measures like "acceptable daily intake level" and "maximum allowable concentration," for example, while judges overseeing toxic torts in the US have been known to accept only scientific evidence as unbiased, uncontroversial evidence, as opposed to evidence of corporate intimidation of scientists or plaintiffs' personal encounters with a given toxicant.[8]

While today's toxicologists might scoff at their predecessors' revision-ist histories and misleading maxim of "the dose makes the poison," my discursive and ethnographic research suggests that the *magical authority* of the discipline's founders remains deeply embedded into toxicology's analytical logics and, in turn, carries authoritative force through public policy and regulation. I further suggest that these hauntings threaten to undermine even the most well-intentioned efforts at leveraging toxico-logical data for environmental justice.[9] Just as viewers do not fully know the concoctions contained by the apothecary jars in Goldstein's cho-sen image, people (inclusive of scientific and lay communities) do not fully know the potency—or malignancy—of chemical industry potions. What is more, industry-aligned toxicologists' romanticized nostalgia for late medieval alchemy serves to recast synthetic toxins as more palatable, even quaint, if somewhat mystical.[10] The textbook toxicologist, meanwhile, holds court as the authoritative, slightly mysterious, expert and paternal wizard. Despite some practitioners' fantastical confidence, toxicology is seriously limited as a method of knowing toxicity, as the following critical analysis of toxicological methods will illustrate.

"Trained Judgement"

When I began research for this project, I expected toxicologists to defend the surety of their methods and subsequent toxicological findings. What I found instead was that toxicologists are among the first to admit, disarmingly so, that their discipline is inherently uncertain. Toxicology "is like forecasting the weather," one of my more politically conservative interviewees declared.[11] The core US toxicology textbook *Casarett & Doull's Toxicology: The Basic Science of Poisons* likewise stressed the predictive quality of toxicology from the very beginning. For example, in 1975, Casarett wrote, "Chief among the roles of toxicologists, whether they be academically, commercially, industrially, or governmentally employed, is that of *prediction*. . . . The assessment of hazard and *the rational projection* of effects in a population are such overriding functions of toxicology that an alternate definition might be '*the science that defines limits of safety of chemical agents.*'"[12] What stands out most to me in this passage is how the "overriding function" of toxicology is to make chemicals safe, to scientifically rationalize "safe use," or "harmless ways of using substances," via toxicologists' "rational projection."[13] While Casarett writes of *limits* of safety, and further acknowledges that toxicants bring hazards, he, and the discipline of US toxicology overall, nevertheless assume that safety and chemical agents can be compatible and, moreover, that toxicologists can rationally predict effects—"the science that *defines* limits of safety." Postwar US society can have it all.

Many intellectual fields may be characterized as uncertain and interpretive, oftentimes by design or definition, such as quantum physics or semiotics, for example. What concerns me, and I hope you too, dear reader, is that toxicologists recognize their field's "chief role" as "that of prediction" and yet position the discipline as The Authority when it comes to chemical regulation, in far too many cases enabling and rationalizing chemical deployment. As my "like forecasting the weather" toxicologist interviewee somewhat irritably explained to me, "Uncertainty doesn't mean we don't know enough to make a decision [about regulating chemicals]—we can act in the face of uncertainty."[14] Ironically, advocates of the precautionary principle, which assumes a toxicant *is* hazardous in the face of uncertainty, likewise agree that uncertainty does not preclude decision-making. But from a precautionary perspective, the decision would be to *halt* production and deployment of the uncertain substance. However, those who interpret toxicological findings more on the safe side have dominated the field since its inception. For as this chapter describes, toxicology cannot truly demonstrate safety; toxicologists can only predict and project safety, or *define* safety, and have historically done so in ways that support the "industrial renaissance," as described in the previous chapter.

Founding US toxicologist Harold C. Hodge admitted to the unprecedented challenges presented by the mid-twentieth century's torrent of uncertain and dangerous toxicants, and indeed leveraged this "unforeseen toxic catastrophe," as he put it, to underscore the great need for expertly trained toxicologists. He wrote reprovingly in his foreword to the first edition (1975) of *Toxicology: The Basic Science of Poisons*:

> Occupational toxic exposures are systematically controlled in many large industrial companies that have developed excellent industrial hygiene and preventive medical practices; small companies frequently cannot afford such services. Nor is the end in sight in the efforts to forestall some unforeseen toxic catastrophe; studies are currently projected on hundreds of compounds, tests of unprecedented breadth, variety, and duration. . . . Today, unrealistically large demands for trained toxicologists are being created by sweeping new federal legislation designed to safeguard against poisonings. Contemporaneously the toxicology training programs of the National Institutes of Health, which had made a promising start in developing specialists, are being terminated despite the obvious discrepancy.[15]

Even with their heavy reliance on "the dose makes the poison," which I problematize later in this chapter, US toxicologists readily admit that the strongest toxicology studies are still only predictive and, further, that chemical production vastly outpaces the scientific process, the "excellent industrial hygiene practices" of "large industrial companies" notwithstanding. This ongoing historical legacy (which was not inevitable, but rather the result of deliberate and specific decisions wherein toxicants were made legal even before and without knowledge of their hazardous effects[16]) is normalized into the present, as is the need for toxicology specialists, who are positioned as humanity's best hope and greatest defense against "some unforeseen toxic catastrophe."

For example, in the eighth edition (2013) of *Casarett & Doull's*, Michael A. Gallo (the Manhattan Project enthusiast featured in my previous chapter), reiterates the paramount importance of training expert toxicologists "to make reasonable predictions." Echoing Casarett's "chief roles" passage from 1975, nearly forty years later Gallo writes, "The contributions and activities of toxicologists are diverse and widespread. . . . They are involved in the recognition, identification, and quantification of hazards resulting from occupational exposure to chemicals and the public health aspects of chemicals in air, water, other parts of the environment, foods, and drugs. . . . In doing so, they share . . . the responsibility for using this information to make reasonable predictions regarding the hazards of the material to people and the environment."[17] In typical *devil trick* fashion (see chapter 1), Gallo coolly lists the wide variety of toxicants people are regularly exposed to as if this hazardous state of affairs is to be expected. Toxicants are proliferate and hazardous, exposures are ubiquitous and unavoidable, and toxicologists are actively contributing, responsibly making reasonable predictions.

Perhaps because so many toxic catastrophes—the "unforeseen" in Hodge's foreword—have occurred between 1975 and 2013, Gallo reads considerably more defensively than Casarett when he describes toxicology as authoritative in terms of toxicant knowledge. While my industry-friendly interviewee insisted that "uncertainty doesn't mean we don't know enough to make a decision," Gallo goes further, insinuating that any nonscientific (read: feminized and racialized) knowledge of toxicants is inferior:

> Toxicology, like medicine, is both a science and an art. . . . For example, the observation that the administration of 2,3,7,8-tetrachlorodibenzo-p-dioxin

(TCDD) to female [laboratory] rats induces hepatocellular carcinoma is a fact. However, the conclusion that it will also do so in humans is a prediction or hypothesis. It is important to distinguish facts from predictions. When we fail to distinguish the science from the art, we confuse facts with predictions and argue that they have equal validity, which they clearly do not. In toxicology, as in all sciences, theories have a higher level of certainty than do hypotheses, which in turn are more certain than speculations, opinions, conjectures, and guesses.[18]

This passage could also be interpreted to mean that only highly and specifically trained toxicologists are to be entrusted with, or are *entitled* to, the task of accurately predicting toxicity. (Tellingly, a number of [in]famous women poisoners of bygone eras, who reportedly poisoned their own or others' husbands, are featured in early toxicologists' selective historical accounts, as discussed in the next chapter.)

Gallo's "science and art" defense of TCDD, a noxious metabolite of Agent Orange, called to my mind the concept of "trained judgement," coined by history of European science scholars Lorraine Daston and Peter Galison to characterize the scientific approach of late nineteenth and early twentieth century Europeans.[19] Trained judgement, Daston and Galison posit, is in contrast to (and an outgrowth of) the "truth-to-nature" European scientific orientation of the late eighteenth and early nineteenth centuries, as well as the "mechanical objectivity" approach of the mid-nineteenth century. Whereas truth-to-nature sought an idealized illustration of a given object, a lily flower, for instance, that would teach naturalists to categorize and identify all individual lilies based on the ideal form, "mechanical objectivity" turned to photographic renderings that would instead more realistically and comprehensively capture the many imperfections of different, individual specimens, ostensibly erasing any interpretation on the part of the scientist-viewer. In Daston and Galison's analysis, the scientific atlases from the mechanical objectivity period evidenced a certain anxiety, "a nervousness before the charge that the [pictured] phenomena were not actually out there, but instead were mere projections of desires or theories."[20] As an antidote to said nervousness, "trained judgement" rejected both the idealized drawings of truth-to-nature and the anti-interpretive photography of mechanical objectivity, rather more confidently seeking a unique mixture of *both* mechanized measurement *and* interpretive representation.[21] Late nineteenth and early twentieth century Euro-American scientists firmly believed in a new "scientific self" who could be taught—just as toxicologists can be trained—to confidently merge the objective with the subjective, or the science with the art, in Gallo's terms.[22] My critical analysis of toxicological methods, further below, reveals the ways in which toxicologists "define limits of safety of chemical agents," illustrating toxicology's interpretive yet expert moves: the *magical authority* of US toxicology.

Daston and Galison further note that this shift, from the supposedly impersonal and "blind sight" of mechanical objectivity to the taught-to-be-intuitive sight of trained judgement, occurred alongside the western European and US eugenics movements. "Racial-facial" atlases became quite popular in the late 1920s and 1930s, even among scientists and students who did not self-identify as eugenicists but nevertheless believed humans could be categorized into different "biological races" and that viewers could accurately determine a person's race with a mere glance at the face.[23] Indeed, proponents of the trained judgement approach often used racialized examples to justify their support for this new method, whether they were physicists, surgeons, or biochemists. One set of researchers celebrated a published compilation of brain images, for example, by exclaiming that this scientific atlas "permitted them to sort out electroencephalograms as confidently as they would distinguish 'Eskimos from Indians.'"[24] "Ways of seeing," Daston and Galison somberly add, "become ways of knowing."[25] Such racialized—and gendered—facets of trained judgement are no less central to toxicology.

"Intuitive Toxicology"

By the late twentieth century, US toxicologists themselves had adopted the term "intuitive toxicology," recognizing the "inherent subjectivity" of "even our best scientific methods."[26] However, the relatively reflexive toxicologists who coined the term "intuitive toxicology" did not go so far as to interrogate or historicize toxicological methods and other presumptions of US chemical risk assessment.[27] Indeed, research consultants Nancy Neil, Torbjörn Malmfors, and Paul Slovic designed their 1990s survey of Society of Toxicology members and the lay public with the explicit expectation that lay people would necessarily know less about toxicants and toxicity. As Neil et al. patiently explained in 1994,

> Human beings have always been intuitive toxicologists, relying on their senses of sight, taste, and smell to detect unsafe food, water, and air. *As we have come to recognize that our senses are not adequate to assess the dangers inherent in exposure to a chemical substance, we have created the sciences of toxicology and risk assessment to perform this function.* Massive regulatory establishments have been formed to oversee the use of these sciences for standard-setting and policy-making. Yet despite this enormous effort to overcome the limitations of intuitive toxicology, it is becoming increasingly clear that *even our best scientific methods still depend heavily on judgments* in order to infer human health risks from laboratory data on animals. Many observers have acknowledged the inherent subjectivity in the assessment of chemical risks and have indicated a need to examine the intuitive elements of expert and lay risk judgments.[28]

In this introductory paragraph, Neil and colleagues acknowledge that toxicology is inherently uncertain and subjective (if superior to human senses), as did their predecessors in *Casarett & Doull's Toxicology*, and for this reason contend that toxicological "intuition" merits closer examination. But the magical authority (and devil trickery) of toxicology has already set in, as Neil et al. unreflexively frame their survey questions around extant toxicological precepts like "the dose makes the poison," as if these fundamentals of the science somehow preexist human society, appearing without anyone's judgement, intuition, or politics.

> Each [survey] question was designed, whenever possible, according to a guiding hypothesis about how experts and "lay toxicologists" might respond. For example, *perhaps the most important principle in toxicology is the fact that "the dose makes the poison."* Any substance can cause a toxic effect if the dose is great enough. Thus, we expected experts to be quite sensitive to considerations of exposure and dose when responding to questions on this topic. In contrast, the often observed concerns of the public regarding very small exposures or doses of chemicals led us to hypothesize that *the public* would have more of an "all or none" view of

toxicity and *would be rather insensitive* to concentration, dose, and exposure (thus equating exposure with harm).[29]

The condescension with which these researchers write about "the
often observed concerns of the public" in 1994 echoes founding US toxicologist Harold C. Hodge's complaints about overly dramatic anti-DDT
activists in 1975 (see chapter 1). Notably, however, and unlike Hodge,
Neil et al. are not necessarily industry-friendly toxicologists. In their
discussion of survey results, they highlight three (of several) important
findings. In terms of "the dose makes the poison," Neil and colleagues'
hypothesis that "lay toxicologists would be rather insensitive" was confirmed: "The public is much less sensitive than the experts to considerations of dose and exposure. . . . They generally tend to view chemicals
as either safe or dangerous, and they appear to equate even small exposures to toxic or carcinogenic chemicals with almost certain harm."[30]
Their 1994 survey results also suggest that "men and more highly educated persons were somewhat less concerned about chemical risks" and
that "toxicologists working for industry saw chemicals as more benign
than did their counterparts in academia and government."[31]

I believe this rather insensitive public would be vindicated today, as
the purportedly unscientific interpretations of low-dose toxicity turned
out to be true, though I would wager a large bet that a 2024 survey of US
toxicologists and the general public would still show men to be less concerned about chemical risks and would still find that industry toxicologists view chemicals as more benign than their academic and regulatory
counterparts.[32] Of course, I am not suggesting that this single survey
accurately and comprehensively captures US scientific and public opinion on toxicants and toxicology. Rather, I quote this paper on intuitive
toxicology at such length because it shows how the magical authority of
toxicology, established firmly in 1975 with the first US toxicology textbook, persisted into the late twentieth century (and continues into the
twenty-first, as I discuss further below).

Prominent US toxicologists then and now offer their trained judgement, or confidently rely on their "intuition" and "art" to determine everything from "harmless ways of using substances" to "juvenile models
for chemical warfare exposure" in (differently) noninnocent ways, while

marginalizing nonscientific knowledge of toxicants as overly subjective or otherwise inadequate. For example, Elaine M. Faustman and Gilbert S. Omenn, two prominent US chemical regulation experts and regular contributors to *Casarett & Doull's*, describe the process of engaging non-scientists and overexposed communities in policy deliberations rather disparagingly:

> Typical [toxic exposure] problems compared in local projects are indoor air pollution, outdoor air pollution, alteration and/or destruction of terrestrial ecosystems, drinking water contamination, aesthetic degradation of the landscape, changes in land use patterns, and non-point-source pollution from everyday activities. *The community participants express their preferences in a mostly qualitative process* that leads to ranking and prioritization. There is also an effort to identify *cultural and social aspects of living circumstances that might put certain population groups at higher risk* through subsistence fishing, poor nutrition, or coexisting exposures; this element is called environmental justice [*sic*]. . . . *Increasingly, toxicologists and other regulatory scientists are being drawn in to these value-laden and sometimes emotionally charged community-based risk assessment and risk management processes.*[33]

The toxicity assessments of "community participants"—who are held responsible for their experiences of toxic environmental exposure via their "subsistence fishing" or "poor nutrition" practices—are "value-laden" and "emotionally charged," whereas the trained judgements of the toxicologist are expertly intuitive. Readers of this textbook passage are also led to sympathize with the toxicologists and other regulatory scientists who are increasingly "being drawn in" to the apparently irrational dramas of community-based risk assessment. Environmental justice (EJ) movements, which are erroneously defined in the excerpt quoted above, would perhaps rank lowest on Gallo's hierarchy from toxicologic fact to lay opinion, as EJ concerns appear to derive from "mostly qualitative" and "cultural and social aspects." Environmental justice is not in fact "an effort to identify cultural and social aspects of living circumstances that might put certain population groups at higher risk" but rather an effort to identify polluters and their racist ideologies that put certain population groups at higher risk.[34] Nevertheless, dominant toxicologists commend their own discipline for being "both a science and an art" (and commend toxicologists, presumably, for being both scientists and artists).

Industry toxicologists' embrace of only privileged subjects' intuition is perhaps unsurprising, but my research suggests this toxicological exceptionalism is not only a feature of "industry goons," as one of my environmental health scientist colleagues calls them. Among my most committed, anti-toxics advocacy interviewees was a nonprofit staff scientist well aware of industry corruption and regulatory leniency—"When was the last time the [US] government got rid of a toxic chemical?!" she demanded at one point during our hour-long conversation—who nevertheless believed that toxicology builds the foundation, forming "the base" of anti-toxics campaigns; "Good science has to be what drives the advocacy," she insisted.[35]

But where does good science come from in this context?[36] Early US toxicologists especially not only relied on their epistemic entitlement and masculinist prerogatives as socially and economically privileged, predominantly white men, but also their racially and sexually mediated intuition, (re)producing what Black feminist astrophysicist Chanda Prescod-Weinstein, alongside critical race theorists, aptly names "white empiricism."[37] Importantly, as I soon learned upon commencing this research project, US toxicology does not claim to thoroughly know toxicants. Instead, in a scientific sleight of hand, US toxicology concedes that synthetic chemicals are inherently uncertain *and* alleges to be the most authoritative source of knowledge about such indeterminate substances. (Relatedly, Prescod-Weinstein finds that her white physicist colleagues easily accept their fellow white men's speculative physics as empirically valid and cutting-edge, but when Black women physicists such as herself engage in such creative and innovative analyses, their work is dismissed as subjective, without rigor, and unscientific.) In sum, the highly predictive and uncertain methods of toxicology are positioned and widely accepted as less subjective, and hence more reliable, than the lived experiences of exposed communities or the critical research of scholar-activists.[38]

Paul Slovic, one of the coauthors of the 1994 intuitive toxicology article cited above, coauthored another, similar paper that same year. This second paper reports on a national survey focused explicitly on "Gender, Race, and Perception of Environmental Health Risks."[39] Building from two premises, evidenced by extensive previous US-based research— namely that "[men] tend to judge risks as smaller and less problematic than do women" and that "people of color are subjected to higher levels of exposure from many toxic substances"—research consultants James Flynn, Paul Slovic, and C. K. Mertz surveyed a random sample of 1,512 English-speaking people residing in the US via phone. The authors summarize their "two new and important results" as follows: "First, non-white males and females are much more similar in their perceptions of risk than are white males and females. Second, white males stand out from everyone else in their perceptions and attitudes regarding risk."[40] Flynn and colleagues argue that biological reductions of risk perception (in terms of gender) are invalidated by the finding that nonwhite men and women perceive risks similarly, and yet cannot ignore how "white males stand out from everyone else in their perceptions" about risk, or express significantly less concern.

The researchers ask, almost incredulously, "Why does a substantial percentage of white males see the world as so much less risky than everyone else sees it?" (Hmm, curiouser and curiouser.) They subsequently answer their own (rhetorical?) question: "Perhaps white males see less risk in the world because they create, manage, control, and benefit from so much of it. Perhaps women and nonwhite men see the world as more dangerous because in many ways they are more vulnerable, because they benefit less from many of its technologies and institutions, and because they have less power and control." While I take issue with Flynn and colleagues' categories of white male versus everyone else,[41] I do think they are on to something here. Perhaps unwilling to continue poking the white supremacist heteropatriarchal capitalist dragon they had approached,[42] Flynn et al. diplomatically and academically retreat: "However, our survey data do not allow us to fully test these alternative explanations. Further research is needed, focusing on the role of power, status, alienation, trust, and other sociopolitical factors, in determining perception and acceptance of risk."[43]

Encouraging as this recognition of power may be—openly questioning why "white males see the world as so much less risky than everyone else"—such critical thinking within toxicology tends to stop as soon as it starts. For instance, Neil and colleagues were surprised by another batch of results from their survey of Society of Toxicology members: "Among the most important findings in this study was the great divergence of opinion among the toxicologists themselves about fundamental issues in [chemical] risk assessment and, in particular, *the high percentage of toxicologists who doubted the validity of the animal and bacterial studies that form the backbone of their science*."[44] Magical authority cuts multiple ways. US government, industry, and academia position toxicology as the authoritative knowledge source regarding toxicants and toxicity, despite the science's widely accepted (and normalized) uncertainties, while toxicologists themselves question their own predictions and projections and yet pursue their toxicological studies as if there is no alternative.

Let us now peer behind the toxicological wizard's curtain, noting more precisely how toxicologists "define the limits of safety of chemical agents" and "make reasonable predictions regarding the hazards of the material to people and the environment." The following critical analysis of toxicological methods begins, as does the core US toxicology textbook, with Paracelsus.

"Father of Toxicology"

> What is there that is not poison?
> All things are poison and nothing (is)
> without poison. Solely the dose
> determines that a thing is not a poison.

This Paracelsus "quote," printed in a format evocative of poetry, stands solemnly as the epigraph before each voluminous edition of the primary US toxicology textbook, *Casarett & Doull's Toxicology: The Basic Science of Poisons*, from 1996 through 2019 (spanning the five most recent editions), and is referenced repeatedly throughout all nine editions (1975 to 2019) of this tome of encyclopedic proportions. The eighth and ninth editions (2013 and 2019, respectively) even include a lively cartoon to drive home the point (figure 2.2). Captioned "Dose and Dose Rate matter," this rather bizarre drawing depicts a mildly angry-looking, old-fashioned white factory worker wearing blue coveralls and a British-style flat cap hanging out of a brick building's window, slowly pouring

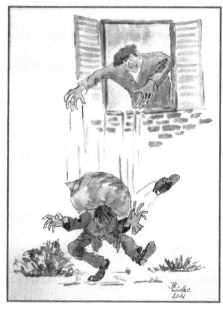

Figure 2.2: "Dose and Dose Rate Matter." Klaassen 2019.

some sort of grain, or perhaps pesticide, out of a burlap sack. The sack's contents trickle down onto another white man, this one wearing a baseball cap perched at a jaunty angle, standing below the window. The man standing beneath the window smiles gleefully yet maniacally as the sack's contents rain over his outstretched arms. Directly beneath this drawing is another of the same two men in the same setting, but this time, rather than slowly pour the sack's contents over the other man's arms, the man hanging out the window is shown rather abusively throwing the entire, full sack down on the man below, who is thus crushed by the heavy load, his baseball cap popping clear off his head due to the force of the impact. I'll say more about dominant toxicology's tendency toward such aggressive, violent, and masculinist humor in chapter 3.

Contemporary toxicologists have also published several celebratory articles on toxicology's favorite Renaissance man, such as "Paracelsus: Herald of Modern Toxicology" and "Paracelsus: In Praise of Mavericks."[45] Several of my public-health-leaning interviewees confirmed, meanwhile, that the dose-response relationship was repeatedly emphasized in their toxicological training, despite its outdatedness. My weed scientist accomplice, featured in the next chapter, characterized contemporary toxicology's use of dose-response as follows: "'The dose makes the poison' is something that people say, but I think that it's like a shutdown kind of statement, and it's almost always in the context of like, 'You, as a consumer are being exposed to this [pesticide, but] . . . your exposures are so low it couldn't even be detected'—stuff like that."[46] Another environmental toxicologist interviewee, who specializes in EDCs, the sort of substances that may be more harmful at lower doses than at higher ones, shared a similar reflection: "Yeah, I would say ['the dose makes the poison'] is probably outdated and it also, it may—I can see that being used in a way to kind of downplay the effects of, kind of, low dosage toxic effects, or pollutants. Because if people just think it takes a large dose to do anything it's like, 'oh, well the ocean's big, we can just dump it into that,' which has been a strategy that we're still using, I think."[47]

I posit that founding toxicologists curated a Eurocentric history of their emergent discipline, beginning with this late medieval, early Renaissance forefather, to add solidity to, and imbue reverence for, such an inherently uncertain science. Presenting modern toxicology as a noble descendant of the maverick work of a Renaissance man such as

Paracelsus lent this nascent science a distinguished legacy, positioning Euro-American men as the rightful heirs of such age-old knowledge.[48] And yet US toxicologists' pedestalizing of Paracelsus and misquoting of his dictum lays bare their ignorance of Paracelsus's life's mission and the true meaning of his sixteenth century words. Troubling "the dose makes the poison" tenet of toxicology not only requires reexamination from molecular and mechanistic standpoints, such as those by biologist Bruce P. Lanphear and historian Sarah A. Vogel, but also from a critical feminist science and technology studies (STS) perspective, offered in what follows.[49]

Allow me to summarize a basic toxicology experiment rather briefly and somewhat crudely, then equally briefly and crudely summarize how EDCs complicate the dose makes the poison, before more carefully examining the historio-cultural emergence of this toxicological tenet. Most toxicological experiments are conducted on rodents. Early designs of a toxicological "kill 'em and count 'em" (their turn of phrase) experiment went something like this: lab-bred rats or mice were exposed to gradually ascending doses of a given toxicant, and their bodily responses to each dose were recorded, either by observation of the living rodents' suffering or by killing the rodents, ideally after a full two years of exposure (if they hadn't died already), and dissecting them to inspect their internal organs. Such toxicological experiments hence made three major extrapolations: (1) from rodent to human; (2) from high dose (given to a rodent) to low dose (that a human may be exposed to); and (3) from short-term (length of study) to long-term (length of human life). Historically, if toxicologists could not see a toxic effect, it didn't exist. This is what toxicologists mean by a "threshold" dose, or threshold dose-response curve. The threshold, discussed in greater detail further below, is the point at which a toxic effect becomes observable. Before and below the threshold, the toxicant has no apparent effect and therefore may be labeled safe.

Basic toxicological experiments assumed that higher doses will necessarily lead to worse toxic effects. By this logic, lower doses were also assumed to be safer doses (particularly below the threshold, or where no toxic effect is observed). EDCs complicate this dose-makes-the-poison presumption because EDCs appear to be *more* harmful at *lower* doses. How can this be? One reason has to do with timing; for instance, a developing fetus exposed to a tiny amount of a toxicant, an amount that may indeed prove harmless to a fully grown adult, can experience an adverse toxic effect because developing fetuses, as one might expect, are extremely sensitive to hormonal (among other) perturbations. EDCs can also be *less* harmful at *higher* doses. How is this possible? Here, one possible reason has to do with EDCs' ubiquity. Estrogen-like synthetic chemicals are ubiquitous in our environments in large part because of their use in industrial agriculture (not to mention hormonal birth control).[50] When the body's hormone system is constantly bombarded with estrogen-like toxicants from the external environment, the body's estrogen receptors may become overwhelmed and even blocked by all the synthetic versions, such that, ultimately, the synthetic estrogen is unable to reach or otherwise access the receptor (conversely, such blockages can cause harm because the real estrogen is likewise unable to access the receptor). I will return to dose-response curves and how EDCs complicate them; for now, please keep this rudimentary version of a toxicology experiment in mind.

Paracelsus in Context

Paracelsus's real name was Theophrastus von Hohenheim, which he reserved for his medical texts. The pseudonym Paracelsus became attached to his more political-astrological and alchemical works, including the treatise in which he wrote "The *Dosis* alone makes a thing not poison."[51] Theophrastus von Hohenheim was a prolific writer, authoring everything from populist pamphlets in German to "sprawling manuscripts" in Latin,[52] nearly all of which were not published until after his death. Some historians posit that he did not choose the name Paracelsus, and further that he did not particularly like this Latinized title.[53] To be consistent and concise, however, I too will refer to this somewhat mythical figure as Paracelsus. Importantly, in sixteenth-century Europe, there was nothing unusual about a practicing physician who also dabbled in astrology, but Paracelsus spent his life battling entrenched ideas and powerful men in medicine, religion, and alchemy alike, a lifelong struggle I will revisit at this chapter's end.

Second, and more crucially, toxicologists removed "the dose makes the poison" from the context of its 1538 text, "The Third Defence

Concerning the Description of the New Receipts." This brief pamphlet was one of seven defenses (in this series) that Paracelsus wrote against establishment physicians, whom he deeply despised for their elitism and, in his view, hopelessly outdated and inadequate remedies. These seven defenses were written in a convoluted (both at the time and certainly to later readers) sixteenth-century Swiss-German vernacular, interspersed with the occasional Latin word. Only much later were they fully translated into Latin, once his manuscripts began to be published posthumously in the late 1500s. The Latin translation reads *Sola dosis facit venenum*, commonly translated into English as "Solely the dose determines that a thing is not a poison" and frequently paraphrased as simply "the dose makes the poison."[54] The English translation I accessed was completed in 1941, on the 400th anniversary of Paracelsus's death.

> If you [establishment physicians] wish justly to explain each poison, what is there that is not poison? All things are poison, and nothing is without poison: the *Dosis* alone makes a thing not poison. For example, every food and every drink, if taken beyond its Dose, is poison: the result proves it. I admit also that poison is poison: that it should, however, therefore be rejected, is impossible. Now since nothing exists which is not poison, why do you correct? Only in order that the poison may do no harm. If I too have corrected in like manner, why then do you punish me?[55]

Paracelsus's punishing contemporaries were appalled by his use of salts, minerals, and metals to treat disease; the practice of ingesting anything other than organic matter (namely plants and herbal extractions) to cure illness was blasphemous at the time. Early twentieth-century toxicologists and contemporary practitioners interpret the phrase to mean synthetic chemicals are *less* harmful in lower doses, thus rationalizing their use and fending off toxicant detractors.

My critical reading finds Paracelsus to be a rather inappropriate figure for modern toxicology to appropriate, for reasons I will return to at the close of this chapter. In any case, this brief pamphlet was somewhat insignificant in terms of the massive corpus of Paracelsus's writings, a minor aside with which modern toxicologists nevertheless remain captivated. The most recent, extensively researched biography of Paracelsus spends scarcely a paragraph of its 300-plus pages on this particular pamphlet. Biographer Charles Webster clarifies,

> The importance attached to dosage [in Paracelsus's alchemical writings] resulted in the ultimately famous dictum of Paracelsus that all things are poison and nothing is without poison; it is the dose alone that frees a thing from its poisonous nature. This statement said what it meant, as indicated by the clarification that all nutriments are poisonous if taken in the wrong amounts. However, *the context of this dictum indicates that Paracelsus's main objective was to insist on the modification of poisons by their chemical correction and not primarily by their dose.* Consequently, it could be argued that Paracelsus was only to a limited extent the anticipator of the modern dose-response relationship.[56]

While Webster is not critical of the dose-response relationship itself, being a historian of late medieval Europe rather than of modern US toxicology, he is arguably the most qualified scholar today to clarify that Paracelsus was *not* arguing that small amounts of poison are necessarily innocuous. What is more, based on Webster's close readings of Paracelsus's copious texts, in accordance with his belief that "nothing is without poison," Paracelsus would likely have modified substances, rather than their quantities, to ensure safety and efficacy.

Unsettling Dose

In addition to toxicologists' misinterpretations and misappropriations of this particular paragraph, in the centuries that have passed since Paracelsus's lifetime, scientists of various taxa have learned that the dose-to-poison relationship is not so simply delineated. Carcinogenic chemicals, for instance, do not become more or less carcinogenic in larger or lesser amounts—they are considered carcinogens at any dose. Dose-response "curves" for carcinogens are thus usually plotted as straight lines, ascending from the zero point on an *x-y* axis (see figure 2.3), or perhaps as gently sloping lines, but in either case, with no threshold, or no safe dose. Recall that the threshold marks the dose at which a toxic effect is observable (by the toxicologist) and that before or

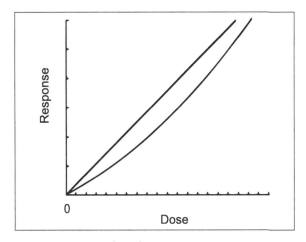

Figure 2.3: Linear and Nonlinear Carcinogenic Dose-
Responses; No Threshold Dose. Courtesy of the author.

beneath the threshold, a toxicant may be deemed safe. *Non*carcinogenic
chemicals are thus said to have threshold dose-response curves.

In the early 1990s, scientists sounded the alarm over the newly labeled
endocrine-disrupting chemicals (EDCs), toxicants which mimic naturally occurring hormones and, again, may be more harmful in smaller
doses than in higher doses, depending on the timing and duration of exposure, rather than the quantity.[57] As opposed to the presumably more
typical threshold dose-response curve to which Paracelsus's adage is applied, EDC dose-response curves are often graphed in a U-shape (see
figure 2.4 for threshold curve; see figure 2.5 for EDC curves).

Before toxicology existed as an academic discipline in the United
States, early practitioners' "trained judgement," as described above,
emerged from their educations in the more established disciplines of
biochemistry and pharmacology. Hence, founding toxicologists borrowed the concept of a threshold dose from pharmacology's conception
of a therapeutic dose. Pharmacologists, or "drug discoverers," as I later
heard some self-identify (we'll meet one such practitioner in the next
chapter), determine how much of a pharmaceutical is enough to be effective, meaning therapeutic, *before* becoming toxic (figure 2.6). Toxicology, by contrast, is a science definitively interested in the "toxicological

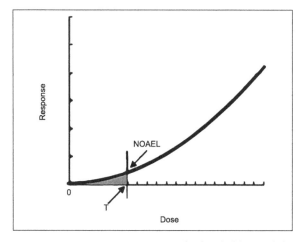

Figure 2.4: Dose-Response Curve with Threshold Dose (T) and No Observed Adverse Effect Level (NOAEL). Courtesy of the author.

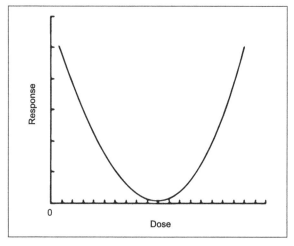

Figure 2.5: Non-Monotonic Curves More Typical of EDCs. Courtesy of the author.

potential" of chemical agents, as Gallo put it in 2013. Importantly then, for toxicology, "effective" *means* toxic, just not *too* toxic. The dose makes the poison.

The toxicological assumption that no harm is done because no response is observed illustrates precisely the sort of magical authority

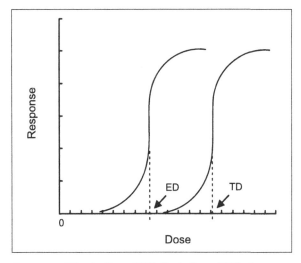

Figure 2.6: Effective Dose (ED), Toxic Dose (TD). Courtesy of the author.

that not only enabled widespread and unevenly distributed chemical contamination but also delimits today's toxicology. Blissfully ignorant, perhaps, of their overprivileged social positions and the partiality of their visions, early toxicologists asserted that their particular perceptions and mathematical calculations ought to be accepted (by US regulators and regular residents alike) as the rigorous, "rational projection" of trained judgment and intuition, as science and art.

Grandfathered In

Setting aside, for a moment, the magical authority exemplified by the threshold dose, one might ask "How did early US toxicologists convince government officials to accept their shaky science as the foundation for federal and state legislation, thereby enabling the widespread deployment of such unknown and unknowable poisons?" In the early and mid-twentieth century, there was arguably little US government resistance or regulation to begin with; the powers that be were generally already aligned with synthetic chemical manufacturers. Frederick R. Davis's historical account shows that founding US toxicologists were almost exclusively funded by the US Department of Defense, which in turn contracted out chemical firms such as Dow and DuPont.[58] Whatever paltry environmental or workplace safety regulations that did exist were the hard-won result of grassroots struggles by factory and farm workers, as well as early public health advocates and environmentalists. By the time the Clean Air and Water Acts of the 1970s were written, for example, tens of thousands of toxic chemicals had already been introduced to the market and were thus grandfathered in, pun intended.[59]

Yet toxicologists still sought scientific legitimacy. Early toxicologists' considerable efforts to present their discipline as a distinguished practice with an impressive pedigree, boasting several highly revered historical characters, suggests to me there was in fact a great deal of unresolved anxiety about the inherent uncertainties of this unstable science. In other words, despite enjoying limited resistance or questioning by government officials from the late nineteenth century onward, US toxicologists still labored to legitimize their highly conjectural new discipline as sturdy and robust: the authoritative arbiter of chemical concerns. I suggest it was in seeking to alleviate their anxieties, about the unknowability of toxicants' effects, that founding US toxicologists turned to the security and familiarity of Eurocentric and patriarchal historiographies.

Pace that anonymous STS reviewer who dismissed my work with "of course toxicologists are bad historians," I draw attention to early US toxicology's misuse of mythical characters like Paracelsus because contemporary, influential toxicologists—those authoring textbook chapters or informing public policy, for instance—uncritically repeat these nostalgic narratives. This myopia produces cumulative effects, not simply delimiting what toxicologists ask and can therefore answer, but also what legislators can legislate, what regulators can regulate, what courts can adjudicate, what consumers can navigate, and what EJ activists can corroborate. By contrast, if toxicologists—and their STS critics—better historicize and expand the purview of toxicological questions, we might also expand the possibilities for EJ futures, a challenge I venture toward in this book's conclusion.

Let us now turn to how exactly toxicologists determine the threshold dose, derive "toxicological potential," and "define limits of safety": the dose-response relationship.

The Dose-Response Relationship

The dose-response relationship is a dynamic derived from Paracelsus's dictum that remains *the* central tenet of toxicology. To quote founding US toxicologist Louis J. Casarett once again, "The concept of this relationship is the most fundamental and pervasive one in toxicology."[60] In the ninth and most recent edition (2019) of the much-expanded *Casarett & Doull's Toxicology* textbook, this relationship is reaffirmed as "the foundation" as well as "the bedrock of modern toxicology."[61] Meanwhile, for his "concise encapsulation," Paracelsus "deserves the laurel crown and the oft-cited appellation, 'Father of toxicology.'"[62] Below, I critically reexamine the dose-response relationship as it is understood by practicing toxicologists then and now.

Early toxicologists primarily relied on rodent experimentation (and continue to do so today, though efforts at reducing the use of live animals for biomedical studies have been underway for quite some time; more on laboratory animals in chapter 5).[63] One method required dosing rats or mice with gradually increasing amounts of a toxicant until 50 percent of this ill-fated rodent population died, termed the "lethal dose at 50" and scientifically notated as LD50. Scientists, including toxicologists, somewhat derogatorily refer to this method as "kill 'em and count 'em."[64] After determining the LD50 of several toxicants, toxicologists created an index of toxicity, allowing them to compare toxicities across substances, ranging from 1 "practically nontoxic" to 6 "supertoxic" (see table 2.1).[65]

Toxicologists typically test only one chemical substance at a time, for a properly controlled experiment. One of the most prestigious toxicologists I had the opportunity to interview, a former director within the World Health Organization's International Agency for Research on Cancer, explained in response to a question of mine (regarding chemical interactivity) that testing multiple toxicants at a time, in what are called cumulative risk assessments, are not necessarily required and can be expensively superfluous.[66] For the purposes of regulation (and litigation), it is enough, this public health expert made clear, to show that one toxicant in the mix is harmful.

To be sure, even founding toxicologists recognized LD50 as a rather crude measure. Casarett subsequently observes, "The use of common

TABLE 2.1: Indices of Lethality. Casarett and Doull 1975, 23.

Summary of Classification Placing Toxicants Into Categories Related to Their Relative Toxicities

Toxicity Rating	Commonly Used Term	Probable Human Lethal Dose, 70-Kg (150-Lb) Man	
6	Supertoxic	<5 mg/kg	A taste; <7 drops
5	Extremely toxic	5–50mg/kg	7 drops–1 teaspoonful
4	Very toxic	50–500 mg/kg	1 tsp–1 ounce
3	Moderately toxic	0.5–5 g/kg	1 oz–1 pint or pound
2	Slightly toxic	5–15 g/kg	1 pint–1 quart
1	Practically nontoxic	>15 g/kg	>1 quart

expressions of toxicity (moderately, slightly, etc.) and (common) dimensions of the total dose (taste, teaspoonful, etc.) enhance the usefulness of this classification in recognizing acute intoxications."[67] Working backward from death, using words and measures one might expect to find in a comic book ("supertoxic") or cookbook ("a taste"), rather than a science textbook, toxicologists are instructed to (intuitively?) derive "a measure of lethality somewhere between two extremes" based on this alarmingly—in my view—simplistic classification table, the common terms of which reportedly enhance its usefulness.

Meanwhile all lethality measures are derivatives from the normative response of the average healthy adult (white) male human, a central figure who is himself an extrapolation from statistical averages. Casarett permits that lethality "is inadequate as an index for the protection of health." However, he also makes clear that the classifications and indices may be relied, indeed depended, on to generate enforceable standards for safety evaluation and regulation: "As the health and safety of man is one of the major concerns of toxicology, . . . guidelines are determined by the probable duration of exposure to the toxicant and an estimate of the dose to a target site based on knowledge of the rate of absorption and elimination of the material. The guidelines set limits of exposure at which there is a reasonable assurance that there will be no deleterious effects."[68] Note the caveats and value judgements in this description of safety standards: *probable* duration, *estimate* of the dose, *reasonable* assurance. Toxicologists-in-training are then introduced to official, regulatory terminology: "The term used to express a safe level is the maximal allowable concentration or the maximal atmospheric concentration (MAC). The levels are derived from animal experiments and human experience and are set by known chronic toxic effects or by odor or relatively minor nuisance effects. Deleterious effects are insignificant at exposure levels below the MAC for eight hours a day, five days a week over a working lifetime."[69] This passage also illustrates the centralizing force of industrial and capitalist economic logics throughout early toxicology, as regulatory applications of toxicological studies revolve around the presumed "eight hours a day, five days a week over a working lifetime."

To flesh out the bare bones of LD50, toxicologists further derived such measures as the "effective dose at fifty" (ED50), at which 50 percent of the experimental population shows a toxic response (other than death) to the toxicant administered, borrowing again from pharmacology's conception of the therapeutic index (see figure 2.6). From the effective—toxic but not fatally so—dose at fifty, toxicologists then derive the threshold dose for the default man.

Crossing the Threshold

The threshold seems an apt metaphor for a science so enamored with Paracelsus, a figure bestriding the late Middle Ages and the early Renaissance and, moreover, one who took his astrological philosophies as seriously as his medical practices.[70] Indeed, the concept of the threshold in modern physiology (and psychology) has become so commonplace that it is no longer connotative, but denotive.[71] The secondary definition of threshold, according to the *Oxford English Dictionary*—listed after "the sill of a doorway," "the line which one crosses in entering," and "the beginning of a state or action"—is "In technical language, a lower limit." The definition continues:

(a) Psychology: esp. in threshold of consciousness. . . . In Physiology and more widely: the limit below which a stimulus is not perceptible; the magnitude or intensity of a stimulus which has to be exceeded for it to produce a certain response.

(b) The magnitude or intensity that must be exceeded for a certain reaction or phenomenon to occur.[72]

In specifically toxicological terms, "a threshold . . . by definition represents a dose below which no response is observed."[73] As mentioned, toxicologists have since determined that certain toxicants may be harmful at any dose, including carcinogens and the more recently identified endocrine-disrupting chemicals, which, somewhat counterintuitively, tend to be more harmful at lower doses than at higher ones.

Toxicants that have not (yet) been categorized as carcinogenic or endocrine-disrupting are considered to have threshold doses, from which are derived the No Observed Adverse Effect Level, or NOAEL. Readers of *Casarett & Doull's Toxicology* are taught that NOAELs may be converted into the regulatory requirements of Reference Doses (RfD) and Acceptable Daily Intake (ADI) levels by dividing the NOAEL by the Uncertainty Factor (UF) times the Modifying Factor (MF) = NOAEL/ (UF * MF). If you are confused by this toxicological jargon I have made my point. Mathematical equations make magical authority seem more rational, and secure, than it is.

Regulatory agencies such as the US Department of Agriculture and the World Health Organization use RfDs as "estimates of a daily exposure to an agent that is assumed to be without an adverse health impact on the human population," while they use ADI levels to define "the daily intake of chemical, which during an entire lifetime appears to be without appreciable risk on the basis of all known facts at that time."[74] "All known facts" include this magical space below and before the threshold dose, where all too frequently no *observed* effect is interpreted by the (intuitive?) toxicologist—and subsequently by the law—to mean no harm done. In figure 2.4, the threshold dose is point T, along the *x* axis. The NOAEL, short for "No Observed Adverse Effect Level," marks the last moment/dose before an adverse effect, or toxic response, is first observed.[75] I have shaded in this liminal space and moment before and below the threshold and NOAEL.[76] Moving up the *y* axis, the percent of the experimental population (or the statistical mean of multiple experimental populations) showing an adverse response to the dose—an adverse response which is now perceptible to the intuitive toxicologist, having crossed the threshold—likewise increases along the *x* axis. In plainer terms, this graphed, slightly curved line shows that the higher the dose, the greater the toxic response, but only after that initial threshold has been breached: the dose makes the poison, once having crossed a threshold. Or: a little toxicant never hurt anybody.

Founding practitioner and textbook coeditor Louis J. Casarett repeatedly emphasized toxicology as a science of prediction and probability, assuring toxicologists-in-training (and other readers) that toxicology's quantitative and conceptual tools stiffen the soft grounds of inquiry and rationalize the interpretive practice "of expressing the toxicity in ways that permit judgment about the safety of the substance, especially in man."[77] Casarett continues, "We can define safety in terms of the probability that a substance will not produce damage under specified conditions and hazard, the reciprocal of safety, in the same terms. . . . *The task, then, is basically one of prediction* of the qualitative and quantitative impact of a substance. . . . In toxicology there looms a basic assumption, at least tacit, but sometimes explicit. This assumption states that one can design and critically execute a series of experimental procedures to arrive at a definition of the probable hazard to man and the magnitude of the hazard."[78]

Let us move more deliberately through the "basic assumption" that Casarett glides over: "that one can design and critically execute a series of experimental procedures to arrive at a definition of the probable hazard to man and the magnitude of the hazard." As this excerpt shows, founding US toxicologists considered themselves capable of knowing chemicals, and further, they asserted that government officials (and, by extension, the lay public) should trust toxicologists' powers of prediction (intuition would come later) in order to derive lawful applications of their predictions. Here again we have magical authority.

Thus even explicit acknowledgment of the layers of assumptions and laboratory limitations built into toxicology—"like forecasting the weather" as one of my interviewees memorably summarized—did not prevent its founding (nor contemporary) practitioners from arriving at actionable definitions such as "maximum allowable concentration" and "acceptable daily intake" level. Toxicological findings are still presented as authoritative despite how tenuous toxicological experiments are in terms of measuring toxicants' harmful outcomes.

Such magical authority remains intertwined with the devil trick; dominant practitioners position toxicology as not only authoritative but also disinterested, even while its architects acknowledge, if casually, the socioeconomic basis for its substances of study. For example, offering no comment on whether toxicants *ought* to be produced, Casarett offhandedly remarks: "By far the greatest number of toxicants stem from the industrial and commercial pool of synthetic chemicals. Thousands of new chemicals are produced each year and many of these reach biologic systems directly or indirectly."[79] While conventionally trained scientists might argue it is not for toxicologists to opine on the substances they are testing, clearly safety evaluations and risk assessments of such slippery synthetics cannot be conducted without a significant measure of judgement, however expertly trained. (In any case, Casarett certainly does not hesitate to editorialize on matters pertaining to those whom he patronizingly terms "the distaff set," as I will elaborate in the next chapter.)

Throughout, contributors to this first edition of *Toxicology: The Basic Science of Poisons* choreograph chemical toxicity into measurable, knowable, stable phenomena, even as they define the discipline as inherently predictive and interpretive. Of course, I am not arguing that toxicology *should* somehow be definitive or disinterested and that Casarett and colleagues were simply doing it wrong. My point, along with other critical feminist STS scholars, is that scientific inquiry is never neutral—even the concept of objectivity is historically contingent[80]—and that practitioners' situated knowledges matter, especially when the "view from nowhere" generates sizable harm somewhere.[81] As one of my interviewees, a toxicologist working for a national environmental nonprofit, put it, "There's a tolerance for risk when it's not your risk."[82]

Toxicology's core tenet of the dose-response relationship thus emerges from a series of predictions, as trained expert and intuitive toxicologists extrapolate from high doses administered to rodents, to low doses that "man" would be exposed to "under specific conditions." The calculations required for such conversions are linearly listed in table 2.2.[83] The intuitive toxicologist further extrapolates from short-term (average laboratory rodent life expectancy is two to four years) to long-term (average human life expectancy, circa 1975, was sixty-eight to seventy-six years), mathematically manipulating the results of, say, a two-year rodent study (the gold standard of toxicology) into threshold doses, and, in turn, acceptable daily intake levels and maximum allowable concentrations and reference doses, for an averaged human.

TABLE 2.2: Comparative Toxicity by Species and Size. Casarett and Doull 1975, 22.

Comparison Of Dosage By Weight And Surface Area (100 Mg/Kg) Dose

Species	Weight (G)	Surface (Cm2)	Dose By Weight (Mg)	Dose By Surface (Mg)	Ratio
Mouse	20	46	2	2	1
Rat	200	325	20	14	1.43
Guinea pig	400	564	40	24	1.65
Rabbit	1500	1272	150	55	2.74
Cat	2000	1381	200	60	3.46
Monkey	4000	2975	400	128	3.12
Dog	12,000	5766	1200	248	4.82
Man	70,000	18,000	7000	776	9.08

On top of these multilayered predictions and extrapolations and statistical calculations, we may also add the wide variety of toxic effects a toxicologist can see and measure (setting aside what is invisible or unmeasurable). Tetraethyl lead, for instance, which is used to prevent gasoline and other fuels from knocking in machinery, can cause severe acid burn on the skin—an acute effect—and eventually impair kidney function without having touched the kidney—a chronic effect. Importantly, as historian Linda Nash observed, "In the toxicological model, only those conditions that could be linked quantitatively to a specific chemical exposure (e.g., a measurable level of airborne lead dust in the workplace) and a known physiological effect (e.g., elevated levels of lead in the blood stream) could constitute chemically induced disease. Felt conditions of illness that could not be diagnosed in the laboratory were dismissed, while diagnosed conditions that could not be traced to a specific chemical exposure were attributed to other causes."[84]

Again, what surprised and disarmed me most about toxicology is how ambivalent its own practitioners are regarding toxicological methods. Writing in 1975, Casarett admits that the dose-response relationship— the most fundamental concept in toxicology—is an entirely uncertain one (if "reasonably" so):

To arrive at a quantitative and precise statement of the relation between a toxic material and an observed effect or response . . . one must know with *reasonable certainty* that the relationship is indeed a causal one. . . . *One is usually in some doubt* about the identity of the specific toxic agent or the true dose to which the organism has been exposed or the site and relative specificity of the response—or all of these. In its most strict usage, then, the dose-response relationship is firmly based on the knowledge or a *reasonable presumption* that the effect is a result of the known toxic agent(s).[85]

Casarett readily admits "one is usually in some doubt" about the toxicant, the dose, the exposure site, the toxic response, or all of the above, and yet toxicologists can claim to know what people need to know about chemicals in order to avoid harm. This is what I mean by toxicology's magical authority.

Thus far I have drawn primarily from the first edition of what would become the core US toxicology textbook, *Toxicology: The Basic Science of Poisons*. What about contemporary practices, one might ask? How does *Casarett & Doull's* teach toxicology today, after specialists in genetic toxicology and the emerging science of epigenetics reveal how harmful effects of chemical exposure can be latent for several generations, while advances in endocrinology have shown that even short exposures to low (formerly known as "safe") doses during critical developmental stages can prove debilitating, if not fatal?[86] Relying on "the dose makes the poison" is gravely misleading in such cases, which are not at all anomalous.[87]

When I showed the 1975 "Comparison of Dosage by Weight and Surface Area" table to an environmental health scientist active today, she dismissed such taxonomies as laughable. And yet in the ninth edition of this dominant textbook, one 2019 descendant of this funny 1975 table appears as "Conversion of Animal Doses to Human Equivalent Doses (HED) for a 60-kg Person Based on Body Surface Area" (table 2.3).[88]

Putting aside questions about toxicological experimentation on micro-pigs versus mini-pigs, among other model organisms listed in 2019, let us recall why one would need to calculate an equivalent dose, assuming such equivalencies exist, between a man and, say, a marmoset. Toxicological experiments on animals are designed, and measures

TABLE 2.3: Equivalent Doses Between Species. Klassen 2019.

Species	Divide Animal Dose (Mg/Kg) By
Mouse	12.3
Hamster	7.4
Rat	6.2
Ferret	5.3
Guinea pig	4.6
Rabbit	3.1
Dog	1.8
Monkey	3.1
Marmoset	6.2
Squirrel monkey	5.3
Baboon	1.8
Micro-pig	1.4
Mini-pig	1.1

and indices of toxicity are calculated, to create reference doses, or legal allowances, for human exposure, rationalizing the continued release of tens of thousands of synthetic chemicals, even without comprehensive toxicological data, into our environments—comprising an inescapable and infinitely interactive presence.[89]

While toxicologists themselves admit such reference doses and legal allowances are somewhat arbitrary, or at least based on prediction, modeling, and "reasonable certainty," I posit that these official terms and calculations work to *conceal* the inherent uncertainty of toxicology, presenting toxicological findings as the solid results of so-called hard science. These scientific facts then become supposedly neutral justification for regulatory frameworks such as acceptable daily intake levels and maximum allowable concentrations.[90] Monsanto, for instance, as well as the US Environmental Protection Agency, has repeatedly pointed out that consumers' everyday exposures to glyphosate (Roundup) through food consumption are well below regulatory limits and therefore safe.[91]

To be sure, toxicology in 2019 is more advanced and nuanced than in 1975. But my research suggests that the "residues" of mostly class-privileged white male and mostly proindustry practitioners' presumptions and predictions have sedimented into today's toxic planet.[92] As mentioned, by the 1976 passing of the US Toxic Substances Control Act, over 60,000 synthetic chemicals already circulating were grand-fathered in, as it were—assumed to be safe based on toxicological evidence deemed naïve, if not ridiculous, by today's scientific standards.[93] Moreover, even though historical dose-response experiments and other toxicological judgements have unintentionally, if irresponsibly, generated widely harmful consequences, contemporary toxicology and subsequent chemical regulation remains rooted in these questionable logics.[94] Chemical regulation continues to rely on toxicological experimentation, and toxicological experimentation continues to rely on the "intuitive" toxicologist's "reasonable presumption" that "the relation between a toxic material and an observed effect or response . . . is indeed a causal one." How might this magical authority be limiting toxicological practice today, particularly by those scientists who align themselves with environmental advocacy and justice movements? I address this question more directly in the second part of this book. The remainder of this chapter reviews how founding toxicologists' questionable logics work their way well into the twenty-first century.

"Everything Comes Down to a Calculation"

My reading of core toxicology texts concurs with public health historian Linda Nash's analysis of toxicology's normalization of toxic exposure. However, my ethnographic research with toxicologists suggests they are no longer "reproducing the world in the image of the early 20th century factory," as Nash wrote.[95] The toxicologists I interviewed had turned their scientific attentions entirely to harm reduction, relying on toxicological measurements not necessarily because such figures might allow them to assess toxicants' effects more accurately but rather because these quantifications provided a basis on which to hold both polluters and regulators to account. Four of my public-health-leaning interviewees reflected on this:

> We're playing the [chemical] industry's game of catch-up! . . . Scientists do not know everything.[96]

I would like to see more common sense [in toxicology], a lot of times we're crunching numbers and dancing on the heads of pins. . . . We tie ourselves up trying to do these precise calculations . . . if a chemical is bioactive, it's bioactive.[97]

The whole way the [chemical regulatory] system is set up is backwards—we're chasing something that's already happened, it's like trying to get a cat back in the bag. We're already contaminated, people are invested. . . . We need decision tools regarding amounts for clean-up, etc. . . . There are many areas where you need a number—it's too big of a problem.[98]

Better epidemiological data is a failure of public health. . . . Why wait for a cancer study in people? . . . The procedural arguments win in court . . . industry wants the same thing but they live in a statistical world; everything comes down to a calculation . . . we don't have numbers for human suffering . . . When I started this job [at an environmental nonprofit], I felt like suing people was mean. I feel differently now. I love the law! We're suing for environmental statutes.[99]

Just as industry-friendly toxicologists readily admit their methods are uncertain, predictive, and judgmental—"both a science and an art"—environmental-health-aligned toxicologists readily admit that toxicology and chemical regulations are inadequate for the urgent tasks of reducing human and ecological suffering. Yet all but one of my thirty-three interviewees, spanning the political spectrum, could think of no alternative to using toxicology to know toxicants (for the purposes of chemical regulation). What is more, while all my interviewees admitted toxicology's inherent limits and noted the pitfalls of industry influence, none went so far as to situate US toxicology's historical emergence, or to critically revisit toxicological knowledge production in a socio-historical light. Hence many of Nash's observations in 2008 remain sadly true today: "The assumptions that underwrite our reliance on chemical-by-chemical standards are derived from . . . the power-laden environment of the early industrial factory. [These] historical contexts . . . should warn us against the easy assumption that what we need most is 'better science' or less uncertainty."[100]

Magical Thinking at the End of Time

US toxicology textbook authors certainly paid attention to historical narratives, even if student and practicing toxicologists tend not
to. The ninth edition (2019) of *Casarett & Doull's Toxicology* was published just as I was wrapping up the greater portion of my archival and
ethnographic data collection. I had to submit a special request to my
university library to order this hefty and expensive hardcover. Naturally
I was the first patron to borrow the book, and the brand-new binding
cracked satisfyingly when I slowly opened the shiny front cover. Sure
enough, the Paracelsus "dose makes the poison" epigraph greeted me,
as did the accompanying cartoon featured in the eighth edition (2013)
(see figure 2.2). However, the obligatory, introductory history chapter
was, for the first time since 1975, substantially rewritten by new textbook
contributors Philip Wexler and Antoinette N. Hayes.[101]

In 1975, Casarett and other founding toxicologists described the discipline as defining "limits of safety of chemical agents"; in 2019, Wexler
and Hayes claim that toxicology arose to "prevent, mitigate, and treat"
the purportedly unanticipated consequences of massive, toxic chemical exposures. Remarkably, both the 1975 and 2019 editions stress the
"unforeseen" nature of "toxic catastrophe." Recall that in 1975, Hodge
assured readers, "Nor is the end in sight in the efforts to forestall some
unforeseen toxic catastrophe; studies are currently projected on hundreds of compounds, tests of un-precedented breadth, variety, and duration."[102] In 2019, Wexler and Hayes somewhat less confidently reassure
that "humans are smart but vulnerable. We need to be prepared for
countless unforeseen events that could compromise our health and
well-being."[103] As ever, prominent US toxicologists elide the politics
of chemical production and distribution of harms in their historical
curations—the devil trick (see chapter 1). After several glossary terms,
Wexler and Hayes preface their 2019 rendition of toxicological history
with a curious caveat: "History is *about* the past; it is not the past. The
past is passive, objective, all encompassing. History is active, subjective, and selective. The further back in time that we look, the more
problematic it is for us to reach, in the present, conclusions about
what happened in the past. Examples, particularly from ancient eras,
described below, will show how tales accepted without question are

currently being re-examined and revised, and remind us that history is also relative."[104]

I read this cautionary entry paragraph as both a critique of the toxicology historiographies presented in previous editions, and as a preemptive against future (and present) toxicology critics. In contrast to previous editions, Wexler and Hayes's "Toxicology in Antiquity" section covers regions other than Western Europe and the United States—namely, Ancient China, Ancient India, Ancient Egypt, Ancient Greece, and Ancient Rome—but only back in time ("Ancient") and only in brief, altogether comprising less than three pages. Tales from the European Middle Ages, Renaissance, and the modern Global North (focusing on the United States) take up the next twelve pages. Paracelsus remains a central character, celebrated for his "incalculable contributions" on occupational exposures especially, even if Wexler and Hayes knock his pedestal down a few notches: "Inevitably we reach the point where we address the incalculable contributions of the unorthodox medical revolutionary, Theophrastus von Hohenheim, called Paracelsus (1493/94–1541). . . . He was a wanderer and iconoclast, and strongly tied to the alchemical tradition. . . . History, though, has vindicated many of his teachings. In addition to his medical works, he was a keen observer and investigator of toxic effects of various agents and wrote a treatise about their effects upon miners."[105]

The discipline of toxicology appears more humble, even regretful, in this 2019 edition. Meanwhile scientific concepts such as endocrine disruption and epigenetics have prompted a more integrative, systems approach to toxic exposure, complicating understandings of the dose-response relationship in crucial ways. And yet toxicologists in the twenty-first century still accept toxicant production and chemical exposure as inevitable and apolitical, as if there is no alternative, and still position the dose-response relationship, however magically derived, drawn, and contested, as central to and definitive of toxicology.

Paracelsus remains the "father of toxicology" as well. But which of his teachings has "history vindicated," specifically? I find that Paracelsus both suits and does not suit modern toxicologists' purposes. He may be a fitting progenitor in the sense that he advocated for the use of inorganic substances, but the similarities between his sixteenth-century practices and those of modern toxicology end there. Paracelsus's salt, mineral, and metallic remedies were not necessarily to enable miners to continue mining, nor to justify their occupational exposures to harmful elements. His unconventional treatments were meant as just that—curatives to *treat* illness, rather than rationale for disease-causing agents. Further, it is a far cry to associate the therapeutic effects of mineral baths, for instance, with the supposedly not *too* toxic consequences of synthetic pesticide exposure, among other economic poisons. (Recall that "economic poisons" is an outdated but arguably more accurate term for toxicants deemed hazardous yet necessary, including pesticides and chemical weapons.)

Modern toxicology's adoption of "the dose makes the poison" works to relativize and abstract all forms of toxicity. Where a particular poison comes from or who becomes poisoned, never mind who profits, is relegated far outside this scientific practice. Toxicology's statistical metrics of dose and response are calculated for clinical, comparative purposes— recall the lethal dose at fifty (LD50) and terms of relative toxicity in tables 2.1 and 2.2—while the politics of and preconditions for bodily harm are elided at best, celebrated at worst (e.g., Gallo's spin on the Manhattan Project "creating a fertile environment").

On another material level, though he was by most accounts a skilled (if uncertified) physician, Paracelsus was neither successful nor accepted during his lifetime. He repeatedly and deliberately railed against establishment medicine, disgusted by powerful physicians' corruption and disdain for the peasantry, thus sabotaging any hopes of a stable medical career or lucrative publishing prospects.[106] Paracelsus wrote legions of cheap, popular pamphlets in German, as opposed to his more distinguished contemporaries' highly specialized, expensively illustrated atlases in Latin, because he was on a self-imposed mission to bring healing (and Lutheran Reform) directly to the people. I imagine he would be greatly dismayed, if not outraged, by modern toxicology's claims on his "dose makes the poison" defense. As historian of European science Massimo Mazzotti put it, Paracelsus was specific about the "we."[107]

Industry infiltration into toxicology and chemical regulation is an open secret, and over the course of my research I ran up against industry representatives at every turn. Corporate scientists dominated the toxicology conferences I attended, for example, which due to their overwhelming presence often looked and felt more like tradeshows than academic meetings. Industry toxicologists such as Daniel Goldstein, the self-styled apothecary historian and Monsanto retiree with whom I began this chapter, make lucrative careers defending in court—via the rational, authoritative force of toxicology—the production and promulgation of harmful toxicants. Surely Paracelsus would not approve.

I can only guess at Goldstein's purpose in aesthetically aligning himself with early Renaissance apothecaries (he did not respond to my repeated requests for an interview). Does he mean to gesture at how far science has progressed since these fanciful beginnings? Is his banner image meant to elicit a sense of tradition and authority, implying that toxicology descends from a respectable, well-established genealogy of learned, rational men? I suggest such romantic images of antique vials work to cushion and normalize the unknowable and now unavoidable violence of synthetic chemicals.

Nevertheless, the "end of time" historical moment during which I write this book makes Paracelsus a more appropriate "herald" than conventional toxicologists might ever have imagined. And my interviewee's quip that toxicology is "like forecasting the weather" seems more apt now than when I first heard it. The coproduced, unforeseen catastrophes of massive chemical deployments and extreme climate events are both increasingly volatile and obscenely uneven. Theophrastus von Hohenheim likewise suffered and worked his way through an exceedingly dark and difficult historical moment. Peasant rebellions and then-heretic followers of Martin Luther were brutally crushed by the powers that be while European conquests of what they called the New World exacerbated extant disparities and forged new, enduring inequities. Incurable, miserable diseases like syphilis and plague were rampant, and Paracelsus's unpropertied, lowly situated parentage doomed him to a hand-to-mouth existence, despite the occasional publication success. He and many other practitioners of his era believed they were at the precipice of the end of the world. It was only his religio-astrological faith that sustained his mission to reject the old order, even though it hurt him tremendously to do so.[108]

Today, struggling through the "unforeseen toxic catastrophe" brought about by the very substances early toxicology helped rationalize, many people believe we are experiencing the end times and, for numerous Indigenous peoples, encountering yet another apocalypse. Perhaps revolutionary toxicologists, and comrades in other(ed) fields and epistemologies, may only sustain our resistance to "toxic disturbances" and their vested interests by drawing on the magic of our imaginations.[109] Future toxicologists need not abandon Paracelsus, then, but be more true to his rebellious, anticorruption, pro-poor, perhaps even astrological, legacies. Knowledge seeking *is* magic seeking, in a way, and with times as polluted and unjust as these, magical thinking may very well be the *only* way to break out of the molds that have been cast for us but not by us.[110]

I contend that the toxicologist's contributory role can no longer simply be the development of ever more precise measurements. Measuring exposures and toxic effects remains important, but toxicologists would do well to make explicit the elisions of this scientific approach, and by doing so, intentionally contribute to racial, reproductive, and environmental justice efforts to reduce the harm done by tens of thousands of legally and irresponsibly unleashed effluents, many of which are here to stay. Rather than use toxicology to rationalize chemical production, or to "define limits of safety of chemical agents," current and future toxicologists might leverage this scientific approach for a reckoning: who has allowed such manufacturing and deployment, who has suffered as a result of these uneven distributions, and how may we best care for those most exposed, without further stigmatization? To whom is a daily intake level acceptable and by whom is a maximum concentration rendered allowable?

Toxicology is rife with uncertainties: the inherent limits of semicontrolled laboratory studies; the extrapolations from rodent to Man to Other; the invisibility of cognitive and other internal impairments; the latency of disease and unknown future consequences; the impossibility of studying all chemicals in interaction in every possible body and space over infinite time. "The basic science of poisons" cannot tell us what we need to know about toxicants in order to evaluate their safety, or even to thoroughly anticipate their dangers. Furthermore, toxicology never has been and never will be neutral. A practice of toxicology grounded in historical, social, and political context, by contrast, might relinquish at last its European medieval historical fantasies and look elsewhere for guidance. I myself feel compelled to chant a mantra recently offered by Black feminist theorist Saidiya Hartman: "Care is the antidote to violence."[111]

Before returning to the radical potential of care, discussed more extensively in chapter 4, in the next chapter I turn to the hypermasculinity of a subdiscipline of dominant toxicology: weed science.

3

Toxicant Masculinity

So, yes, let's take the figure of the feminist killjoy seriously. Does the feminist kill other people's joy by pointing out moments of sexism? Or does she expose the bad feelings that get hidden, displaced, or negated under public signs of joy? Does bad feeling enter the room when somebody expresses anger about things, or could anger be the moment when the bad feelings that circulate through objects get brought to the surface in a certain way?
—Sara Ahmed[1]

Weed Science Bros

I was inappropriately dressed. Having mistakenly assumed that this professional assembly of weed scientists and pest control advisors would be like other academic conferences I have attended, I wore my characteristically high-femme, business casual attire, complete with handbag, jewelry, and rose gold sandals. Suffice it to say I did *not* blend in with the agricultural-chemical crowd. As I walked toward the outdoor area where the morning session was about to begin, I immediately noticed how discordant my appearance was. The vast majority of professionals participating in this annual weed science conference, numbering around 250 attendees, were sporting work boots and dungarees, despite the day's forecast of heat at 100 degrees Fahrenheit, paired with company-branded polo shirts and outdoor recreation-style hats. Most participants presented as burly, white men, but there were a fair number of people who presented as white women, as well as a smaller handful of folks who presented as women and men of color. The conference emcees all appeared to me to be white, Euro-American men and women, with the exception of one man who self-identified as Middle Eastern.

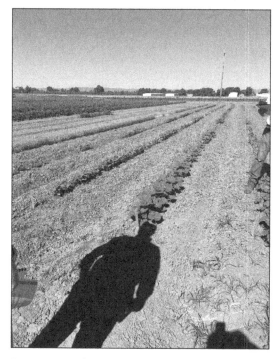

Figure 3.1: Weed Science Bros. Photographed by author.

Without putting too fine a point on it, everybody but me was ruggedly dressed, and appropriately so, as the morning's activities soon revealed. I turned to watch the friend who had given me a ride drive slowly but surely away and accepted that there was nothing to do but embrace my markedly out-of-place aesthetic. Laughing compassionately at myself, I took a deep breath and strode toward the growing gathering of weed science bros with as much unassuming confidence as I could muster. Once I began introducing myself as a *social* scientist, any perceived oddities regarding my dress (literally) seemed to be explained away. Generally, the other conference participants responded to my misfit appearance and ingenue questions rather like they might interact with a colleague's awkward teenager at an office holiday party. Not babying exactly, yet still paternal. Perhaps my rookie mistakes were endearing. In any case, I went with it.

Herbicidal Gallows Humor

I offer this seemingly superficial anecdote about (femme) affect as a way of communicating the hegemonic masculinity of the weed science space.[2] For of course it was not simply my footwear—poorly chosen for treks from outdoor experimental field site A to outdoor experimental field site B—that made me uncomfortable, but rather the scene's overriding man-boy vibe, complete with mud-spattered trucks and power tools. These conventionally boyish preoccupations were highlighted at the expense, I thought, of deeper and broader agricultural and environmental issues. The following vignettes from this day of generatively uncomfortable ethnographic fieldwork illustrate what I mean by *toxicant masculinity*.

Sensitive readers may also note some devil trickery at work here, as conceptualized in chapter 1. Toxicant masculinity and the devil trick are indeed difficult to tease apart, and the presence of one certainly does not preclude the other. In fact, toxicant masculinity, the devil trick, and magical authority all reproduce and coconstitute one another. One might understand the devil trick and magical authority as both symptoms and reinforcements of toxicant masculinity, as this chapter will illustrate.

I mentioned in this book's introduction that pesticide brand names alone provide much fodder for critical feminist analysis. Allow me to relist some of those names here: Prowl (pendmethalin), Regiment (bispyribac-sodium), Stinger (clopyralid), Outrider (sulfosulfuron), Mission (flazasulfuron), Cadre (imazapic), and, my personal favorite, Macho 4.0 (imidacloprid). Midway through my ethnographic work, I gave just such a research talk for a feminist history working group within a large, public university. Unbeknownst to me, a weed scientist was in the audience; he wrote to me after the event. I panicked slightly when I read the opening lines of his email: "I'm writing primarily to out myself as someone that does the research that you critiqued in the second half of your seminar." Agrochemical corporations are notorious for harassing environmental health researchers in the physical sciences, never mind queer feminists in the humanistic social sciences. But as my eyes continued scrolling down the electronic page, my tensed body began to relax. He wrote, it turned out, to *thank* me for my talk, and to share his own discomfort with the masculinism and militarism of the industrial agriculture world in which he works. He also thoughtfully provided two more pesticide brand names to add to my list: Battlestar (fomesafen) and Gunslinger (formerly known by its main ingredients, Picloram+D, or picloram and 2,4-D). (The toxicant 2,4-D was a component of Agent Orange, one of the highly toxic herbicides deployed by the US during the Vietnam War, the lingering effects of which are still burdening Vietnamese civilians and US veterans today.[3])

The subsequent research assistance generously offered by this weed scientist conspirator, so to speak, was invaluable to my analysis at multiple levels. At the most basic yet crucial level, he helped me gain access to weed science spaces and learn of weed science cultural norms I might otherwise have missed as an outsider. On a more conceptual yet material level, his own stated discomfort with the masculinist and militarist slant of the discipline, and hence his willingness to participate in my critical project, shows that there are liberatory cracks working through weed science's tough facade. Like toxicologists more broadly, weed scientists too have wrestled with some of the inherent contradictions of their discipline since its inception, explicitly addressing, though not necessarily with enough concern, their field's reliance on chemical manufacturers' funding, for example. As the unusually reflexive yet well-published weed scientist Robert L. Zimdahl writes, "It is worthy of note that the first president of the Weed Society was from the chemical industry, an indication of the close association between academia, government, and industry that continues to the present."[4] What is more, "all of the early U.S. weed science textbooks, those published in other countries . . . , and those written more recently devote more than a third of their content to herbicides and chemical weed control." Zimdahl continues, "Herbicides and chemical weed control have shaped weed science and have in large measure been responsible for most of its achievements and many of its problems."[5] Chemical corporations' deep pockets and accordingly extensive influence are so ingrained into the training and application of weed science that this industry presence remains largely unquestioned among educators and practitioners—it is indeed entirely expected and normalized. As an outsider to weed science in more ways than one,

I found the unmistakable but unremarkable presence of chemical corporations at university research sites quite jarring.

Even at public US institutions, in particular those colleges and universities established by the Morrill Act of 1862 and the Hatch Act of 1887—"to establish and maintain a permanent, effective U.S. agricultural industry through the provision of federal funds to create an experiment station associated with the land-grant college of agriculture in each state"[6]— the outsized influence of private corporations in weed science research is widely accepted as the status quo. As Tim,[7] my weed scientist interlocutor, informed me, "The [public] research that [weed scientists] are paid to do by the chemical companies shows up two years later on the pesticide label."[8] (Pesticide is an umbrella term that also includes herbicides, fungicides, and rodenticides. All herbicides are pesticides, but not all pesticides are herbicides.) While the ties that bind toxicant industry and toxicant science are so intertwined as to be virtually inseparable, I submit that defectors and resistors within weed science, from more established practitioners like Zimdahl to the newer generation of practitioners like Tim, demonstrate the dawning of a new day in agricultural extension and ecotoxicology. What if certain plants were not categorized as weeds, for starters, and hence not positioned as the pests whose deaths by pesticides are thus rationalized by particular interests?[9] I will return to Tim, my unexpected yet welcome weed science informant, and the openings his participation portends, later in this chapter.

At the weed science conference I attended, toxicant masculinity (macho 4.0?) manifested most clearly when pest control advisors, as they are known in the industry, commented on the toxic effects of pesticides that their field-based experiments reveal (experiments which are generally designed in order to help *register* pesticides, not to restrict or prohibit their use—controlled, rather than banned, as founding US toxicologist Harold C. Hodge might say). Throughout this practitioner-oriented meeting, agriculture industry professionals, including presenters and attendees, frequently employed and seemed to enjoy a dark sort of sarcasm, or gallows humor, if you like. For instance, one presenter repeatedly joked about how certain crops on our site visits were scheduled for "torturing with herbicides" (Macho 4.0, it just so happened). We were also forewarned, with just the slightest hint of sadism, that portions of test vineyards "will look they've been hit with a flame thrower." This particular presenter also adopted a callous yet clinical tone that reveals weed science ways of knowing: "Here you'll see some *nice injury symptoms*" (emphasis added). Similar to Michael A. Gallo's disturbing twist on the devil trick, wherein toxic catastrophes are recast as scientific advancements (see chapter 1), pesticide experts reframe the damage done by toxic chemicals as fascinating experimental results.

Weed scientists' mere visual assessments of herbicide toxicity tests also struck me as strange, if not presumptuous. Surely there are limits to scanning one's eyes across a small test plot on which several different chemicals were sprayed side-by-side, limitations which thus might exclude considerations of soil health, interchemical reactivity, pesticide drift, or longer-term plant health and viability, among other potential concerns. Farmers may indeed know their crops quite intimately by sight, and may have the experience to connect certain visual cues with nonvisible symptoms, but the pest control advisors offered frequent caveats, mansplaining with magical authority, one might say, such as "Injury on [fruit] doesn't always correlate with yield damage."[10]

Walking through test crop rows, portions of which, we were forewarned, "will look like they've been hit with a flame thrower," conference attendees carefully examined varying degrees of horticulture torture (figure 3.2). I overheard at least one practitioner concur with the presiding pest control advisor, rejecting a grower's complaint that this particular herbicide might inflict serious damage on the produce to be harvested, by declaring "[These symptoms] don't look bad at all!"

At one point, as I tread lightly between heavily sprayed experimental crop rows, sweating profusely under the day's high heat, a state Department of Pesticide Regulation (DPR) staffer strolled just ahead of me—we both saw a small brown lizard, common to this region, dart across our chemically saturated path. The DPR person joked, "Well *he* doesn't seem to be affected!" I replied, smirking slightly, "As far as we know . . ." The pesticide regulator laughed and responded, in a gently mocking tone, "Yeah, he could have had three heads, he ran by too fast!"

The (de)merits of exclusively visual assessment aside, any (in)visible harms done to other animal and plant life, never mind the people assigned the deadly work of spraying the toxicants or harvesting such pesticide-saturated produce, went entirely unmentioned. My

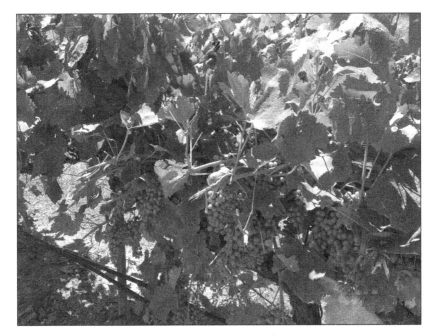

Figure 3.2: "Nice Injury Symptoms." Photograph by author.

observations corroborate those of other critical scholars, who have similarly found that industrial agriculture's heavy reliance on pesticides remains imbricated with its white supremacist approach to racialized labor. Pesticide advocates frequently respond to "labor issues" with increased chemicals and more mechanization, rather than paying living wages or complying with occupational health and safety requirements.[11]

Who's Afraid of Autonomous Weeders?

Indeed, the first and last time that farm laborers were explicitly mentioned at this day-long weed science conference was during the presentation featuring a white European entrepreneur's "autonomous weeder," a tractor-sized machine with robotic arms that apparently loosen the undesired plants (weeds) growing around desired plants (crops), ostensibly making it easier for a human laborer following behind the machine to uproot the loosened weeds. The pest control advisor who opened the autonomous weeder presentation, representing the public half of the "public-private partnership" that sponsored this event, began by explicitly stating two problems. The first problem, he announced, was the lack of chemical solutions (pun intended?) for fruit, vegetable, and nut crops: "We don't always have new herbicides but we have new technology." The second problem he proclaimed was worker safety: "I invited OSHA [Occupational Safety and Health Administration, a state agency] to view this demonstration but they didn't come." His irritation with OSHA did not end there, as he further complained to the audience that "[this US state], *unlike forty-nine other states*, requires that a human attendant be within ten feet of an autonomous weeder any time it is in operation" (his emphasis). Representing the private half of the partnership was a heavily accented, white European operator and entrepreneur, who followed up with assurances that this robotic weeder could help address "problems with work force." Whether those problems were health, (im)migration, or wage-related was left implicit. Or, alternatively, precisely whose labor problems—the employer's problem of paying laborers, or the laborers' problems of workplace hazards and potential loss of work—were not specified.

In any case, at this point in the demonstration I noticed I was one of only a few attendees still paying attention. Several of the agrochemical corporate representatives, sprinkled generously throughout the audience, I should emphasize, seemed to have lost interest, and were huddled several yards away, well out of earshot, seeking shelter from the punishing sun in the long, narrow shadow cast by the chartered conference bus. They did not seem the least bit threatened by the possibility of an autonomous weeder replacing their pesticide products. As the unusually critical practitioner and historian of weed science Zimdahl dryly notes, "Weed science has been strongly influenced by [pesticide] technology developed by supporting industries, employed in research by weed scientists, and, ultimately, used by farmers. Weed scientists similar to scientists in many technological disciplines have not sought historical reflection."[12]

The significantly smaller crowd of conference attendees who remained close to the machine watched it—or "he," as the operator repeatedly gendered the machine—with great curiosity but little excitement, crouching down to examine how well it/he had weeded the rows of young plants in the experimental field site. To my untrained eye, the weeds looked barely disturbed; at most the robotic arms had loosened the soil around the weeds, such that some so-called problematic human laborer might have an easier time pulling up the plant pests by hand. I too wandered away from the presentation, seeking relief both from the oppressive heat and the equally deflating thought that larger investments were being made in such techno-optimist machines as robotic weeders than time-honored methods of chemical-free farming. To quote Zimdahl yet again, "The dilemma of developing a discipline that claimed to be an objective science based on the study of a subjective class of plants is clear but has not been questioned. . . . What was implicit but never made explicit in any definition or in the minds of weed scientists was the fact that weeds are products of the way agriculture is practiced."[13]

On the blissfully air-conditioned bus back to the conference center, I found myself seated next to a corporate-employed chemist, who struck up a conversation by asking "Are you learning anything?" "Yes!" I responded, a little too enthusiastically. "Well that makes one of us," he replied, rolling his eyes. I invited him to share his specific complaints. He explained that he wanted more context and background before each field-based presentation—namely, which weeds are of concern to which crops and why? And which pesticides work and which do not? "What do you mean by *work*?" I asked. I sought this clarification because I was genuinely unsure whether a pesticide "working" (from the viewpoint of a pest control advisor) also meant that the chemical did not harm either the cultivated crop or the human applicator and harvester. He answered me promptly and simply: "It kills the pest."

Toxicant Masculinity

I conceived of the idea of *toxicant masculinity* months before this weed science conference, as it happened. The concept occurred to me while driving home from the Society of Toxicology conference discussed in chapter 1. After the event, my poster coauthors and I naturally spent much of our one-hour journey home debriefing about the day, particularly the moment when our poster was being judged by one of the conference presenters, a pharmaceutical industry representative who emphatically identified himself as "a drug discoverer, *not* a toxicologist."

Our project leader, a young but highly accomplished woman of color, had been explaining to him our use of the Ten Key Characteristics of Carcinogens, a standard biomedical framework which we applied in our literature review of certain herbicides.[14] As she began to detail the key characteristics that our study revealed, Dr. Drug Discoverer interrupted her to scoff, dismissively, "Well, if you look hard enough you'll find any of these [key characteristics in any given chemical compound]," implying that this World Health Organization–approved framework was absurd. My fierce yet highly-attuned-to-hierarchy junior colleague paused for a moment, having been rudely interrupted, and stared at our poster judge intently and yet blankly for just a fraction of a second. I could almost see her brilliant brain scanning possible responses, weighing her relatively inferior social position against her professional reputation, the expectations of her hovering advisor, and the etiquette of the conference environment. Skipping only the slightest moment of a beat, she quickly resumed her explanation, gently stressing that *she* had not come up with these key characteristics, but rather that they were a standard across biomedical fields. (No doubt that as a highly educated, young woman of color, she is well-practiced in the emotional labor required to make middle-aged white men feel less threatened by her presence and intelligence.) He impatiently motioned for her to get on with explaining the specific results of our systematic review, then scribbled some notes on his poster-judging card before striding to the next board.

The entire exchange lasted no more than two minutes, but it came up on the car ride home. My colleague was not the least bit surprised by this instance of toxic masculinity (or epistemic entitlement, as feminist philosopher Kate Manne might call it), and this was when I pondered aloud about "the toxic masculinity of toxicology." These sorts of interactions with toxicologist men at toxicology conferences, or in toxicology-related conversations on campus, and so on, happened to my interlocutor all the time. She also noticed how regularly her advisor, another woman of color in toxicology, was condescended to by predominantly white men in the field. Yet she casually shrugged off this instance as annoying if predictable, noting how successful her advisor is all the same, in terms of academic publications and scientific accomplishments, and the conversation soon moved on to other toxicology gossip. (Yes, that's a thing.) But the idea of *toxicant masculinity* stuck with me. The weed science conference I attended later that same year only threw these masculinist tendencies into sharper relief.

Mansplaining and epistemic entitlement are certainly not unique to US toxicology, but there are particularities to toxicant masculinity that are worth excavating here, as masculinist presumptions about "harmless ways of using substances" have all too often resulted in devastatingly gendered effects, from the women disproportionately harmed by the toxic, multigenerational effects of thalidomide (a sedative prescribed to pregnant women for morning sickness) and DES (a synthetic estrogen prescribed to women simply for experiencing menopause) to the undue burdens placed on individual pregnant women to protect the unborn from toxic exposures, as well as the predominantly women caregivers who shoulder the lion's share of the extra care work required for overexposed children and other family members who struggle with exposure-related illness and disability.[15]

Once again, founding US toxicologists' historiographies shed light on the origins of toxicant masculinity, which lives on today not necessarily in cavalier dismissals of potential harms, although that tendency certainly remains prevalent, but in patriarchal premises that undermine even *anti*-toxics science, advocacy, and policymaking. Let us return to the authoritative US toxicology textbook *Casarett & Doull's* for a moment, where important distinctions are set between who is entitled to and may be entrusted with poison(ing), versus who conspires and poisons with murderous intent.[16]

"A Conspiracy of Women"

Founding US toxicologist Louis J. Casarett, whom we met in chapters 1 and 2, deliberately distinguished the professional, clinical, and rational science of poisons from history's conniving, political, and emotional acts of poisoning. Casarett marked this distinction by othering women—largely of Western European but also occasionally of Greco-Roman and African descent—and by othering prehistoric and non-European men, all of whom he grouped under the term "primitive." The following excerpts from the opening chapter of the first, 1975 edition of *Toxicology: The Basic Science of Poisons* (coedited by Casarett and John Doull) reappear almost verbatim up through the eighth edition (2013) of the textbook. Thus begins the budding US toxicologist's history lesson: "Toxicology predates man and, in a variety of specialized and primitive forms, has been a relevant part of the history of man. . . . Earliest man was well aware of the toxic effects of animal venoms and poisonous plants. His knowledge was used for hunting, for waging more effective warfare, and, probably, to remove undesirables from the small groups of primitive society."[17] Such narratives make explicit US toxicology's typically more implicit masculinism and white supremacism, as European and later Euro-American scientists are positioned as the superior humans who domesticate and rationalize the unruly, feminized, and animalized poisoners of pre-Enlightenment eras and non-European peoples.[18] Moreover, founding toxicologists' claim that toxicology (magically) "predates man" also serves to naturalize toxicants, as if these newly synthesized chemicals are mere extensions of, or rather improvements on, plant toxins and animal venoms.[19]

Without citing any anthropological scholarship (though, admittedly, English-language anthropology circa 1975 might not have been any less white supremacist or patriarchal), Casarett "maintains that [science] here only imitates or carries out the inevitable demands of nature," to quote feminist theorist and activist Kate Millett's classic critique of social science texts.[20] Casarett describes modern toxicology as "a relevant part of the history of man," invoking an imagined prehistory to justify men's invention of toxicants as an inevitable response to natural demands: "His [toxicological] knowledge was used for hunting, for waging more effective warfare, and, probably, to remove undesirables from the small groups of primitive society."[21] While Millett was applying these feminist critiques to the social sciences, her scathing analysis may be extended to the natural sciences as well—just replace "sociology" with "toxicology": "Thus sociology examines the status quo, calls it phenomena, and pretends to take no stand on it. . . . Yet by slow degrees of converting statistic to fact, function to prescription, bias to biology (or some other indeterminate), it comes to ratify and rationalize what has been socially enjoined or imposed into what is and ought to be. And through its pose of objectivity, it gains a special efficacy in reinforcing stereotypes."[22] More recently, anthropologist Juno Parreñas has written about "Man the Hunter" from a postcolonial feminist perspective: "Man the Hunter was narrated in the first world as a carrier of technology, specifically tools, which he used to colonize the world through expansive human migration. Colonization is a subtle yet significant concept insofar as it implies that occupying land and exploiting its use is a natural way of being."[23] Likewise, the way that founding (and settler colonial) US toxicologists narrate their historiography implies that synthesizing and deploying toxicants to harm other people—"for waging more effective warfare" and "to remove undesirables"—is a natural way of being.

Moving swiftly through the pre-Christian Levant and early medieval Europe, Casarett spends an exorbitant amount of time and space detailing how unethically, if effectively, women made use of poisons, from the time of "Antiquity" to the "Age of Enlightenment." First, he remarks on the ancient Roman era, writing, "It was during this period that a conspiracy of women to remove those from whose death they might profit was uncovered, and similar large-scale poisoning continued from time to time until 82 B.C. when Sulla issued the Lex Cornelia."[24] Note in this summary how it takes an authoritative man, Sulla, to rein in "a conspiracy of women" and enforce a hierarchical social order via the Lex Cornelia. (Lex Cornelia is a somewhat ambiguous term, referring to any ancient Roman law sponsored by an official belonging to the family of Cornelius. Sulla, or Lucius Cornelius Sulla Felix, was one such official, a Roman army general and dictator known as "the first man of the republic to seize power through force."[25] Needless to say, none of this broader context is provided in Casarett's historiography.)

Casarett continues briskly on to the European Middle Ages:

> In less organized but more colorful ways, the citizens of Italy in the Middle Ages also practiced the art of poisoning. A famous figure of the time was a lady named Toffana, who peddled specially prepared arsenic-containing cosmetics (Agua Toffana). . . . Toffana was succeeded by an imitator with organizational genius, a certain Hieronyma Spara, who provided a new fillip by directing her activity toward specific marital and monetary objectives. A local club was formed of young, wealthy, married women, which soon became a club of eligible young, wealthy widows, reminiscent of the matronly conspiracy many centuries earlier.[26]

Casarett's patronizingly sexist tone—"A local club was formed of young, wealthy, married women, which soon became a club of eligible young, wealthy widows, reminiscent of the matronly conspiracy many centuries earlier"—shifts only slightly, and the general sentiment remains, when he turns to European Enlightenment sorceresses:

> A paragon of the distaff set of the period was Catherine de Medici. Catherine, although not so thoroughly fabled as her Borgia relatives and ancestors, was in tune with her time, a practitioner of the art of applied toxicology. . . . *As appeared to be all too common in this period (or any period), the prime targets of the ladies were their husbands.* However, unlike others of an earlier period, the circle represented by Catherine (and epitomized by the notorious Marchioness de Brinvilliers) depended on direct evidence to arrive at the most effective compounds for their purposes. Under guise of delivering provender to the sick and the poor, Catherine tested toxic concoctions, carefully noting the rapidity of the toxic response (onset of action), the effectiveness of the compound (potency), the degree of response of the parts of the body (specificity, site of action), and the complaints of the victim (clinical signs and symptoms). Clearly, Catherine must be given credit as perhaps the earliest untrained experimental toxicologist.[27]

Casarett begins here to delineate the science and "the art of applied toxicology," in direct contrast to "primitive" human warfare, "conspiracies" of women, and "colorful" young, wealthy, murderous widows. This notion of toxicology as both a science and an art lives on, as detailed in my chapter 2. Weed scientists too, claim their practice as "a science and an art," and grant themselves a magical authority with concomitant toxicant masculinity. For example, Zimdahl quotes a prominent weed scientist writing in 1982: "Properly understood, *insect control as a science and an art* should be seen to touch our deepest assumptions about the proper role of political power, our methods of organizing socioeconomic activity, and *our sense of man's role in the cosmos.* . . . Insects may be small and invite contempt, but efforts to deal with them evoke all of the most deeply held beliefs about what it is to be human."[28] Weed scientists today, who are largely if not exclusively employed via industrial agriculture, continue to approvingly cite one of their forefather's quips that "It is not wrong to propose that there are only three ways to begin to farm: patrimony, matrimony, and parsimony."[29] As Zimdahl himself ultimately concludes, "No one disputes that weeds have been present as long as other pests, but they have not been studied as long. The major figures in early weed science all completed their education and developed their careers in the twentieth century. *Available descriptions of the history of weed science and the dominant rhetoric do not include views from outside the discipline because they are often regarded as negative and emotional and, therefore, unscientific.*"[30]

Despite Catherine de Medici's apparent meticulousness and prescientific experimentation, and despite her relative wealth, privilege, and power, Casarett makes clear that as a woman, "Catherine," whom he has relegated to "the distaff set" and further marked as inferior by repeatedly, casually referring to her by her first name, cannot be the Medieval figure from whom modern US toxicology derives its (magical) authority. Women "perhaps" make excellent poisoners, even "untrained experimental toxicologist[s]," like Catherine de Medici, but they are emotional, conniving, and greedy—certainly not the sort mid-twentieth century toxicologists would choose to lend credence to their nascent discipline. Founding US toxicologists' medieval progenitor of choice is rather Paracelsus, as discussed in chapter 2.

Women Are Sorceresses, Men Are Scientists

Casarett's tales of witchy women poisoners continue, but I will spare my readers these additional sexist narratives, condensed and only slightly updated versions of which remain through to the 2013 edition of the textbook. I highlight these excerpts to show the white masculinist and myopic worldview of US toxicology's founding fathers. From my standpoint, Casarett's renderings of Toffana, Hieronyma Spara, and Catherine de Medici, among other conspiratorial women Casarett profiles but whom I did not include here, bring to mind the research of such scholars as Black feminist theorist Angela Y. Davis, Black feminist historian Darlene Clark Hine, Marxist feminist Silvia Federici, and feminist historian of science Londa Schiebinger, to name a few.[31] Such critical histories attend to *why* so-called witches or hysterics practiced poisonings or feigned mental illness—namely, to resist oppressive patriarchal and racial relations. Women throughout history have pretended to be psychotic to escape the legalized rape of marriage, have taken abortifacients to prevent their unborn children from being sold into slavery, have been caricatured as conniving simply because powerful (and not so powerful) men found these women's medicinal knowledge threatening to the prevailing social order. Did the women Toffana served seek money or emancipation? Did La Voisin poison 2,000 infants or save 2,000 women from unwanted pregnancies? One man's poison is another woman's antidote.

Casarett also profiles many (in)famous men who systematically poisoned their political rivals, but his tone is markedly different. For example, "It has been postulated that arsenic was the poison with which Agrippina killed Claudius to make Nero the emperor of Rome. This postulate is supported by the later use of the same material by Nero in poisoning Britannicus, Claudius' natural son. The deed was under the direction of Locusta, a professional poisoner attached to the family."[32] Unlike his language reserved for ladies—careless, matronly conspiracy, untrained, the distaff set, and so on—Casarett avoids condescension when describing poisoner men of the past and tends to provide more historical context and less editorializing for their motives. Socially and economically privileged men are not only *entrusted* with poisoning, this dominant toxicology textbook implies, but moreover are *entitled* to do so. Having set the toxicological scene, in the next section I return to my ethnographic research sites, illustrating how toxicant masculinity persists into the present.

Dramatized Dangers

Despite, or perhaps because of, my outsider status and blatant incongruence in nearly every toxicology space I entered, from lecture hall to conference center to agricultural field (but not environmental nonprofit!), I experienced my own share of toxicant masculinity. I tried my best to leverage various interlocutors' dismissals and condescension, playing dumb and strategically employing my own emotional labor so that interviewees might relax their guard. But throughout my life I have never been able (or willing?) to shrug off patronizing and borderline hostile treatment by hegemonically masculine men as readily as my colleague did after Dr. Drug Discoverer's rude dismissal, for instance.

Interestingly, the vast majority of my expert interviewees were women. And notably, the only two people who responded with irritation

and impatience to my interview questions, even though they had provided their informed consent, were two of four men (compared to
twenty women) I interviewed in the earlier days of my ethnographic
research. (This interview count does not include the nine members of
the toxicology lab I embedded myself within later in the course of my
data collection, five of whom were men and all of whom were respectful,
see chapters 4 and 5). The two toxicologist men who treated me rudely
during our interviews occupied opposing ends of the toxicological political spectrum; one was a world-renowned and revered expert in public
health and chemical regulation, known for testifying on plaintiffs' behalf
in toxic torts. The other had been a political appointee of a Republican
US president, among other powerful and prestigious positions, and was
known to side with industry in various chemical controversies. I cannot be sure what prompted these interviewees' hostility and impatience,
and their attitudes during our approximately hour-long interviews may
very well have had nothing to do with me. (I did overhear one speak to a
woman in the background with incredible derision, so maybe he's simply
misogynistic, or rude to everybody.) However, it is also quite possible
that I was spoken to with such palpable irritation for some combination
of the following reasons: because I am a woman, because I am not a
biological scientist, and because I raise questions about toxicology's validity and effectiveness. The "don't worry your pretty little head" tone of
Casarett & Doull's became more like "you don't know what you're talking about, sweetie" in direct conversation. Put another way, Hodge's gendered complaint of 1975—"The dangers of the indiscriminate overuse
of pesticides have been so dramatized that some beneficial substances,
irreplaceable at present, are banned rather than controlled"[33]—could
easily have been uttered today.

Zimdahl's analysis of Weed Science Society presidential addresses
over several decades reveals parallel themes, wherein powerful weed
scientists

> claimed that most pesticides whose use had been suspended by regula-
> tory action had been suspended in response to public outcry or misuse
> rather than on the basis of what [they] called "valid or verified scien-
> tific data." . . . [Weed Science Society] presidents and the audience they
> addressed were overwhelmingly supportive of the view that herbicides

could be used with confidence when they were used properly, that is, according to label directions. . . . Presidential emphasis thus continued to
be on the essentiality of maintaining and improving production and on
*the problems caused by the perceived emotional, non-scientific claims of the
environmental community.*[34]

An important element of this gendered, don't-be-so-dramatic dismissal by US toxicologists is related to the dominant tendency to elevate
natural science over all other(ed) knowledge systems, including social
sciences.[35] As glossed in the introduction, I focus on the toxicant masculinity exhibited by these interviewees' responses not as individual
indictments but rather to demonstrate how the dominant culture of US
toxicology may be characterized as toxicant masculinity.

"How Big Could the Risks Be?"

The industry-friendly interviewee who responded quite harshly to my
questions about the inherent uncertainty of toxicology, whether in terms
of its methods or the chemical substances themselves, did not disagree
with my summation—toxicologists are quick to point out how uncertain
their discipline is (it's an art *and* a science!; see chapter 2)—but became
noticeably irritated as if anticipating that I would point to this uncertainty as a reason to not rely on toxicology for the purposes of chemical
regulation. Toxicology is "already very artificial," he insisted, acknowledging its inherent limitations, "but we can't wait for the epidemiology
so what's the alternative? How big could the [chemical] risks be that
are still out there? There would be a lot more introspection in toxicology if so many bad things were happening." He further declared that
"academic labs' [studies] are less rigorous than a company study," and
he repeatedly stressed that "it's an *interpretation* issue . . . *interpretation* of the data is *not science* . . . science doesn't *say* things. Motivated
researchers are misrepresenting what we know."[36] When I pressed him
on this last point, alluding to the tobacco industry tactic "doubt is our
product,"[37] he paused, sighed in mild exasperation, and conceded that
"some have weaponized uncertainty."

Note the devil trickery here as well; toxicants are recognized as potentially harmful but positioned as inevitable: "We can't wait for the

epidemiology so what's the alternative?" Environmental health scientists frequently recite the mantra "Good epidemiology is a failure of public health" (I heard this phrase uttered, verbatim, by at least three different interlocutors during my ethnographic research), which I thus presumed to be the sentiment in this interviewee's comment as well. Epidemiologists study toxic exposures, among other health issues, that have *already* occurred or are ongoing outside of any controlled experiment (or beyond the control of the scientist), measuring and following populations who bear the burdens of environmental toxicants because of their occupation, for example, such as factory and farm workers, or because of some historical event, such as wartime exposures to chemical weapons. "Not waiting for the epidemiology" in this context means not deliberately exposing humans to specific doses of toxicants over time and then establishing a scientific conclusion as to whether the toxicant, or dose, is harmful. Toxicology is thus understood here as *preventing* hazardous exposures because its lab-based animal experiments, however uncertain, allow scientists and regulators to *predict* how a human might respond to a given chemical substance. Recall the "juvenile model for chemical warfare exposure" presentation I described in chapter 1. Of course, ironically, and as any environmental justice activist and advocate will testify, human and other(ed) ecologies are in fact exposed to tens of thousands of hazardous chemicals that scientists know next to nothing about.[38] One could argue the transnational chemical industry and its governmental enablers have enrolled the entire planet, without our informed consent, in a massive and massively uncontrolled experiment. Yet this industry-leaning toxicologist, who was employed by a university, incidentally, confidently dismissed such evidence: "How big could the [chemical] risks be that are still out there? There would be a lot more introspection in toxicology if so many bad things were happening."

Both he and the other irritable male toxicologist I interviewed identified "political interference" as the problem, as opposed to toxicology's inherent uncertainties. For example, the same academic and industry-friendly toxicologist previously quoted recalled his time at the US Environmental Protection Agency (EPA): "Most interference [in chemical risk assessment] is from the political side. . . . [Working at the EPA] is probably no different from [working for] a [chemical] manufacturer."[39] He did not mean this lack of difference in the sense that EPA is necessarily industry-aligned, as anti-toxics advocates contend, but rather in the sense that EPA is as motivated and interested as industry. His reflections echo Michael A. Gallo's equivalencies between the laboratories of such corporations as Dow, Union Carbide, and DuPont and those of the US government (where everyone cares equally about worker safety; see chapter 1). One of the state-level regulators I spoke with at the Society of Toxicology conference nervously reiterated to me several times during our fifteen-minute conversation that "we get sued from all sides."[40] Government regulators do indeed seem to be caught between the goals of public health and the mandate of economic growth, however a critical race feminist analysis reminds us that the state is no neutral actor (see the introduction). Chemical industry insists that government regulators are overly activist (read: emotional and unscientific) while anti-toxics advocates argue that these same regulators are overly sympathetic to industry (without necessarily questioning the certainty of toxicological findings). As one lead toxicologist for a national non-profit scoffed, "EPA does have people who go [work there] for the public good, but many work for industry. The idea that it's an activist agency is hysterical. . . . It is *not* a radical organization, that couldn't be further from the truth. EPA is highly influenced by what industry is saying."[41]

The prestigious public health researcher who also responded quite impatiently to my interview questions used the word "interference" as well, in the context of chemical manufacturers presenting obstacles to "sound science" and meaningful regulation. He further maintained, in response to a prompt of mine regarding the role toxicologists play in chemical policy, that sociologists and political scientists are useful insofar as they can shore up toxicological findings (of the right practitioners, presumably). "Social scientists are needed for public relations and communications [but] ought to allow the science to move forward without political interference."[42] Again, this knowledge hierarchy, wherein the natural sciences are positioned as superior and more truthful than all other(ed) knowledge claims, is not unique to toxicology. Yet I wish to underscore here how *sexualized and racialized* these ideologies are: the rational, serious, masculine business of toxicology and chemical regulation belongs to the "hard" sciences, while the political interference and feminized dramatization of toxic exposures are relegated to the "soft" science of sociology, if not the nonscience (or nonsense?) of activism.

I did not always experience toxicant masculinity as aggressive, nor did I experience toxicant masculinity from men exclusively. The three people I spoke with who worked for major chemical corporations (two informally interviewed at a conference, the third formally interviewed via phone) all displayed different strains of toxicant masculinity, while remaining exceptionally kind and courteous. One such interviewee was friendly and patient when I abruptly and awkwardly approached him at the weed science conference described earlier, having made a beeline toward him from across the outdoor experimental field station when I spotted a particular chemical corporation affiliation on his nametag. Nevertheless, when I asked him to comment on the International Agency for Research on Cancer's (IARC) 2015 classification of glyphosate (Roundup), the most ubiquitous herbicide on earth, as a probable human carcinogen,[43] he confidently asserted—in a jaw-dropping display of chemical gaslighting—that science has not associated *any* pesticides with *any* cancers, though he allowed for some neurotoxicity. I did not object to his patently false conclusion out loud, but I thought of the throngs of epidemiologists, and toxicologists too, who have gathered evidence to the contrary; suffice it to say *several* pesticides are strongly associated with *several* cancers. Black feminist astrophysicist Chanda Prescod-Weinstein notes, as quoted in the epigraph to chapter 2, that the difference between epistemic injustice and epistemic entitlement is "resistance not just to testimony but also to empirical fact."[44] I submit that this kind of blithe yet confident, wholly inaccurate assertion is a prime example of not simply white epistemic entitlement (similar also to mansplaining, per philosopher Kate Manne), but also chemical gaslighting.[45]

The chemical industry employee I interviewed formally via phone, a woman, was easily the most patronizing of all my interviewees. Despite knowing that I was, at the time, a PhD candidate at a prestigious US research university, she spoke to me as if I were a young child, even pausing at several points during our interview to ask if she should spell-out the "big words" she was using. And even after having introduced myself as a scholar of environmental studies, she described well-known figures like Rachel Carson (of *Silent Spring* fame) and Norman Borlaug (of Green Revolution infamy) to me as if I would not have heard of them.[46] She also distilled and simplified the toxicological studies I asked her to elaborate on as if I could not possibly handle the complexity of the science, summarizing glyphosate studies, for instance, as follows: "You can dose animals with very high doses and it doesn't bother them . . . cancer is a DNA problem; glyphosate doesn't bother cells."[47]

This particular interview was studded with (fake) gems; I highlight only a few excerpts and affects here to emphasize that the performance of toxicant masculinity is not limited to men, imbricated as it is with a more generalized, Euro-American scientific supremacy. Per toxicant masculinity: if you are not a toxicologist, you simply do not understand and are not qualified to reach conclusions—never mind write dissertations or regulations—on toxicants. As this chemical industry interviewee bemoaned herself, there are far too many "naive recommendations from powerful people" when it comes to pesticide regulation, echoing Hodge's 1975 complaint that "the dangers of pesticides have been so dramatized that some beneficial substances, irreplaceable at present, are banned rather than controlled."[48] The next section turns to US toxicology's masculinist compulsion for chemical control more specifically.

Boys Will Be Boys

In her provocative book *The Tragedy of Heterosexuality*, sociologist Jane Ward notes how heteropatriarchy forges erotic bonds between straight men. Because (straight) women have been historically caricatured and socially positioned to be troublesome, demanding, inferior to, inexplicable, irrational, and useful only in service to men, (straight) men have historically devoted much more energy to spending quality time and nurturing meaningful relationships with their man peers. "Straight men," Ward writes, "have created countless rituals, games, art forms, traditions, and spaces designed to explore and pursue their own pleasure, typically in the company of other men."[49] Ward cites examples such as the twenty-first century "man cave," which may be understood as a more recent iteration of nineteenth century hunting lodges or gentlemen's clubs—including faculty clubs—of the twentieth century.[50] To this list of homophilic, masculinist spaces and rituals, I add two more: the Shed, a mainstay of US land grant university campuses,[51] and the Weed Contest, an annual pesticide science tradition (read: hazing).

Scholars and advocates have well-documented the direct links between chemical weaponry and US pesticide development and deployment.[52] However, with some notable exceptions—namely Carol Cohn's "Sex and Death in the Rational World of Defense Intellectuals," published in 1987, and Traci Brynne Voyles's "Toxic Masculinity: California's Salton Sea and the Environmental Consequences of Manliness," published in 2021—relatively few researchers have attended to the distinctly masculinist, homoerotic character of US toxicology's preoccupation with military-might-cum-agricultural-control. As I argue throughout this book, identifying US toxicology's inherent masculinism—toxicant masculinity—must be fundamental to environmental justice struggles, particularly those that strive to redeem or otherwise leverage toxicological ways of knowing for more liberatory ends. Without this feminist attention to toxicology's masculinist logics, even the most well-intentioned, environmental justice-aligned toxicologists may be limiting themselves, and environmental justice movements, to "the master's tools."[53]

In this section, I rely primarily on my weed scientist informant Tim's descriptions of both the Shed—a central gathering area and workspace of agricultural experiment stations, among other sites of toxicological application—and the Weed Contest, detailed in what follows.[54] In addition to Tim's recollections and reflections, based on his personal encounters in the Shed and as a previous participant in the Weed Contest, my analysis also draws from his photographs of the Shed, generously documented for my benefit, as well as US Weed Science Society webpages, videos, and other promotional material describing this semiannual and multiregional competition.

The Shed

The Shed at Tim's research institution is a simple, drab, decidedly utilitarian structure; a prefabricated steel and vinyl rectangle with garage-like overhead doors. The exterior features rusty work tables, nested piles of plastic five-gallon pails, and a corrugated metal awning. The interior is part barn, part laboratory, where pesticide-spraying tractors and plastic test tubes intermingle. Scattered in numerous organized piles across the open floor are steel canisters, presumably containing toxicants; old

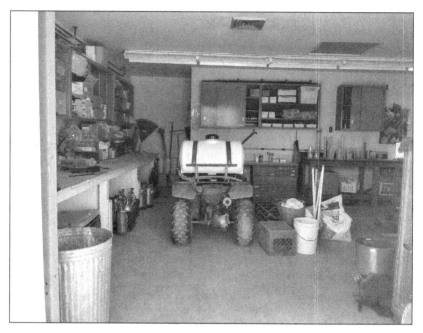

Figure 3.3: The Shed. Courtesy of author.

wooden filing cabinets bearing precarious labels of unknown provenance, presumably for lab and sprayer equipment; several miscellaneous buckets; those ubiquitous, plastic bins commonly referred to as milk crates; and partially used vinyl bags of soil or fertilizer. Overall, the Shed appears cluttered in a well-used, functional kind of way—not an absent-minded or negligent sort of mess but rather one that suggests its various users have many different kinds of tasks that they struggle to stay ahead of. Farm and gardening equipment such as rakes, hoes, and shovels are lined up in an orderly fashion against the back wall, perched inside mud-spattered, hollow plastic cylinders, nailed into the wall for that precise purpose. Echoing this orderly line of tools are vertical rows of plastic funnels and test tubes, hanging upside down to dry on a wall of pegs, also installed for that specific use. Everything is coated with a thin yet unmistakable layer of grime—likely a quotidian yet potent mixture of dirt and pesticide drift.

The interior's grimy, plywood worktables and counter tops are warped and stained, and, like the rest of the shed, they appear hastily and frequently visited as well. Wrenches, bungee cords, and measuring tapes share the dusty surface with WD-40 and an industrial-sized role of disposable, perforated rags. On open shelves installed in the wall above are stacks on stacks of boxes containing single-use vinyl gloves and N-95 face masks, items that became treasured household commodities during the COVID-19 pandemic, which began just as I sought Institutional Review Board approval to observe toxicology labs in person (detailed in chapters 4 and 5).

Pesticide sprayer equipment is easily the most prevalent item. There are spray arms and spray nozzles, backpack sprayers and tractor sprayers, and tool chests full of multicolored nozzles, each color denoting a specific size, neatly stored in its own rectangle of space in the multidrawer toolbox. My eyes are overwhelmed by all the bits and pieces: hoses, buckets, countertop scales, industrial gray, thick plastic aprons, goggles and face shields, clear plastic gallon jars of an eerily yellow-green liquid, weed whackers, more buckets of dirt (?), rolls on rolls of neon tape signaling "caution" in classic yellow alongside hot pink, cobalt blue, and neon green. The cool gray and beige metal filing cabinets that line the wall behind the test tubes and tape rolls seem somber and reserved against all this flashy color. Behind those metal cabinet doors, which according to my informant are typically open shelving units (at least in other sheds he has worked in), are hundreds of neatly organized yet grime-covered glass and plastic bottles, ranging in size, in descending order from top to bottom shelf, from pill bottle to fish tank. Each container holds trademarked blends of differently toxic pesticides. Some are snot-green, some are mud-brown, some are antifreeze-blue. Some bottles evoke antique apothecary glass, recalling the Monsanto scientist's blog header image featured in chapter 2 (figure 2.1), others pass for laundry detergent or dish soap. Despite being covered in a thick layer of grime, each bottle's label is clearly visible.

As haphazard as the shed might appear on first glance, upon closer inspection, I sank into the realization that this is not a safe space for someone who is not expertly trained—in comprehending pesticide labels, in operating farm equipment, in lab safety protocol. The toxicant bottles behind those closed metal doors seemed sinister, taunting me with their eerie silence and deadly poisons. The last thing I noticed was indeed watching me, a plastic, life-sized model of a great horned owl, the

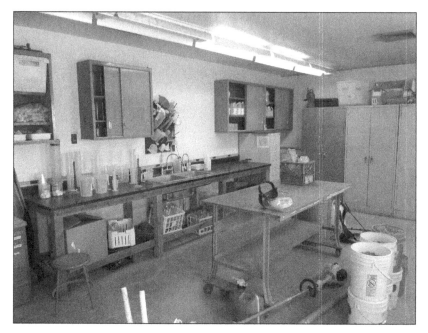

Figure 3.4: Power Tools and Lab Beakers. Courtesy of author.

type farmers and gardeners might install in their field or yard to scare off other "pests." I typically feel an affinity with owls, especially the great horned, whose calls I hear outside my bedroom regularly and find rather enchanting. And of course I have seen these plastic owl figurines before. But everything in the weed shed began to take on a sinister affect; the fake owl's beady eyes glinted in the sunlight, as if to warn me away from the pesticide shelves, sternly looking down on either its contents or my criticisms, or both.

Perhaps I am a bit dramatic, as Hodge might have dismissed me in 1975 (or today), and to my knowledge, no practicing, woman-identified weed scientist has been overtly excluded from the shed. By comparing this workspace to a man cave and offering this description as a facet of toxicant masculinity, I am not claiming that women are unwelcome in weed science. While comprising a minority of the participants at the weed science conference I attended, women were certainly prevalent enough to suggest that they are not all that anomalous in the field. My claim is rather that spaces like the shed reproduce a specific approach to plants and insects in terms of agriculture, rendering them "weeds" and "pests" that must be controlled and exterminated with toxic synthetic chemicals. This control and extermination, moreover, requires heavy equipment and proprietary substances, all of which demand an expertly trained weed scientist, agricultural extension agent, or pest control advisor. Women can certainly do this work, but they must perform these tasks in ways that conform to the white supremacist masculinism of industrial chemical agriculture.

I chatted casually with one young white woman at the weed science conference described earlier in this chapter, asking why she attended the event. In response, she spoke passionately about her older brother, who worked as a pest control advisor and inspired her to join the profession. Having just started out as a chemical corporation employee, she told me how much she loved talking to growers out in the field, helping them troubleshoot problems (with pests) with her expanding expertise. A conventionally attractive, slim, bottle-blond with tanned skin, this young woman and aspiring pest control advisor knew to wear work boots, a short-sleeve polo, and dungarees, unlike clueless me. I noticed she fit right in with her pesticide company colleagues, and I felt a funny mixture of sadness and fascination as I watched her look up, literally and figuratively, to the men who loomed large above her, wearing a practiced, if subconscious, familiar expression of femininized submission-plus-enthusiasm. Maybe, I mused to myself, she yearns for the same kind of power her older brother and senior pest control colleagues wield? The power (cravings) of pest control advisors is the subject of what remains of this chapter.

The Weed Contest

I later learned that I had in fact experienced a miniature, toned-down version of a weed contest at the weed science conference I attended (in a dress, embarrassingly). *The* Weed Contest is specifically for weed science students, from undergraduate to PhD, and is indeed a rite of passage, and pathway to employment, for said trainees. From my perspective it functions more like a hazing ritual, but I am jumping ahead. By contrast, the professional weed science gathering I attended included only a voluntary, low-key weed-identification quiz and "herbicide symptomology" segment, for a bit of weed-scientist-nerd-fun plus show-and-tell. I will start by describing the microcosm of the quiz, then analyze the pièce de résistance that is the US Weed Science Society's annual Weed Contest.

Needless to say, the very terms "weed" and "pest" expose the myopic framing of industrial agriculture. A plant or insect only becomes a weed or pest under specific, human-devised and culturally constructed conditions.[55] Relatedly, the title "pest control advisor," referring to professionals either employed directly by pesticide manufacturers or indirectly by US land-grant universities (in which case they may also be titled "agricultural extension agents") also evidences industrial agriculture's prioritization of profit and yield over environmental health.[56] But while it may be easy, if no less necessary, to point fingers at chemical manufacturers for grossly overpolluting the planet, pest control advisors and agricultural extension agents seem to skirt blame for the very same massive chemical contamination because they are perceived as, and actively maintain their positions as, apolitical, disinterested, objective scientists—"I'm just a technician" one chemical corporation employee demurred to me at the weed science conference. In Zimdahl's critical analysis of his own discipline, he summarizes, "Weed scientists frequently claim that solving social problems is not their responsibility. However, the common claim that modern agriculture, supported by modern weed management practices, saves the world from famine is a claim of a positive social effect. Weed scientists cannot have it both ways. They cannot claim credit for saving the world from famine while denying their social role. The claim that agricultural and weed scientists do not have any obligation to solve social problems is therefore an empty one."[57]

Given that unsettling the supposed innocence, rationality, and apolitical truth of US toxicology is a central aim of this book, I offer the weed quiz, the Weed Contest, and the Shed as manifestations of toxicant masculinity and also to stress the urgency of studying toxicants differently. By cloaking themselves in the virtuous and patronizing mantle of science, pest control advisors and agricultural extension agents not only avoid political accountability, but also enable toxic environmental pollution to proceed as if there is no alternative and as if Man *can* exert control over the widespread, bioactive, economic poisons he has unleashed without Others' consent.

Underreported Broomrape

One of the weeds included in the conference's weed-identification quiz, branched broomrape (Latin name: *Orobanche ramose*) has been characterized by the state in which I conducted this research as an "A-list noxious weed," "parasitic weed," and "quarantine pest." (Yes, those are technical terms.[58]) Plants so unfortunately classified must be reported to regulatory authorities, after which the unhappy grower must first mechanically destroy her crop, then fumigate her field with the highly toxic, and expensive, methyl bromide. This crop destruction and fumigation costs growers at least $6,000 per acre, not accounting for lost profits due to decreased yields or increased labor expenses, according to the agricultural extension agents presiding.

Furthermore, there are zero state financial support programs for growers whose fields are afflicted with broomrape, contributing to significant problems of underreporting. Pest control advisors ominously warned conference attendees that this noxious, parasitic weed is far more widespread than state records indicate and is nearly impossible to eradicate. Presenters then proceeded to demonstrate a new method of (quasi-)control being tested—direct herbicide application plus "chemigation" (wherein chemicals are pumped into irrigation pipes)—to ascertain the effects of such toxic deployments on the desired crop, not the weed itself. Previous experiments have apparently shown that growers must learn to manage broomrape, rather than hope to eliminate it. This tenacious plant has tiny, dust-like seeds that can persist in the soil for decades and seems to have developed complete pesticide resistance (though this last observation was left implicit).

Performing the devil trick (see chapter 1), these weed science presenters offered no alternatives to industrial, petrochemical-dependent agriculture, nor for that matter any acknowledgment of the toxicity of methyl bromide, the fumigant used in an attempt to quarantine broomrape-d fields.[59] According to the US Agency for Toxic Substances and Disease Registry (ATSDR):

Methyl bromide gas easily penetrates most protective clothing (e.g., cloth, rubber, and leather) and skin. Prolonged retention in clothing and rubber boots may lead to chemical dermatitis and severe burns. Skin absorption may contribute to systemic toxicity. . . . Methyl bromide is a neurotoxic gas that can cause convulsions, coma, and long-term neuromuscular and cognitive deficits. Exposure to high concentrations of pure methyl bromide may cause inflammation of the bronchi or lungs, an accumulation of fluid in the lung, and irritation of the eyes and nose. Tearing agents added to methyl bromide to provide warning of its presence can also cause these symptoms, even at very low concentrations. Skin contact with high vapor concentrations or with liquid methyl bromide can cause systemic toxicity and may cause stinging pain and blisters.[60]

Methyl bromide is also a major contributor to ozone layer depletion.[61] (Even when conventional toxicology and epidemiology *do* document toxicants' severe harm to humans, highly hazardous chemicals are still normalized and necessitated as economic poisons.[62])

Other important issues left unaddressed at the weed science conference included how this varietal of broomrape came to present such an "A-list" threat to US commodity and food crops, noxious enough that methyl bromide exposure is deemed preferable, and legally sanctioned by the state, in comparison. Arguably, broomrape's proliferation has much to do with the way the US agriculture system is structured, including its dependency on large volumes of pesticides (generating plant resistance), and landscapes of massive, monoculture fields that require repeated, destructive machine-tilling of the soil.[63] Related strains, such as California and clustered broomrape (Latin names: *Orobanche californica* and *Orobanche fasiculata*, respectively) were viewed quite differently by Native Americans—for example, the Paiute used the plant to treat colds, flu, and other respiratory ailments.[64] Late nineteenth century physicians used another close relation (Latin name: *Orobanche americana*) "to stop bleeding of bowels and uterus, and for diarrhea. Externally, used to treat skin infections caused by Streptococcus, as a poultice or wash for wounds, ulcers, and herpes lesions."[65] I looked up these related plants after the conference out of curiosity, and credit my critical theory training for inspiring such inquisitiveness. How might weed science be conducted differently, *named* differently, or rendered irrelevant, I wondered, if agricultural extension agents were given the freedom and financial support to apply other options besides chemical control?

This by all accounts typical gathering of pesticide manufacturers, pest control advisors, and agricultural extension agents exhibited no such knowledge of nor interest in plants' cultural geographies or medicinal uses, and these lessons do not appear to be part of their standard training. Just like the *Casarett & Doull's Toxicology* textbooks I analyze throughout this project, any historical context that weed scientists provided was only to underscore the duration of a given weed's or pest's persistence, such as field bindweed (Latin name: *Convolvulus arvensis*; colloquially: orchard morning glory), which Eugene Woldemar Hilgard, one of the founding fathers of California agricultural extension, reportedly detested. On an official university extension blog, one weed scientist reports, "Native to the Mediterranean region and Western Asia, field bindweed is presumed to have been brought to the United States (in 1739) as a seed contaminant. The species moved westward and was officially documented in the state of California (San Diego County) in 1850. By the first quarter of the twentieth century, EW Hilgard (The Weeds of California, 1891) and FT Bioletti (The Extermination of Morning-glory, 1911) had proclaimed the species to be the most troublesome weed in the state."[66] Note the use of the passive voice in this agricultural extension report, similar to the toxicology texts I analyzed previously: "Field bindweed is presumed to have been brought to the United States (in 1739) as a seed contaminant." What postcolonial science and technology studies (STS) and critical environmental scholars term biopiracy, bioimperialism, colonial botany, imperial ecology, or bioprospecting is narrated here as a depoliticized yet malevolent appearance "as a seed contaminant."[67] This passage neutralizes settler colonialism *and* presents organisms from the Mediterranean and Western Asia as contaminants to the settler colonial nation of the United States in the same breath.[68] At the weed science conference I attended in 2019, the agricultural extension agent presenting on the troubles of bindweed, for which glyphosate is "the least poorly effective," being the only herbicide that "controls inconsistently" (as opposed to "controls not at all"), stressed to us audience members that "the name [*Convolvulus arvensis*] *literally* means 'to entwine fields'" (his emphasis), without recognizing the possibility that the settler-colonizers who thus named the plant embedded their partial vision directly into their classificatory structure and nomenclature.[69]

Conference organizers included a total of fifteen plants in the morning's weed-identification quiz activity—prizes included experiment station-produced food products and branded baseball caps—but no one among this gathering of pest control advisors successfully identified all fifteen flora. A staff member from the state Department of Pesticide Regulation won with a high score of thirteen. In closing, the overriding message of the weed quiz was that certain plants belong and certain plants do not, providing the context and conditions within which pesticide use makes perfect sense and, furthermore, is entirely necessary. Together, industrial agriculture and US toxicology make a medicinal and practical plant like the orchard morning glory into the contaminating and troublesome bindweed, constructing a battle in which pest control advisors enthusiastically enlist and step into formation, ready to serve.[70]

A Fraternity of Weed Science Bros

Before turning to the higher stakes version that is the Weed Contest, allow me to situate my concept of toxicant masculinity in theorizations of hegemonic masculinity more broadly, which are particularly relevant to my analysis of pest control advisors. Historian Gail Bederman chronicles the emergence of a distinctly "United Statesean" type of hegemonic masculinity, which she terms "primitive masculinity."[71] In brief, Bederman's archival research shows how turn of the twentieth century, privileged white men managed much of their settler colonial anxieties of illegitimacy through sexuality. (Other postcolonial historians offer complementary analyses.[72]) Wealthy white men felt emasculated in comparison to the displaced and dispossessed men around them who had no choice but to labor with their bodies or were otherwise looked down on as closer to nature, and hence uncivilized and primitive, including poor white men, hypersexualized Black men, and perhaps especially the "noble savage"—Native and Aboriginal peoples. Privileged settler-colonizers' turn to what we might call white collar jobs today—that sitting-indoors-behind-a-desk-all-day kind of postindustrial capitalism—left these elite US men feeling as though their manhood, alongside their muscles, was wasting away. President Theodore Roosevelt, profiled at length in Bederman's work, serves as a prime example.[73]

Roosevelt was born a sickly and frail child, and as he pursued public office, he began overcompensating for his weak constitution by performing an extreme, robust, tough, and sporty sort of masculinity, evidenced by his vociferous advocacy of eugenics and hunting-as-conservation, as well as his publicity photographs and stunts, such as shooting adult male lions on the African continent. Primitive masculinity, in Bederman's analysis, gave elite white men the best of both worlds. Having caricatured and appropriated what they saw as other(ed) men's threatening masculinity and mystical closeness to nature, colonizers in the United States merged a rugged enjoyment of the outdoors with white supremacism, branding themselves civilized yet virile sportsmen, conservationists, and, wouldn't you know it, scientists. For as historian of science Jenna Tonn similarly documents, turn of the twentieth century colonial zoology morphed into a sort of settler biology, wherein explorer men relocated from exotically dangerous wilderness sites to indoor, urban, northeast US laboratories—"the boys in the lab," as Tonn calls them.[74] The privileged white men of Tonn's archive exerted special effort to *not* be viewed as effeminate because their scientific study no longer required arduous, colonial treks across exoticized lands and seas, but instead left them hunched over microscopes for years on end.[75]

Several scholars and practitioners have since commented on the white bro culture of STEM (science, technology, engineering, medicine) that persists into the present, from geology to physics.[76] Weed science is no exception and in fact may provide one of the starkest examples. Weed scientists are scientists, but unlike the "boys in the lab" of Tonn's work, they conduct outdoor experiments in harsh conditions, operate heavy and increasingly complex machinery, and, to top it all off, get to drive trucks and sport steel-toed work boots. One of my toxicologist interviewees fondly recalled his experiences in aquaculture for precisely the reasons summarized above—"it was manual labor in a way that I enjoyed."

> I've worked construction, my dad's a plumber, an HVAC guy, so I did a lot of construction work on job sites before, so I was familiar with, you know, manual labor. It was a lot of that. But it was manual labor in, in a way that I enjoyed, not like laying concrete or shoveling, you know, digging ditches, it was like going towards, like, I thought it was the best of both worlds, you know? I got to work with my hands, I got to work outside, I got to work with . . . something I'm really passionate about. And so, this was a really unique experience for me, and I didn't think anything like that existed. You know, I did not want to work on a farm-farm, a traditional farm. . . . I wish there was a way where I could have a job that would allow me to go in the field and collect my samples and then come back in the lab and analyze and that's what I really want to do so, a bit of both, outdoor hands-on work and but also doing something really exciting with that, not just like ecology where, you know, you go out there and you observe and you count some things and you move some things around, you find patterns, but actually bringing that stuff in, analyzing it, whether it's DNA or RNA and really kind of looking under the hood, to see what's going on. It's pretty cool.[77]

This stated desire for *both* "outdoor, hands-on work" *and* high-tech, computer-driven analyses to "really look under the hood and see what's going on" well-encapsulates toxicant masculinity. In the case of weed science, perhaps the Shed is the new man cave. Or toxicant masculinity is the new primitive masculinity?

Feminist killjoy though I may be,[78] I am certainly not against having a bit of fun on the job. I myself have enjoyed many a mud-spattered ride in a pickup truck for work purposes. However, there is an undercurrent of white supremacist, masculinist compulsions to control and categorize across weed science, and toxicology more widely, that frequently spills over, bubbling to the surface in pesticide names like "Gunslinger" and "Battlestar," or plant names like "broomrape," for that matter, as well as flippant observations like "torturing with herbicides," "nice injury symptoms," or such technical terms as "noxious, parasitic, A-list pest." Let us now turn to how the homophilic, protomilitary, fraternity-like culture of hegemonic masculinity manifests in the Weed Contest.

Spraying and Hazing

There are four regional weed science societies (WSS) across the United States, three of which sponsor an annual weed contest: the Southern WSS, North Central WSS, and Northeastern WSS. The Western WSS does not sponsor its own contest but student members of the Western WSS may enter into the other WSS contests upon invitation. Each contest, which my weed science informant (an able-bodied, heterosexually coupled, socially privileged white man, incidentally) described as "demoralizing" and hazing-like, functions explicitly as a networking event and recruitment strategy for pesticide manufacturers.[79] Contests are "proudly sponsored" via "public-private partnerships" between land-grant universities and transnational chemical corporations such as Bayer (the Germany-based firm that bought the US-based Monsanto in 2016).

For example, a slickly produced promotional video on the North Central WSS website opens with a Bayer representative, sporting the same company polo shirt uniform prevalent throughout the weed science conference I attended, eventually cutting to a Kansas State University professor one-third of the way through the one-minute, forty-five-second clip.[80] The video shows several groups of three- or four-person student teams working studiously beneath a man's narrating voiceover, recorded in a down-home-country-yet-coolly-professional tone, chock-full of weed science slang like "plant path" (short for plant pathology).

The student teams featured in the video consist of young men and women, all of whom appear white and all of whom sport matching short-sleeve polo shirts, with their respective university logos where a professional's corporate logo would be, almost like scrimmage shirts for their postgraduation life—training tops?—paired with jeans or khakis. These contestants are shown furrowing their brows and sweating nervously during the "Written Calibration" portion of the contest, a paper-based exam, then studiously pouring carefully measured pesticide mixtures into special plastic cylinders and vials, evoking the stereotypical laboratory chemist at his bench, pouring gurgling potions into beakers and test tubes (see my chapter 2). Another scene from the video depicts the Shed, where contestants gather to display their expert knowledge of pesticide spray nozzles and hoses. As the North Central WSS Weed Contest rules state, for this portion of the contest, "questions may be related to all aspects of herbicide application. Potential topics may include (but are not limited to) sprayer calibration, application volume, load ticket calculations, active ingredient calculations, adjuvant rate, area calculations, metric and English unit conversions, ability to use a pesticide label, nozzle nomenclature and selection, sprayer pressure, droplet size, drift reduction techniques, etc."[81]

And this is merely for the "Written Calibration" segment of the event (50 points). The "Team Sprayer Calibration," worth 200 points, is where contestants must demonstrate their "ability to calibrate and properly operate a research backpack sprayer." Per the contest rules:

> Each team will be given a basic (easily solved) written problem that will be calculated during this session. The answers to the question will provide the parameters (application volume, recommended droplet size, etc.) to which a CO_2 backpack sprayer is to be calibrated. Each team will be expected to choose the appropriate nozzle tips, speed, and pressure for accurate calibration and application. Each team will be asked to deliver a designated number of gallons/acre or liters/hectare over a given length or area demonstrating proper sprayer use. Scoring will be based on accuracy of calibration and application. . . . Once time is stopped, no further adjustments can be made to the sprayer. The calibrated sprayer is then used by a contestant to spray a predetermined area with the judge watching for proper boom height, speed and uniformity of spray pattern. Following the application evaluation, each nozzle will be checked for accurate output. Variation in output up to ±4% variation per nozzle will be allowed. As an example, if the correct nozzle output is 150 ml/15 sec, the acceptable range will be 144 to 156 mL/15 sec.[82]

Other components of the contest include Weed Identification, similar to the informal weed-identification quiz I witnessed but with twenty-five plants (out of a possible seventy-five) instead of the fifteen I observed, and for between 100 and 300 points (depending on the size of the student team). The "Herbicide Application Technology" component consists of the written calibration and team sprayer calibration tests described above. Third on the contest rules list is the "Identification of Unknown Herbicides," where students must identify specific herbicides used based on the toxic effects exhibited by plants, as opposed to identifying the weeds that must be "tortured" with herbicides. Naturally these written contest rules do not use such terms as "tortured," like I had overheard during my ethnographic fieldwork, but more clinically and scientifically state that "students [must] demonstrate their ability to identify herbicide mechanism of action and active ingredient based on symptomology seen on treated plants and selectivity among different species."[83]

The culminating event of the Weed Contest, and the portion used most directly for chemical company recruitment according to my informant Tim, is the "Problem Solving and Recommendation" segment. Here, judges and contestants engage in role-play scenarios, acting as real-life growers and real-life pest control advisors who must "think on their feet,"[84] as the Bayer representative stated in the promotional video, to "troubleshoot a plant production problem in a field (agronomic, horticulture, turf) or non-crop situation and recommend an effective solution to that problem."[85] The rules go on to specify that "this event is to be presented and handled in a 'role-playing' situation. The student will be asked to assume the role of an extension, sales, or research person when dealing with the client. Any commodity (corn, soybean, wheat, vegetable, turf, etc.) or scenario (such as herbicide injury, weed resistance, agronomic errors, etc.) is eligible to be the focus of the Problem Solving and Recommendation event. . . . The top performer within each situation will participate in a common scenario (not used in the preliminary round) to determine the overall winner."[86] Contestants are judged on the following: "25 points—How the student approached the farmer. 45 points—Assessment of situation; determine the problem. 15 points—Recommendation for current year. 15 points—Recommendation for next year (or future years)."[87] Note the equivalencies and interchangeability between "the role of an extension, sales, or research person."

These written descriptions, and even the promotional video, do not adequately capture the intense, competitive, and masculinist energy of the event, which Tim recalled as a demoralizing hazing. I felt some of this energy during my own embodied experiences at the weed science conference but rely primarily on Tim's impassioned recollections of weed contest experiences. He reported, further, that "every fourth year, there is also a 'Weed Olympics' which has students from all over North America (really U.S. + one university in Ontario) and supersedes the regional events. Each of the regional contests probably attracts twenty to thirty 4-person teams from ten to fifteen universities which are almost entirely 1862 land-grant institutions. My impression is that most teams study together for at least a few hours a week beginning after their spring semester ends, though there are stories that get passed around where teams practice much more than that (especially from Texas A&M and University of Arkansas)."[88]

Importantly, my queer feminist critique of toxicant masculinity is not simply about the aggressive, homophilic affect of such spaces, it also calls attention to the deep, enduring industry infiltration into weed science as an epistemology and practice. Like US toxicology textbooks but even more overtly, these multiregional and semiannual weed contests clearly demonstrate how pesticide manufacturers' interests define the methods, tools, language, and questions of weed science, providing both the problems of and solutions to weed persistence and herbicide resistance. US public university educations are a direct conduit into pesticide corporations' research and development, in terms of both human capital and intellectual property. Recall Tim's observation that "the research [public university weed scientists] are paid to do by the chemical companies shows up two years later on the pesticide label."[89]

Folded into such toxicant masculinity, of course, is the devil trick (chapter 1), wherein pesticides, and the US industrial agriculture system that demands such toxicants, are presented as inevitable and desirable. Moreover, pest control advisors perpetuate the vicious cycle wherein industry-defined problems and solutions remain cloaked under the mantle of objectivity, disinterestedness, and quantification. Toxicant masculinity likewise reproduces the magical authority (chapter 2) of toxicology, as "extension, sales, or research" persons make authoritative claims regarding their products' efficacy at controlling weeds, despite mountains of evidence to the contrary.[90] Weed science is a serious business.

Confronting the Limits of Toxicant Masculinity

Zimdahl, whose uniquely critical history of weed science—an exception that proves the rule—I relied on heavily for this chapter, cynically notes,

"Self-scrutiny was not part of the curriculum. . . . Weed scientists . . . have focused on finding short-term solutions to the economic, environmental, and ecological problems of modern agriculture without acknowledging the argument that long-term solutions may be possible only when the capitalist, profit-driven character of the agricultural system has been recognized and addressed."[91] He also offers some offensive, white man's burden sort of pronouncements, for example: "If weed scientists in developed countries turn their backs on the needs and potential wrath of the poor, many of whom are women, and the unpleasantness of a crowded world while focusing on past successes and the technological dreams of future successes, catastrophic consequences that can now be seen in the rear view mirror may be close and unavoidable (sanctuary for terrorists, spread of drugs and weapons, political extremism, immigration by refugees to developed nations, and spread of disease)."[92] And yet he later avers, "The excessive magnitude of our [US] technological power demands humility."[93]

Meanwhile, my unexpected research accomplice and weed science informant Tim suggests that the weed science of the mid-twentieth century is increasingly irrelevant and failing to resonate for contemporary practitioners. However readily they may seem to adopt and advocate for the use of pesticides, weed scientists are easily among the most cognizant of the hazards generated by economic poisons, not the least of which is ever-increasing weed resistance, because ever more pesticide-resistant weeds require ever more pesticide applications. One conference attendee I sat with at lunch, for example, assured me that all growers want to stop using chemical pesticides, but feel trapped economically. Historically, however, weed scientists have tended to see "the growth in herbicide use as clear evidence that more weed scientists [are] needed,"[94] just as founding US toxicologist Harold C. Hodge celebrated how tens of thousands of new synthetic chemicals generated the discipline of toxicology: "The recognition of pressing toxic hazards called scientists to tasks that sooner or later transformed them into toxicologists."[95]

Rather than uproot the problem, in other words, dominant toxicology and weed science teaches its practitioners to remain stuck in the proverbial and literal weeds, barely managing the symptoms in an endless loop around the toxicant treadmill, at unsustainable speeds that are nevertheless no match for weed resistance. This book's outro gestures at radical alternatives to the myopic worldviews of weed science and dominant toxicology. The next two chapters, 4 and 5, comprise my critical feminist analysis of and collaborations with toxicologists in a different set of field and laboratory sites, where I turn my focus toward the messy complexities of endocrine disruption, feminist intervention, and animal liberation.

4

Fuzzy Family Feelings

An environmentalist genetic toxicology is one that seriously attends to basic questions of biology but also maintains an activist orientation toward environmental health research. Such a science will recognize that answers to the questions that molecular biology asks are not in themselves solutions to environmental problems and that conflating the two is often a recipe for political inaction—an environmental hazard of a different sort.

—Scott Frickel[1]

Missed Opportunities

It was my first year as a PhD student and my first semester as a teaching assistant. I was particularly excited for this discussion section with my twenty, twenty-something undergraduates because I was teaching Giovanna Di Chiro's "Polluted Politics? Confronting Toxic Discourse, Sex Panic, and Eco-Normativity."[2] In her contribution to the edited volume *Queer Ecologies: Sex, Nature, Politics, Desire*, Di Chiro critiques the heterosexist rhetoric of renowned integrative biologist Tyrone Hayes, among other endocrine-disrupting chemical (EDC) scientists. Hayes happens to be a beloved—at least by his students; the institution has been less kind[3]—professor at the very same university where I was then funding myself through my doctoral program by working as a graduate student instructor. Hayes is well-known for his charismatically unconventional teaching and lecturing style. For example, dressed in flamboyant scarves and pink silk suits, he memorably performs an "Atrazine Rap," describing how this synthetic chemical produced by Syngenta Corporation alters frog sex.[4] Such arguably queer performances notwithstanding, Di Chiro calls out Hayes's research for fueling the "heteronormative sex panic" around so-called gay frogs, as Hayes's lab describes atrazine-exposed male frogs who have sex with other male frogs (in the laboratory) as "demasculinized" and "feminized."[5] To be sure, Hayes is not alone in using these terms to describe EDC-exposed animals.[6] Sometimes feminization refers to a physiological effect, such as the presence of ovarian tissue in testes. Other times, EDC scientists (and advocates) use demasculinization to describe animal behaviors, such as same-sex sexual acts and same-sex couplings, in terms of care for offspring.[7] In any case, after enthusiastically delivering a mini-lecture on queer feminist science and technology studies (STS) critiques of the heterosexism permeating EDC-related research on animals, I triumphantly turned toward my students expecting to have blown their heteronormative brains. Perhaps because Hayes happens to be such a charismatic figure on campus, my students simply stared at me, looking mildly horrified, and said nothing. After an awkward silence, one of my more politically engaged students, a young woman active in the local food justice scene, spoke up: "But the frogs," she declared, incredulously, "they *are* suffering" (her emphasis).

Deflated, I meekly muttered something about how yes, some frogs exposed to atrazine via Hayes's experiments were born with physical differences, such as missing or extra limbs, that may generate some degree of discomfort. However, I continued (with my confidence shaken), Hayes's observation that atrazine-exposed frogs with testes attempting to mate with other frogs with testes—a same-sex sexual act that Hayes links to EDC exposures—ought not be interpreted as a necessarily harmful outcome of chemical pollution. Same-sex sexual acts are regularly recurrent across the animal world and frogs in particular happen to "sex-reverse" in the wild, irrespective of EDC exposure.[8] Needless to say, the discussion did not unfold as I had imagined, in part because my students' quizzical response took the wind out of my righteous sails. The challenge of communicating this nuance—how to galvanize political action against chemical poisoners without either stigmatizing the poisoned, putting environmental health researchers on the defensive, or minimizing the harms of toxic pollution—has troubled me for the near decade since that morning in a college classroom. (I should add, as one of my toxicologist interlocutors pointed out to me, that in large part because of Hayes's and other ecotoxicologists' research, the European

Union has banned atrazine and the US Environmental Protection Agency [EPA] is considering stricter regulation of the herbicide.[9])

* * *

Critical feminist scholars of toxicity are in a unique and privileged position to collaborate with environmental health scientists, and each of our fields are deeply concerned about the well-being of socioecological systems. This chapter chronicles my experience embedded within a toxicology laboratory at a prestigious research university, a lab renowned for its work revealing the multigenerational, adverse outcomes of toxic contamination in a variety of marine ecosystems. I offered my training in critical theory as a way of guiding these toxicologists away from tacit eugenicism, such as when disability is understood solely as an undesirable abnormality caused by chemical exposure.[10] In exchange, this particular group of toxicologists let me see behind the wizard's curtain, teaching me that scientists who might seem disinterested or insensitive to an outsider like myself, having based my impressions on their published output, are actually rather *enchanted*, in the Max Horkeimer and Theodor Adorno sense, with the natural world, and, moreover, compelled by powerful emotions of care and love for the living, and struggling, more-than-human animals they study.[11] As one senior member of the lab explained to me, "All too often I find it hard to describe my work to non-scientists when so much of what I do seems like I don't care for the organisms I work with (i.e. their eventual sacrifice), but in fact I think I care more than a lot of non-scientists, because I am trying to do something to help save the species! But that may be hard for non-scientists to fully understand."[12]

In the next chapter, I inquire after the latent queerness of toxicologists' enchantments with more-than-human animals. This chapter focuses on forms of intralaboratory care work, gesturing toward the more critical study of toxicants such care work portends. This laboratory care work, I submit, marks an exciting and vital entry point for more of what anthropologists Paul Robbins and Sarah Moore term "politically honest" science.[13] (Robbins and Moore critique those biologists who lament the Anthropocene and yet overlook the political economy of carbon emissions. In other words, we humans have not all contributed to climate catastrophe equally, nor are we humans all feeling its effects equally.[14])

In the wake of the 2020 murder of George Floyd, alongside other Black people victimized by police violence in recent years, the members of this esteemed, inquisitive laboratory were explicit about their commitments to environmental health and racial justice, as compared to the scientists in Robbins and Moore's analysis, for instance. Where and how might such stated commitments to social justice imbricate with scientific work on sea-dweller vitality? Before addressing this question, allow me first to clarify what I mean by care work.

Caring in Context

A rich feminist literature exists on the politics of care work, also theorized as social reproduction, reproductive labor, or emotional labor.[15] This scholarship reveals how caregiving roles—raising children, attending elders, preparing family meals, consoling and supporting other people emotionally, providing friendly customer service, and so on—remain all too often uncompensated and expected, if not demanded, of women regardless of their social locations or professional positions. In the context of chemical exposures, legal scholar Dayna Nadine Scott and other researchers have noted how working women and women of color especially not only bear heavier toxic body burdens because of their disproportionate exposure to toxicants (in such items as cleaning solvents, ironically labeled personal care products, and thermal receipt paper, for example), but also bear heavier burdens in terms of the extra care work required *because* of toxic pollution, tending to children, partners, parents, and other loved ones who require additional caregiving due to the adverse health outcomes of chemical exposure.[16]

While critical of the expectation that women naturally perform care work or provide caregiving without compensation, feminists are not necessarily critical of care work itself.[17] Indeed, caregiving is taken seriously as an *antidote* to (chemical) violence.[18] Urban sociologist Manuel Tironi, for example, conceptualizes "hypo-interventions" and "intimate activism" via his ethnographic work with the impoverished community of Puchuncaví. Overwhelmed, psychically and physically, by fourteen industrial complexes, including the largest copper smelting plant in Chile and four thermoelectric plants, the somewhat isolated and immobile (as in, unable to relocate) residents of Puchuncaví resist in what small yet significant ways they can: tenderly applying homemade oint-ment to a loved one's toxicant-induced rashes, meticulously wiping toxic residues off the plants in their backyard gardens, and so on. These hypo-interventions and gestures of intimate activism will not stop the economic and political structures that produce and enable this toxic, in-dustrial compound, but, as Tironi argues, not every person poisoned by pollution is in a position to become an activist, in the more traditional, larger-scale mode, such as organizing public demonstrations. Tironi's work seems to suggest a form of surrender, as if global-financial power asymmetries and the toxic hazards they unevenly distribute are too enormous and ubiquitous to counteract. While Tironi does not advocate for apathy, neither does he unrealistically expect fence-line communities to resist more aggressively in the profoundly unfair fight against indus-trial polluters. Struggling and surviving under a highly constrained set of oppressive preconditions, the people of Puchuncaví are rather com-mendable for their insistent tenderness, despite personally having little to no hope of prevailing over the petrochemical corporations responsi-ble for their ill-health. The inability to escape toxicity does not preclude caring, loving acts between and among those poisoned, in other words. In certain contexts, care work may indeed be the *only* viable, expectable response to the harmful effects of toxic pollution.

Critical disability scholar-activists add much to feminist analyses of care work as well, prefiguring the concept and practice of "radical care": "a set of vital but underappreciated strategies for enduring precarious worlds."[19] Rather than view the care of individuals and communities living with disabilities as a chore, scholar-activists such as Leah Lak-shmi Piepzna-Samarasinha urge us to understand care work as a collec-tive responsibility and, moreover, as work that can also be pleasurable.[20] Importantly, and in concert with Robbins and Moore's call for more politically honest science, the literature on radical care draws explicit connections between disabling institutions and individualized disabil-ity. Without romanticizing the *need* for care work, or fetishizing care work itself, critical disability scholar-activists underscore how care work can and should be practiced as an act of "solidarity, not charity,"[21] in the sense that care work provides a meaningful and tangible alternative to a dominant paradigm that simultaneously necessitates and neglects, depoliticizes and dismisses, care. As the editors of a timely special issue on radical care write, "Reciprocity and attentiveness to the inequitable dynamics that characterize our current social landscape represent the kind of care that can radically remake worlds that exceed those offered by the neoliberal or postneoliberal state, which has proved inadequate in its dispensation of care. . . . It is precisely from this audacity to produce, apply, and effect care despite dark histories and futures that its radical nature emerges. Radical care can present an otherwise, even if it cannot completely disengage from structural inequalities and normative assumptions regarding social reproduction, gender, race, class, sexuality, and citizenship."[22]

The relatively privileged members of the prestigious toxicology lab I worked with are not, as far as I know, engaged in existential struggles for daily survival to the degree that fence-line communities are, nor am I. Privileged researchers such as ourselves are, however, attempting to produce knowledge for the good of the planet within "unavoidable circumstances" of "structural inequalities and normative assumptions." To what extent might the "intimate and banal details" of laboratory care work point us toward an otherwise study of toxicants,[23] one in which the structural forces that produce and perpetuate environmental racism, heterosexism, and ableism are called to account, while those marginalized and disabled by these very forces are care-fully embraced, rather than operationalized as pitiful victims or monstrous and burdensome abnormalities to be avoided?

Kate Millett's observations on the patriarchal family structure are also relevant to my ensuing discussion of laboratory care work, not only because I (rather brazenly) evoke the title of her 1970 work *Sexual Politics* for my own book's title, but also because the institution of the scientific laboratory struck me as deeply patriarchal, complete with Principal Investigator (PI)/Head of Household on whom all lab/family members are financially dependent.[24] (Importantly, as critical race feminism illuminates, a PI can *not* identify as a man and still the laboratory structure can remain masculinist.) Reflecting on the failures of previous sexual revolutions, inclusive of women's liberation, Millett writes, "Only the outer surface of society had been changed; underneath the essential system was preserved undisturbed. Should it receive new sources of support, new ratification, new ideological justification, it could be mobilized anew. Patriarchy could, as indeed it did, remain in force as a thoroughly efficient political system, a method of social governance, without any visible superstructure beyond the family, simply because it lived on in the mind and heart where it had first rooted itself in the conditioning of its subjects, and from which a few reforms were hardly likely to evict it."[25]

As my lab mates and I discussed over several months, surface-level commitments to diversity, equity, and inclusion (DEI) by some university administrators and scientific elites are unlikely to generate the long-term, meaningful changes needed to make laboratory research and its public applications more justice-oriented, because "underneath the essential system [is] preserved undisturbed."[26] Nevertheless, my close readings of salient moments in our lab meetings, a few of which were rather uncomfortable, if generatively so, and one-on-one interviews suggests that these thoughtful scientists (en)counter the confines of their discipline with small yet mighty acts of care.

Fuzzy Family Feelings

In the thick of the coronavirus pandemic, I began attending the weekly meetings of a toxicology laboratory that investigates multigenerational changes wrought by EDC exposures. Like many scientific research laboratories, during the early months of the pandemic most lab work shifted to remote modalities—primarily in the form of the now (in)famous Zoom meeting—except for the at-minimum physical interactions required, such as for keeping experimental lab animals alive. During my remote field work, this highly renowned, research-focused, or "R1," public university lab consisted of a core group of nine members, including the PI, Ben.[27] It was these nine members whom I spent the most time with and interviewed individually. Being an academic lab, membership numbers fluctuated as students entered the program and graduated over time, or as funding became available and unavailable, particularly for postdocs. During the two consecutive academic terms (approximately twenty weeks) I attended meetings, I met two alumni of the lab; a postdoc who was on his way out to accept a more permanent position just as I was joining the group, and another postdoc who visited her former colleagues to report on her experiences as a scientist working to inform environmental policymaking. Two undergraduates joined later in my remote field work as well, both of whom I opted not to interview because of our relatively short time together. I did, however, interview a professional research collaborator of the lab, Chris, an employee of the US EPA.

Almost immediately, I observed how this lab, under Ben the PI's mentorship, proudly maintained both professional and personal relationships with its graduates. Members seemed to consider the lab like a family (or perhaps the family they never had), with Ben at the helm as the benevolent, paternal, head of household—an affect only accentuated by the fact that the lab manager, Katie, also happened to be the PI's spouse. (I soon began affectionately referring to her in my field notes as "lab mom.") Ben and Katie would regularly host lab meetings at their home, outdoors, in observance of COVID-19 protocol, celebrating the end of each academic term for example, with dinner (pizza), drinks (beer), and dessert (ice cream)—the US college student meal de rigueur—over chill, streaming music and lively conversation. My feminist proclivities led me to approach this sense of lab-as-family as necessarily burdened by heteropatriarchal baggage, but it was not long before I too began to take comfort in the parental caring of the husband/PI and wife/manager team.[28] They clearly cared about their highly achieving students' quality of life, encouraging and modeling such behaviors as taking time off for physical exercise and spending time with loved ones, while also making sure students and postdocs had access to the office space, working conditions, and equipment necessary to produce quality scientific work, including everything from noise-canceling headphones to ergonomic desk chairs, as well as making sure lab-related chores were evenly distributed among members.

I would not go so far as to suggest that this caring, if heteronormative, scientific lab dynamic is typical of R1 universities in the United States, and yet I do wonder about the extent of its atypicality. Perhaps natural scientists are more caring and emotional (as opposed to disinterested and rational) than their outward-facing research publications would have critical feminist STS scholars believe. To be sure, there is an element of self-selection here—only an already open-minded lab would welcome a critical feminist, with the explicit purpose of studying *them*, into their midst. I offer the following close readings of several ethnographic vignettes and interviews with lab members to illustrate how I came to understand lab work as care work, or what I call *fuzzy family feelings*. Whether during direct discussion of feminist STS criticism, regular check-ins about the lab's experimental animals—a task that lab members themselves referred to as "fish care" (discussed further in chapter 5)—or more philosophical reflections on the role of toxicology in environmental justice and climate crisis more broadly, these toxicologists showed extraordinary care for one another, for the more-than-human animals they experimented on (while also, nevertheless, experimenting on them), and for the earth's diversity of ecosystems that are so distressingly under siege.

"If Diversity is So Important, Where is It Now?"

I approached this particular lab at the suggestion of a close colleague in the biological sciences, who knew that Ben worked on EDCs and was an exceptionally kind human being, as far as PIs of R1s go. After having been politely but firmly turned down by three other PIs working on EDCs, I was hopeful that my colleague's personal recommendation would help. Thankfully it did; Ben was quite welcoming. I presented my ethnographic intentions honestly, if vaguely (by necessity), to his entire lab: I sought to better understand how toxicologists, including scientists in adjacent fields who regularly use toxicology, know what they know about EDCs. In true scientist feminist/feminist scientist fashion, I did not claim to be a neutral observer and committed to presenting my scholarship to the lab, taking my turn alongside all other members.[29] I openly acknowledged that my very presence would shift the dynamic of the lab, and made note of such shifts to the extent possible in my field notes. Because the lab members knew I was researching permutations of sexism and racism in toxicology, I sensed they were more self-conscious than they might otherwise have been during discussions that were explicitly about (in)equity.

For example, before I had presented my critical feminist STS research to the lab (I purposely chose a date later in the term), lab members admitted that they were curious about my intentions, and that this curiosity alone catalyzed new conversations. As one junior member, Bruno, revealed to me, "Before you gave your talk, I think this was some time after you were introduced to the lab—even just that introduction and kind of integration of your work into our lab sparked conversations between me and [two other lab members] and just really got us thinking about these things [relating to diversity, equity, and inclusion in the natural sciences], and even just, just having a presence, like, *you, there*, kind of really sparked some of those conversations."[30] Bruno's generous and thoughtful observation about my sheer presence in the group—*"you, there"*—making a positive difference is encouraging in and of itself. What if all toxicological labs integrated critical theorists into their weekly discussions? What would toxicological knowledge production look like, and how might it move differently through the world, if critical feminist thought and practice were present and at play from the beginning? If the study of toxicants was simultaneously the study of society and critical theory?

Bruno also, hesitatingly, expressed his frustration and disappointment with his university's surface-level response to diversity in education, what he perceived as a bare-minimum and self-serving effort, in direct contrast to the in-depth, sustained conversations we were now having in lab meetings. I quote this interview at length to underscore both its form and content.

> I've always felt like, like with applications—like when I applied to [this university] I had to write a diversity statement. Then the first day of the first class of my [term] was like a dedicated hour about diversity . . . The point that I want to say isn't that I disagree with it, it was more like, *if [diversity] is so important, where is it now? Why is it just—it, it just seemed like it was done to fit some quota.* That's my impression. *It felt like a way for maybe the university to remove themselves from blame.* I don't know if that's the right word to say and that may be the completely wrong perspective but that was just my perspective. It seemed very surface level and—not that the content was surface level but more like how it was presented was surface level. I—like, *to contrast that with your talk, and kind of just with Ben and just this collaboration overall—it's the opposite of that. And that's what I think the maturation of this should be, is conversations like this [interview], or conversations like you had with us a few weeks ago* and—I never got that anywhere else, and it's just strange to me that [an institution] can say that diversity is a priority, but there's no conversation really about it. . . . And with the [institutional] talk about diversity, *no one ever talked about diversity of* ideas *and that was something else*

that kind of struck me [about your presentation in lab] because diversity is important, but I think people bring a diversity of ideas. And that has never been brought up, ever, in a diversity talk or a diversity statement, which just seemed interesting to me, to omit that. So in that regard, I would say, *how [DEI efforts have] been handled or implemented, often leaves me wondering what the true intent behind it is* because I feel like there's a very real need for diversity. There's a very real need for representation. But it just seemed like, maybe, that—in my opinion, it didn't seem like it was being incorporated or integrated enough, and that was kind of my issue with it. . . . It's never a one-on-one conversation, it's an, it's like an emotionless email, and you've got to take this [diversity] training and you do it once a year and everybody does it to get it over with. And we all kind of complain about how dumb it feels to do it.[31]

I could not help but notice how haltingly this highly astute and generally well-spoken, emerging young scientist expressed himself when it came to topics outside his formal training. The number of caveats, qualifications, and apologies in his response suggest to me that while he feels strongly that his institution's stated concern for the importance of diversity is disingenuous (his word)—as evidenced by their one-hour, once-a-year presentation and "emotionless email" regarding a requisite diversity training course—he hesitates lest his words be misconstrued as critical of the value of diversity itself. He clearly believes in the importance of integrating diverse peoples and perspectives throughout lab discussions and practices. I found his enthusiasm for the kind of sustained, meaningful conversations about diversity, equity, inclusion, *and justice* that I was trying to foster with the lab quite encouraging.

The more meaningful conversation this lab member recalled with gratitude was the mini-lecture I had prepared on critical feminist STS (about twenty minutes in length, for a two-hour lab meeting), introducing lab members to core concepts such as Donna Haraway's situated knowledge, as well as postcolonial critiques of Euro-American taxonomies, contemporary genetics, and dominant research methods more broadly. I was careful to highlight not only my feminist STS predecessors' work on *who* counts as a scientist, but also *what* counts as science, hence the aforementioned lab member's observation that I had emphasized a "diversity of ideas" as well as of people. Next, I summarized my dissertation research on the history of US toxicology in terms of endocrine-disrupting pesticides specifically by way of segueing into the then-current ethnographic project involving the lab.[32] I ended my presentation by floating the following questions: Can contemporary toxicologists overcome toxicology's masculinist and militarist (and eugenicist and imperialist) history? What barriers and opportunities exist in terms of practicing toxicology differently?

I did my best to present these outside critiques of the very science this lab engages in with humility, asking open-ended questions rather than insisting on a particular feminist perspective and furthermore acknowledging that the lab has much to teach me. Judging by lab members' earnest responses to my presentation, my attempts at *not* putting folks on the defensive seemed to have worked. But they did express some frustrations. One of the lab's senior members, Kelly, had remained silent during my twenty-minute presentation (on US toxicology's masculinist and militarist emergence) and the ensuing discussion, but spoke poignantly towards the end of the meeting: "I feel unknowledgeable, this is still so new to me. . . . I don't have much knowledge about the issues we're talking about, I really don't know so much about what was in that article." (I had recommended reading before my presentation Rohan Deb Roy's "Science Still Bears the Fingerprints of Colonialism."[33]) She continued,

> I'm disappointed in myself, I should know more about these things, it's not taught in the classrooms, I have to take time away to do that. . . . It has to come from yourself, you're not being pushed to do it from the outside by the institution. We all want to talk about it and know more about it, but finding the time—it's not in our job descriptions, to take time out to do that. . . . *I'm grateful that Ben is open to taking time away from the science to talk about this*, even labs that think it's important don't have the time to set aside to do that. *We need more push from the institution and better discussions of DEI, it never goes deep enough.* We don't have the knowledge; we have to be led by someone with more knowledge or we need to read more before discussing in order to have conversations to move us anywhere. *It would be nice to revisit this each [term], devote one [lab] session, have a more guided discussion, with some sort of reading, or inviting someone to talk with us*—I don't want to put it on one person in the lab to lead the discussion.[34]

While Kelly's impassioned plea could be read as somewhat defensive, I felt she was soberly reflecting on her own lack of exposure to critical histories of science and calling out research institutions and training programs for deprioritizing such work. As her junior colleague Bruno similarly observed, in the interview excerpted above, "It's just strange to me that [an institution] can say that diversity is a priority, but there's no conversation, really, about it." Given the intense publish-or-perish pressures put on research-focused scientists, especially those as early in their careers as these graduate students and postdocs, "taking time away from the science" to learn more about the racism and heterosexism (among other -isms) permeating dominant science would put emerging scholars such as themselves at a significant disadvantage. "We all want to talk about it and know more about it, but finding the time—it's not in our job descriptions." I also sensed Kelly's response was earnest rather than defensive because of her expressed desire for additional, more structured conversations, again, similar to her junior colleague Bruno, on the oppressive cultural ideologies embedded into scientific disciplines—"It would be nice to revisit this each [term], devote one [lab] session, have a more guided discussion."

"Boring Truth Doesn't Work"

Interestingly, when we returned to what the lab categorizes as DEI discussions later in the second term, the conversation did become a bit more defensive, or at least provocative.[35] Inspired by my presence, I like to think, one lab member, Olivia, took it upon herself to learn more about critical feminist STS, electing to enroll in a seminar on this very subject. She then presented some of what she was learning back to the lab, and I found the group's pushback illuminating.

I happened to interview Olivia shortly before her planned presentation, which felt more like a conversation between colleagues than an interview, during which she confessed to me that she was nervous she did not know the material well enough herself to be presenting it to her lab mates. She also spoke of the difficulty of selecting the right (as in nonoffensive) words in her own writing on EDCs' adverse effects on reproductive development.

Um, so I—actually I'm a second author on a publication and the first word is "feminizing" and I didn't really love that title, but I wasn't the first author so I just kind of, I mean I edited up the paper but I never said anything about the title. But yeah, I think it's like, "Feminized effects of . . ."—I can't remember. I mean, I know the project but I can't remember the title off the top of my head. Um, yeah, I don't know. And [in the critical feminist STS seminar] we were discussing . . . so, if you can identify some of these words, these metaphors, you know, can you go about trying to not use them and trying to change them? We were talking about how to [unclear], especially when they become, like, established terms in the field that everyone uses, and how do you replace them and—yeah, it was a good discussion but, yeah, also difficult to think about. *I was thinking . . . I never said it, but I was thinking, "I wish someone would just tell me—like, give me a list. Here's what you use, what not to use, like, absolutely, I can follow it."* But, yeah, thinking about trying to be the one to determine, you know, what words or terms to replace [feminization or demasculinization] and what to replace them with—like, that would be the challenging part.[36]

Olivia revealed at least two cultural norms of contemporary US scientific training that are pertinent to my analysis here: hierarchy and (standard operating) procedure versus an iterative, participatory process. The hierarchical structure of dominant scientific knowledge production is evidenced by her experience as a junior member in her prior lab, wherein she contributed to an experiment as well as the editing of an ensuing paper and yet did not feel confident (or supported?) enough to voice her concerns over the title of published article on which she remains listed as a coauthor. Second, and relatedly, her desire for a list of accepted terms, and her discomfort with the *process* of determining which terms might be more accurate and less harmful, reflects how the dominant scientific approach in US laboratories seems to favor and encourage procedure—"give me a list . . . absolutely, I can follow it"—rather than process—"How do you replace [established terms]? . . . [It's] difficult to think about."

During our conversation, I tried to be as encouraging as possible, mentioning the oft-repeated assurance that the best way to learn something is to teach it. I also found her nervousness perfectly understandable; I have a PhD in critical science studies and I still feel anxious when presenting critiques of science to practicing scientists. Olivia's position was perhaps more nerve-racking, as the audience in this case consisted of her peers and mentors. How they responded to her, a *bonafide* member of the lab, surely matters more to her level of comfort and security in the group than for me, as I was only a passing interlocutor.

On the day of her presentation, with much self-deprecation and numerous apologies, Olivia bravely taught feminist STS scholar Banu Subramaniam's "Snow Brown and the Seven Detergents: A Metanarrative on Science and the Scientific Method,"[37] following by a mini-lecture on unintended bias in scientific language. Lab members responded positively and empathically to Subramaniam's critical reflections on being a brown, immigrant feminist in white, US masculinist biological science. By this point, I had come to know the lab members well enough to not be surprised by their generous, thoughtful responses to a critical scholar like Subramaniam. Ben the PI, for instance, had mused after my presentation a couple months prior:

> There is a deeply rooted conceit that scientists are the objective counters of things, "only the truth ma'am," that kind of stuff, something I think about and struggle with. Science is different in that it is evidence-based, but to be taken seriously I can't be an advocate—that's emotional, that's not evidence-based. Even though I have these values I can't express them. [Bruno] Latour pointed out that conceit, most famously. Scientists are humans and products of their social environments. . . . Latour argued against that idea that scientists were ever the white-lab-coat-wearing rationalist. Maybe by admitting that conceit they'd do better science.[38]

(If Ben was trying to impress me by name-dropping STS scholar Bruno Latour, he did, though I would have been even more impressed if he had name-dropped a critical feminist STS scholar like Banu Subramaniam.) While I would question Ben's separation of evidence from emotion— "Science is different in that it is evidence-based . . . even though I have these values I can't express them"—under this extraordinary PI's mentorship, this equally extraordinary group of scientists-in-training were among the first to admit the myth of purely objective science (though they were still attached to said myth, as discussed below), and they remained open to feminist and postcolonial critiques of the scientific method.

Notably, however, in the lab meeting during which Olivia nervously presented on her newfound interest in critical feminist STS, a visiting undergraduate, Gregory—who also happened to be the only African American student I encountered in the lab during my short stint as a participant-observer—objected to postcolonial critiques of dominant science. He firmly disagreed in particular with the observation that this way of knowing is not the only way of knowing, and moreover not the most superior way of knowing: "I think science *does* transcend other forms of knowledge, beautifully, and that those aspects of science need to be cherished and preserved."[39] I let Gregory's comment float, curious to see how the others would respond to his defense of dominant science, but this idea that there is a transcendent beauty to dominant science—as well as his implication that its transcendence is under threat—did not come up again until the next meeting, and only then because I brought it up. I decided to ask lab members to reflect on the visiting undergraduate's comment (who unfortunately was not in attendance that day, and he and I never crossed paths again), curious if there was indeed a preference and desire, even if they knew it to be untrue, for science's purity and objectivity.[40] "Agreed," Ben remarked. "There is a beauty to this approach that has led to some deeply profound, foundational knowledge of how nature works . . . this recent-ish method has been amazingly successful in helping us understand how nature works, and there is a beauty to that, something aesthetically pleasing to that. . . . It's pretty cool to make a 'discovery.' . . . You hear that a lot from people who love science, as a way of discovering the world and spending your time."[41]

Perhaps this commitment to science—as an above-the-fray escape from the messy, brutal realities of unjust societies and unhealthy ecologies—is what makes even such reflexive scientists as these bristle at feminist critiques, as the following vignettes illustrate. Ben's comments regarding the aesthetics of scientific discovery, and his junior student's cherishing of such transcendence, brought to my mind feminist historian of science Rebecca Herzig's work *Suffering for Science*. Herzig contextualizes the Euro-American and socioeconomic origins of this idealized, pure scientist, who devoutly, often ascetically, pursues science for science's sake. "Those [nineteenth century] scientists seeking to counteract the siren voices of materialism, commercialism, and utilitarianism elevated [personal] sacrifice precisely because it denied the logic of compensatory exchange. It was the nonreciprocal character of the scientist's labors that assured his separation from the degradation of the modern marketplace."[42] Herzig further documents how the privileged role of science in US society, as it was performed by socially privileged scientists, wandered further and further from practical applications that might improve everyday lives. "Failure is not epiphenomenal to research . . . , it is central to the very definition of the true scientist's endeavors . . . , [one who] belligerently resists all useful scientific work, forgoing both professional publication and therapeutic applications as he takes on obscure [scientific] problems."[43] By contrast, feminist killjoys such as myself, to borrow Sara Ahmed's reclaiming of the term, bring scientists back down to earth, sometimes kicking and screaming.[44]

Things started off promising. Olivia turned from a generative and, I would say, successful discussion of Subramaniam's "Snow Brown" article to share her recent lesson in biased language. She was warmed up now, and seemed considerably less nervous as she excitedly exclaimed to her peers, "This was one of those moments in [the critical feminist STS] seminar that I was like"—she mimed her head exploding—"metaphors can have material consequences!"[45]

As she moved rather quickly through several examples ("invasive species,"[46] "chemical castration," and the "war on AIDS") I sensed Ben in particular becoming increasingly uncomfortable. He was on board with the invasive species critique: "A lot of these terms are tied up with *intent* that doesn't exist in natural systems. There's no intent with an 'invasive' species. That intent is something that's a big problem for scientists. You see all these terrible, bullshit uses of Darwinian evolution in economics, like survival of the fittest . . . anthropomorphizing can really mess things up in both ways . . . migration can also be benign, or beneficial."[47] "Chemical castration" (a problematic turn of phrase I return to in the outro), however, perhaps hit a little too close to home because of the lab's own work on EDCs.[48] While Ben was not in disagreement with the potential offensiveness of such language, he wondered aloud if its use might be a good strategic, political move:

People with mal-intent to misinterpret science will do it regardless, why is it on *us* to be so careful with our language? . . . Powerful interests in society get their message across because they lie, and say dramatic things, so if scientists want to compete, maybe we need to take the Fox News approach, exploit people's fears. It's worthwhile grappling with that. If it's for a good end, reducing pollution, then why not lie about it? Why not exploit people's fear? Why not exploit people's fears of "Black people taking over"? Why not play their game and force *our* agenda?[49]

His students responded with comments like: "Exaggeration creates extremism, that approach would backfire." Ben pressed on:

BEN: How come that [extremism] hurts only the Left, and not the Right?

UPTON [SENIOR LAB MEMBER]: Scientists will lose their moral high ground and it will just be seen as a battle of rhetoric, we have to hold ourselves to a different standard.

BEN: The stakes are too high now, the time for calm, 95 percent sure of blabbedy-blah—the stakes are too high for that. *You're fighting deeply penetrating lies with boring truth, it's not going to work.* That's the argument people make for riots: Black people have been so violently oppressed for so long, so it's time to burn it down, at some point—when do you abandon your scientist's cloak? [Emphasis added.]

I could not help but pipe in at this point, suggesting that this harmful language might alienate the very people who would be essential comrades in said struggle to burn it down, and moreover that exploiting people's fears doesn't necessarily work to motivate legislative action in terms of reducing pollution—US congressmen have strongly repudiated scientists' suggestion that *their* sperm counts are in decline.[50] We were running short on time, however, and Olivia was eager to get through the rest of her presentation, so the conversation moved on. She had continued to militarized metaphors, offering such examples as the "war on AIDS" and "targeted drug delivery," when Ben nearly cut her off in indignation.

Oh, come on. This is getting to be too much. You need to use terms that people understand, and that people can generate some imagery around.

If you had only scientific words then how do you communicate to people outside of science? I think you can easily take this argument of offensive wording off the rails. I get the [critique of the] war on AIDS, but targeting? Really? Those metaphors are pretty accurate and powerful. If one of the consequences is normalizing how bad war is, then I guess it's a negative consequence, but the words are actually quite accurate.[51]

Visibly flustered, Olivia tried to articulate a decisive response, and I wondered if she was as flummoxed by Ben's strong pushback as I was. Somewhat weakly, yet astutely, she countered that "targeted" also implies that the pharmaceutical-chemical *is* that precise when drugs in fact produce a lot of off-target effects, to which Ben responded, "To improve your targeting is both a desire of medicine and war." Apparently unaware that with this comment, he seemed to have simultaneously completely missed *and* succinctly summarized a central point of his student's presentation on (un)intended bias in scientific language, Ben quieted down and our discussion quickly continued to ableism—so quickly that I did not have a chance to jot down Olivia's examples in my field notes—then abruptly ended because we were out of time.

As is his custom, Ben signaled the end of the meeting with words of encouragement to his students, including gratitude for their presence and hard work, and it occurred to me that what I experienced as masculinist, abrasive pushback might not have ruffled anyone else's proverbial feathers. While the other lab meetings I attended did not reach this somewhat heated intensity of discussion, the fact that Ben closed with his usual peptalk suggested to me that he enjoyed the exercise, and moreover that this sort of mildly aggressive debate is normal and acceptable. Gregory, the visiting undergraduate, added just before we all signed out of the Zoom meeting that he was ready to "burn it down" alongside Ben, and everyone laughed together in a heartwarming show of solidarity.[52] Perhaps the truth is not so boring after all.

The Personal is Political ↔ Science is Political ↔ Science is Personal

I found myself in Olivia's shoes about a year later. I had returned to the lab, at their invitation, to discuss a paper I recently coauthored with amphibian biologist and ecotoxicologist Max Lambert, in which we argue that heterosexist language and ideology limits scientific and political progress on EDCs.[53] Max and I illustrated our argument with a particular case of a particular species of frog, *Rana clamitans*, which Max has studied extensively in urban and suburban environments, where frogs are exposed to numerous EDCs. Max, as he had been trained, initially concluded that imbalanced sex ratios—too many females—in these frog populations were a result of these populations' overexposure to EDCs. (Ecotoxicology typically finds that EDCs adversely affect frogs' reproductive fitness, producing not only imbalanced sex ratios but also same-sex sexual behavior and intersex frogs, as glossed in this chapter's opening vignette.) However, after thinking critically and reflexively with queer feminist STS, Max reexamined his data and realized rather that temperature changes, as well as higher mortality rates for males, led to imbalanced sex ratios in these particular frog populations, not the hormonal perturbances from EDC exposures.[54] Max and I built from his specific scientific journey to argue that standardized ecotoxicological terms such as feminized and demasculinized "lead scientists astray," misguiding ecotoxicological research in addition to stigmatizing gender nonconforming and queer human communities.[55]

We likewise built from Max's scientific journey to argue that all biologists would do well to reexamine the assumptions and standardized language of their disciplines, especially when such assumptions and terminology may reinscribe the very same (tacit) heterosexist and eugenicist beliefs that position certain populations to be more exposed to toxicants than others in the first place (in the sense that marginalized communities are more likely to be located near and/or work in toxic sites because social and institutional forces construct these communities as less valuable, pollutable, and disposable[56]). Because the presence of "intersex" frogs and same-sex sexual behavior among frogs is frequently interpreted as an adverse outcome of EDC exposure, Max and I also cited other scientists' biological research showing that intersex frogs can in fact reproduce, and that same-sex sexual behavior is not an abnormal animal behavior and hence not indicative of species decline. Meanwhile, our argument continued, when old assumptions are discarded, new questions arise—such as, Why and how does temperature affect metamorphizing frog sexes? Why are more males dying than females?—that expand biological knowledge more broadly. None of our critiques of dominant ecotoxicology are meant to dismiss the harmful effects of chemical pollution on frogs particularly and the globe generally. Nevertheless, in retrospect, I should have recalled how intensively Ben grilled Olivia, as described above, and prepared accordingly. Instead, feeling nostalgia for the fuzzy family feelings I had frequently enjoyed as a participant-observer with this lab, I barely prepped for the meeting, looking forward to what I was sure would be a productive and encouraging conversation. Indeed, a flood of positive feelings washed over me as soon as I logged-in to Zoom and saw so many familiar faces. I hadn't realized how much I missed my weekly meetings with this brilliant and hard-working community. So confident was I in how smoothly our reunion meeting would run that it never occurred to me to invite Max, who is without question the biological expert between us, to join the discussion.[57]

My elation soon turned to dismay, as "journal club"—this (and other) lab's term for such scientific paper discussions—did not resemble the sort of critical feminist conversations I was more accustomed to in the academic fields that comprise my intellectual home. One by one, each lab member stated their strong disagreements with the arguments Max and I had articulated. The journal club structure and procedure pitted one (me) against ten (them, including three new lab members whom I had not met previously). Rather than engaging in the sort of generous and care-full feminist critique I had naïvely expected, the lab embarked on an adversarial, debate-like discussion wherein I was single-handedly, and repeatedly, defending myself against a crescendo of criticisms (some of which, I reflected later, revealed a lack of reading on their part, with the notable exception of Ben the PI, who had clearly devoted much time and effort to closely reading the paper). Each lab member built on or merely echoed the criticisms shared by their colleagues, further adding to my sense of feeling overwhelmed and overpowered. In short, I felt there was nothing feminist about the encounter and that I had failed at my efforts to catalyze a more justice-centric approach to EDC research.

Lab members' criticisms of the work were variations of the same three themes: (1) It is journalists, not scientists, who are to blame for offensive language; (2) These terms (e.g., "feminized") are effective because they are terms that nonscientists understand. Or, so goes the logic of objection number two, it's necessary to use admittedly sloppy descriptions because nonscientist readers will not respond in the same way to "testes with ovarian tissue" as they will to "demasculinized," for instance. This second objection not only contradicted the lab's first objection (accusing mischievous journalists of misquoting innocent scientists), but was also posed as a challenge, directly to me: "What words would *you* use to get Congress to act?"; (3) Reproductive fitness *is* impaired by chemical exposure and *is* a good measure of declining population health. ("What should we be measuring instead?" they countered.)

I felt flustered, and frustrated, on several levels. I did not want to engage in this debate-like format, which in my view prevents a nuanced conversation and precludes consensus-building, as the debate structure itself forces an oversimplified binary of (we're) right and (you're) wrong. I also happen to be one of those people who needs time to organize her thoughts and articulate a coherent response; I do not perform well under pressure or think and speak quickly. But in refusing, intentionally, to engage in that sort of rapid repartee, I then effectively failed to call on the claims of the article under discussion, one of which is that these measures of reproductive fitness are not direct measures but rather rely on proxies, and that these proxies are steeped in, and reentrench, heteronormative assumptions about normal and natural, regardless of the intentions of the individual scientist. Ben countered later, in his care-full yet critical review of my draft of this chapter, "Nothing is more clear to me [than] that when exposures threaten reproductive fitness, this is bad. We can make that judgement while at the same time care for creatures and people who are exposed."[58] Max and I would agree with Ben that toxic disruptions to reproductive organs can be bad for reproductive outcomes and that we can recognize reproductive harm while caring for those whose reproductive systems have been harmed. Where Max and I disagree with Ben is that the presence of so-called intersex or gay frogs *necessarily* means that frogs' (and, by extension, humans') reproductive fitness is threatened.

Through iterative exchanges between me and interested lab members in the months following this reunion meeting of sorts, it became clear to me that the substance of the paper's feminist critiques did not entirely come through in that journal club moment (and it's no wonder, given its debate-like structure, my particular incapacities for rapid-fire rebuttal, and my relatively weaker grasp of evolutionary biology and ecotoxicology). I will try to be clearer in this chapter, enjoying the luxuries of writing (and a little help from my natural science friends) that allow me adequate time to process and better articulate my response. First, I will briefly restate my positions on objections 1 and 2, as listed above. Then I will elaborate further on objection number 3, which, as I alluded to in this chapter's opening vignette, remains the most challenging queer feminist STS critique for me to effectively communicate to scientist colleagues. In our article, Max and I do not mean to suggest that proxies are always uninformative for toxicology. We argue, rather, that toxicologists (and evolutionary biologists) ought to examine the historical emergence and sociocultural contexts of the particular proxies they take for granted as universal, apolitical laws of nature.

Notably, when I later shared my initial reactions of frustration with the lab, Kelly, one of the senior women members (senior as in academic rank, not years of age) demonstrated the depths of her caring and reflexivity:

> As a lab we may not have done our best here with this discussion. . . . I think a lot of the discussion was directed to you because of our lack of knowledge on the topic and because you were the most knowledgeable in the room about it. . . . *I think the way we go about these debates is extremely scientific, which is why it comes off as harsh sometimes. I think it's something that has taken me a long time to get used to and to not take too personally over time. This type of critique is something that is taught early on in science*, it took me a long time to learn as I felt we were purposely always trying to find a fault or mistake in a scientific paper. . . . I remember the first time I got a review back and I was so distraught! And then my advisor told me that [it was] actually a mostly positive review![59]

I have experienced my fair share of harsh reviews and (un)seemingly personal attacks within social sciences and humanities spaces as well; unfortunately, "this type of critique" is "taught early on" in dominant forms of education outside the biological sciences. (Truth be told, the meanest review I have ever received was from a self-identified feminist scholar reviewing for a self-identified feminist press.) Nevertheless, Kelly's normalization and acceptance of this adversarial, debate-style approach—"It's taken me a long time to get used to and to not take too personally over time"—as well as the defensiveness I sensed in all parties, myself included, is precisely where I would hope feminist STS might intervene.[60] Must journal clubs be this type of "extremely scientific" in order to be valuable, whether in terms of improving inquiry or strengthening analysis? Might scientists instead exchange ideas with less defensiveness and more humility, again, myself included, such that the recipient of critique does not frequently and familiarly experience the process as "trying to find a fault or mistake" and moreover as one that they simply have to "get used to"? Which is another way of saying, rather than training scientists *not* to take criticisms of our work personally, might we acknowledge that our scientific work is always already personal—in the sense that we, being persons, are committed to and invested in our intellectual projects—and remain mindful of those personal attachments both when creating our own and reviewing others' work?

Ben was genuinely surprised by my initial reactions to journal club, which I shared with him and the entire lab in the first draft of this chapter. While we continue to disagree on certain fundamentals, as I will elaborate in what follows, the time and care with which Ben crafted his response to my chapter drafts have left a lasting, positive impression that hopefully extends in my direction as well. As my (auto)ethnographic methods are intentionally iterative, I include lab members' responses to my first drafts as additional data, with their permission, for this revision. Ben wrote, for example:

> I train folks in my lab to be critical of ideas and not the person, and try to live that paradigm myself. I think that we did a good job of that during our meeting about the . . . article, but you clearly felt personally attacked, and because of this I think that many of the legitimate criticisms that we have as ecotoxicologists were either dismissed, ignored, or misunderstood. . . . Of course, the book chapter also evaluates us as individuals—our world view, our biases, our intentions—and that is hard to get used to (as I said before, we are used to criticizing the ideas and not the person, but of course ethnography as a field, and its goals and the rules of play, are quite different). There were many points in the article that made me bristle—some of the criticisms of me and of lab trainees were legitimate,

but many others made me realize that in some important ways we have apparently failed to understand each other (you and me and our group), and we (me and my group) in particular have failed to communicate what we, and our science, is all about.[61]

After reflecting on his comments, I realized that Ben's deliberate, well-meaning paradigm of scientific practice—"to be critical of ideas and not the person," echoed in Kelly's comment that "the way we go about these debates is extremely scientific, which is why it comes off as harsh sometimes"—explains why we have so much trouble bridging disciplinary divides. Having spent the better part of a decade as a feminist critic of science among natural scientists, I find one of the greatest impediments to cocreating a critical feminist toxicology arises from feminist STS versus toxicology's widely divergent views on objectivity. "The personal is political" is a long-running feminist slogan. "Science is political" may easily be considered the tagline of STS. Feminist STS, then, might be summarized as "the scientific is personal." People trained in the dominant sciences, however, are trained to separate ideas from the person, and hence to not take critiques personally, as Ben and Kelly explained to me. While I appreciate, and indeed welcome, Ben's efforts to model how to criticize a scientific paper without making the author of that paper feel personally attacked, I also believe, per my feminist STS training, that oneself and one's science are wholly inseparable. Ben himself, ironically, underscored this very inseparability of oneself and one's science when he explained: "I . . . try to live that paradigm myself."

Importantly, feminist STS does not consider the inseparability of self and science, and its subsequent lack of objectivity, to be a bad thing. As canvassed in this book's introduction, one of the main contributions of feminist STS is that such situated knowledge leads to *stronger* objectivity.[62] Researchers will necessarily create more complete and more accurate accounts of the (natural and cultural) world when they explicitly acknowledge and consider their social locations, inclusive of all the ways their social locations produce their partial visions, which, in turn, shape the research questions they ask, the research methods they embrace, the phenomena they observe, and the scientific conclusions they reach. Put another way, like feminism or eugenicism, evolutionary biology and toxicology too are *ideologies*, reflective and reproductive of historically specific cultural norms. I do not mean to relativize and level these different ideologies as if they are somehow ethically equivalent; it goes without saying that there are enormously important philosophical and material differences between feminism and eugenicism, for instance. Rather, I am attempting to articulate why such an open-minded and thoughtful group of EDC toxicologists still bristles at critical feminist reconsiderations of their field.

Objections on Objectivity: Part A

Let us now return to journal club objections numbers 1 and 2: (1) It is journalists, not scientists, who are to blame for offensive language and (2) These terms (e.g., "feminized") are effective because they are terms that nonscientists understand. Even during this uncomfortable (for me) exchange, I felt confident in my responses to these criticisms, insisting that scientists and journalists alike can do better. To defend one's use of such terms as "feminized" or "chemical castration" because these resonate better with the public (which public?) is not a good reason to employ insulting and inaccurate language, and moreover assumes the public cannot comprehend subtleties.[63] And, arguably, if such terms were truly resonant, then famed EDC scientist Louis Guillette's declaration to US congressmen in 1995—"Every man sitting in this room today is half the man his grandfather was. Are our children going to be half the men we are?"[64]—would not have needed to be followed up by epidemiologist Shanna Swan's book in 2021 (among others), chronicling how "our modern world threatens sperm counts and imperils the future of the human race."[65]

As discussed in chapter 3, prominent US politicians, scientists, and advocates have been fretting about supposed declines in white male virility since at least the nineteenth century, when more rural, manual forms of labor increasingly shifted to more urban, sitting-behind-a-desk jobs—civilization was seen as feminizing. Simultaneously, as immigrant and formerly enslaved populations made social, economic, and political gains in ways threatening to the status quo, elite white men perceived their physical and social power to be slipping.[66] Scott Frickel's history of the study of toxicant-induced mutagenesis likewise found that "genetic toxicology drew rhetorical sustenance from much older preservationist and conservationist discourses . . . . The preservationist impulse to honor and protect wilderness, in particular, is widely apparent in the rhetorical construction of human genes as scarce and fragile resources. . . . Geneticists repeatedly made references to the uniqueness of the human genetic material using language evocative of the . . . early-twentieth-century pastoral spiritualism of John Muir."[67] Frickel also quotes testimony by a genetic toxicologist (Gary Flamm) given before the US Congress in 1971, predating Guillette's by about two decades: "Many scientists, particularly geneticists, are deeply worried whether man's stewardship over his own genetic material might not be tragically inadequate."[68] Which is to say, these heteropatriarchal, eugenicist, and white supremacist concerns are not new, and if frightening powerful men into action by questioning their manhood were an effective political strategy, EDCs would have been banned a long time ago.

Objections on Objectivity: Part B

In that journal club moment and over the course of the months that followed, during which time I processed the meeting alone and with willing lab interlocutors, I found crafting an effective response to objection number 3 (reproductive fitness *is* impaired by chemical exposure and *is* a good measure of declining population health) to be considerably more challenging. Something clicked for me months later, during a conversation in which Olivia, Kelly, and I gathered to discuss the journal club experience together. Kelly, the slightly more senior toxicologist of the two, patiently explained to me, "We [the lab and the author] agree about being cognizant about choosing our words, but still disagree on what phenotypes we should be measuring. *The whole point of biology is reproduction, everything boils down to whether animals are able to reproduce and pass on genes. . . . Biology is messy, we do the best we can with proxies. Biologists try to come up with laws, like physics, but we have so many exceptions to the rules and we kind of just acknowledge that, but still talk about the rules as if that's the main event.*"[69]

Kelly beautifully articulated one of the core, and somewhat willful, misunderstandings between feminist analyses of biology (such as my own) and dominant paradigms of evolutionary biology and ecotoxicology (accepted by this lab).[70] Critical feminist STS in particular rejects the notion that the "whole point of biology is reproduction." Queer feminist STS does, however, concur that "biology is messy."[71] A crucial difference, then, is that traditionally trained toxicologists "try to come up with laws" whereas queer feminist STS approaches to biology (and toxicology) *revel* in the unruliness of nature and try to learn from all the ways that the supposed rules are repeatedly broken. Perhaps the queer biological rule is that there are no biological rules. And yet even this difference may instead be a commonality. Kelly continued,

> We [biologists and toxicologists] are trying to find patterns in biology but also *expecting exceptions* [*emphasis added*], trying to find exceptions to the rule . . . Some populations [of fish] may be more resilient [in response to the same external stressors] than others, so there *is* a reason to ask [*her emphasis*] the same questions of the same populations—*biology just breaks the rules all the time*, [*emphasis added*] which is why it's hard to extrapolate . . . *Personally I'm very interested in the exceptions to the rule in biology* [*emphasis added*].[72]

EDC toxicology too, then, expects and seeks explanations from the exceptions, just as queer feminist STS rejects the notion that certain biological laws are universal truths. The sticking point, or the source of my and this lab's failures to understand one another, appears to be EDC toxicology's unquestioned acceptance of certain biological rules in particular.

From a critical feminist STS perspective, tenets such as "the whole point of biology is reproduction" and "everything boils down to whether animals are able to reproduce and pass on genes" are *beliefs* about biology, not universal rules, that emerge from a specific, spatially and historically located knowledge system. This knowledge system has remained so dominant for so long, particularly in the US context, that it is widely accepted as unassailable truth rather than one of several knowledge systems. Given that toxicologists (among countless other scientific and lay thinkers alike) accept this belief as natural law, as they are trained to do, then it appears perfectly logical—while critical feminist STS interpretations appear totally nonsensical—that proxy measures of reproductive fitness (namely, female-to-male sex ratios in a given population, the presence of intersex individuals, or observations of same-sex sexual behaviors) are demonstrative of the harms caused by EDCs. These evolutionary theories and experimental logics are thus mutually constitutive and self-reinforcing. As Ben reiterated, in his care-full if critical response to my first drafts: "Many of the issues we [as a lab] have with the . . . article remain in the book chapters. . . . The critique about how reproductive fitness is measured and interpreted (language about proxies etc.) is *deeply flawed from a scientific perspective, and threatens the perceived legitimacy of this entire enterprise*, especially if you intend for ecotoxicologists and evolutionary biologists to be at least part of your audience—and this threat is not because evolutionary biologists are ignorant of eugenics and ableism."[73] In turn, I care-fully, respectfully note that Ben's response evidences his *personal* investments in the scientific fields of evolutionary biology and ecotoxicology, not unlike my *personal* investments in critical feminist STS. Understandably, Ben does not want either himself as an ecotoxicologist or ecotoxicology as a field to be labeled eugenicist. But if I, among other scholars, argue that tenets of evolutionary biology and toxicology stem from eugenicism,[74] and Ben *identifies* as an evolutionary biologist and ecotoxicologist, it follows then that my criticisms of science—the ideas—are difficult to disentangle from the scientist—the person (just as I struggle not to take critiques of my scholarship personally).

Again, feminist STS does not consider personal attachments to science to be bad. However, we must acknowledge them and admit how these formations of the scientific self shape our knowledge claims. Thus Ben's claim—that my "critique about how reproductive fitness is measured and interpreted . . . is *deeply flawed from a scientific perspective*," and that this deep flaw "threatens the *perceived legitimacy* of this entire enterprise"—implies that the scientific perspectives of evolutionary biology and ecotoxicology are somehow free of ideology and personal investments, unlike the "enterprise" of my critical feminist STS project, and therefore have greater legitimacy. Contesting the evolutionary biological (and hence ecotoxicological) rule that "everything boils down to whether animals are able to reproduce and pass on genes," as Kelly neatly summarized, necessitates a brief detour into (feminist) critiques of genetics, sociobiology, and behavioral ecology.

Gene Machines

Dominant science's long-standing belief in The Gene as the most explicatory and fundamental source of all life, inclusive of animal *behavior*, has been thoughtfully and extensively deconstructed by several critical STS scholars, as well as feminist and Marxist biologists.[75] I will return to STS critiques of animal behavior as phenotype in the next chapter. For now, I must take this slight detour into genetics, or rather critiques of genetics, because of the linkages between the primacy accorded to genes and the so-called biological rules embedded into dominant conceptions of reproductive fitness. The controversial field of sociobiology enjoyed its heyday from roughly the mid-1970s to the 1990s. However, elements of sociobiology's guiding assumptions (and celebrations of its racist promulgators) persist across biological fields today, including evolutionary psychology and behavioral ecology, for instance.[76]

Sociobiology and its descendants share "the assumption that, insofar as behaviors have a genetic component, then, given their prior subjection to the shaping force of natural selection, they are expected to maximize the individual organism's fitness."[77] What, readers may be wondering, could possibly be wrong or ideological about an organism (involuntarily) expressing its genetic-program-cum-behavior in ways that maximize its evolutionary fitness? Scholarship critical of this theory (not all of it feminist) highlights two central issues. The first is the belief that evolution unfolds through animals' involuntary and compulsory attempts to maximize their fitness. The second, related issue is the belief that genes program behavior. In sociobiology's (and, in a more veiled fashion, behavioral ecology's) capitalist-utilitarian twist on Darwinian evolution, organisms, including humans, are naturally competitive and self-serving by seeking to reproduce in order to pass on their genes, and as such, organisms possess little to no agency because organisms' behaviors, sexual or otherwise, are always fundamentally about maximizing fitness.

Sociologist Eileen Crist compellingly argues that sociobiology and behavioral ecology's view—that every animal's every behavior necessarily stems from a genetically driven compulsion to maximize fitness and reproduce—seriously limits scientific and societal understandings of animal behavior:

Sociobiology enthusiastically embraces the neo-Darwinian view of evolution, according to which the chief mechanism of evolutionary change is that of natural selection acting on the genetic basis of an organism's phenotype—the phenotype consisting of the set of traits that are manifest. Behaviors are considered phenotypes, which, insofar as they vary and have a genetic component, are subject to natural selection. . . . The game of maximizing inclusive fitness runs itself, for its logic is inexorable: the genes that maximize reproduction proliferate and take over because they get reproduced. This state of affairs is portrayed as unconditionally competitive, impersonal, and amoral.[78]

In turn, Scott Frickel's study of genetic toxicology found that "environmentalism provided an ideological discourse in which geneticists could effectively express their evolutionary concerns. . . . The goal of the new eugenics in improving the human genetic condition and the goal of the genetic toxicology movement in preventing further genetic damage were complementary."[79]

Max and I offered a parallel analysis in our article, unsettling dominant ideas about evolutionary fitness by drawing from the critical race and critical disability literatures in particular:

Concepts of biological fitness are inextricable from sociocultural conceptions, even if scientists try to separate them. In evolutionary biology, "fitness" is defined as the probability of producing offspring as a function of differences in reproductive output or survival. . . . However, "fitness" in broader society—including among natural scientists—carries connotations of health, belonging, desirability, and superiority and, moreover, conjures theories of eugenics. . . . Controversy notwithstanding, biologists often assume that adaptive (rather than neutral) evolution is the evolutionary process primarily shaping their study systems, such that certain organisms are understood as well fit for their environment while other individuals are assumed to be strongly selected against, because they are understood as "naturally" less fit. . . . Conversely, STS historians have illustrated how eugenicist ideology evinces a deep anxiety that those labelled unfit, abnormal, and deviant will survive, dragging down superior (if fragile) individuals with them; animal breeders refer to this supposedly natural process as "the drag of the race." . . . While

contemporary evolutionary biologists make concerted efforts to distinguish between evolutionary fitness and more colloquial uses of the term,
cultural understandings and scientific definitions remain difficult, if not
impossible, to disentangle.[80]

The anonymous biologists who peer-reviewed our paper strongly
pushed back against our claim that scientific and colloquial meanings
of terms are inextricable from one another. We wordsmithed enough to
keep this stance in the article's final version, but perhaps Crist's summation will be more persuasive for still-skeptical readers here. Her focus
is on the economic idioms of sociobiology and behavioral ecology, but
her analysis easily extends to the connotations of fitness in evolutionary
biology and toxicology: "Since economic language [or fitness language]
is already operative in the vernacular, sociobiology [or toxicology] *cannot deploy the language without partaking of the extant knowledge of its
meanings.*"[81]

When it comes to EDCs' apparent effects on the reproductive fitness
of frogs, evolutionary biology and ecotoxicology are based on the ideologically, historically, and culturally contingent premise that nonhuman
animal populations exist solely to reproduce. Within this worldview,
any sexual behavior that does not produce offspring is maladaptive and
hence indicative of species and population decline. Moreover, the animals that do produce offspring are understood to be passing on both
their genes *and their behaviors* to subsequent generations. It follows
then, that if evolutionary biology and ecotoxicology interpret same-sex
sexual behaviors as maladaptive genetic phenotypes that will be passed
on, then nonhuman animals' same-sex sexual behaviors are cause for
concern because same-sex animal behavior does not generate offspring
and therefore contributes to species and population decline. Queer feminist STS, among other belief systems, does not view more-than-human
animals as mere gene machines, existing only to procreate,[82] while current and historical evidence strongly indicates that same-sex sexual behavior has existed as long as animals have, thus refuting the idea that
same-sex sexual behavior is evolutionarily maladaptive.[83]

OK, my dwindling readership might still be wondering, but what
about the physiological harms that EDC exposures *do* generate? The
underwhelmed undergraduates from this chapter's opening vignette,

the anonymous biologist reviewers of the journal article under discussion, and Ben and his lab, all returned again and again to some version of this statement—"But the frogs—they *are* suffering"—upon reading queer feminist critiques of EDC science. For example, in Ben's powerful words, "I am deeply confused about why [your] writing repeatedly seems to minimize the actual violence caused by chemical exposures to individuals and populations, with repeated minimization in particular of the insidious reproductive impacts of EDCs. [Your] writing repeatedly seems to conflate the identification of biological/reproductive impacts with the human rights abuses of historically marginalized folks."[84]

While acceding that terms such as demasculinization warrant reconsideration, Olivia similarly, if more diplomatically, reflected:

"Demasculinization" could be a concern further down the line for population decline; proxies and predictions [of reproductive fitness] are the best we can do [as opposed to direct measures]—it's about survival of the species, reproduction is important. But extrapolating from frogs to humans . . . ? Humans do a lot more individual choosing, reproduction is not the main point of our lives, not being able to reproduce doesn't take away from who a person is, although we could imagine a *Handmaid's Tale* type of situation . . . That could be a negative effect. Removing reproductive endpoints would be inconceivable for ecotoxicologists. . . . We are not thinking about how individual frogs are suffering, but rather more about the survival of the species.[85]

This pushback from both Ben and Olivia prompts me to offer two crucial clarifications from my critical feminist STS perspective, the second of which I will expand on in the next chapter. Pointing out the tacit eugenicism of evolutionary biology and ecotoxicology's core tenets regarding reproductive fitness does not amount to a minimization of "the actual violence caused by chemical exposures." On the contrary, exposing toxicology's latent eugenicism (among other prejudicial historical legacies, addressed in this book's chapters 1–3) shows how the violence caused by chemical exposures is even deeper and wider than previously thought! My critical feminist analysis joins increasingly urgent demands to radically shift the focus of ecotoxicology. Critical feminist STS asks biologists to turn away from proxies and predictions regarding animals' reproductive success, with all their unintentional heteronormative and eugenicist underpinnings, as well as all their unavoidable chemical and biological uncertainties. Critical feminist STS asks biologists instead to move toward the undeniable and amply documented evidence of chemical corporations' irremediably destructive effects on all life on earth—destructive effects which don't have to be and frequently are not related to reproduction—precisely because chemical contamination *is* so thoroughly, extensively violent.[86] For those toxicologists who *do* wish to focus on reproductive health (and for good reason), I invite them to model their approach after the reproductive justice movement. Unlike reproductive choice, which narrowly focuses on abortion access, reproductive justice encompasses all the social and environmental factors that are prerequisites for raising healthy and happy families, with dignity.[87] Reproductive justice demands viability of ovaries, testes, and neonates, but also, and crucially, reproductive justice demands access to quality, affordable health care and housing as well as safe, steady employment with livable wages. And so rather than reduce reproductive fitness down to its physiological components (which are still only proxies), toxicologists might expand their conceptions of reproductive success out to its social and political preconditions (which are all-too-concrete realities).

Again, in an effort to be crystal clear, I reiterate that queer feminist STS critiques of EDC toxicology are not meant to minimize toxicants adverse effects, including on reproductive health. Especially, as Ben likewise pointed out, given the uneven distribution of EDCs: poor people and people of color are disproportionately more exposed to harmful toxicants, including *but not limited to* harms related to reproduction.[88] What my critique means to suggest is that toxicologists are getting lost in, or distracted and perhaps even seduced by, the wrong details. Throughout *Toxic Sexual Politics* I have argued that status quo ecotoxicology is not the institutional force that will stop polluting corporations, even with all the authoritative weight of dominant science's objectivity behind it. I offer this argument because my research revealed how ecotoxicology descends from a basic science of poisons that was designed by people who were politically aligned with poisoners. Toxicology measures (and, to some extent, makes) chemical and biological rules and how toxicants break them while omitting who came up with the rules and how the rules may be limiting research questions and skewing results, as well as omitting all the other social and political factors that make specific toxic substances so prevalent and unevenly distributed—social and political factors that are far more reliably documented and evidenced by overexposed communities' lived experiences than by proxies of wild animals' reproductive (or not) sexual antics.

I contend that ecotoxicology's built-in belief, that it is not individual frogs who matter but rather species or population health on the whole, is itself an enduring effect of dominant science, wherein Man is separate from and superior to Animal. Such thoroughly cultural and ideological hierarchies remain cloaked under the objective mantle of sociobiology and behavioral ecology's neo-Darwinian interpretations of evolutionary fitness. As Crist writes, "The impact of the economic idiom on the domain of experience and lived action involves the erasure of an animal lifeworld—an everyday world of experience of activity and leisure, pleasure and pain, abundance and hardship, exhilaration and fear, rivalry and affection. Tropes of the lifeworld are not denied in any direct sense, but simply swept aside, preempted by the absolute priority of reproductive success, its corollary of competition, and the economic idiom that delivers them."[89] Within dominant conceptions of evolutionary fitness, frogs (alongside all other nonhuman animals) don't have sex just for fun or for pleasure, or it doesn't matter whether they do, because frogs merely procreate to pass on their genes and mindlessly, maximally survive as a species. If and when scientific observers of animal behavior believe that frogs only exist and behave to maximize fitness and produce offspring, then these same observers will logically conclude that nonreproductive sexual acts, and nonreproducing individuals, signal population ill-health and species decline.

What is more, the belief that frogs and other animals lack the agency and subjectivity that humans possess, or what Crist refers to above as a "lifeworld," is a belief that stems from the same hegemonic worldview that rationalized the overproduction and uneven dissemination of toxic synthetic chemicals to begin with. In an effort to communicate more clearly than I have in the past, I repeat, I am not suggesting that EDCs do not harm frogs, among countless other organisms, nor do I wish to downplay the insidious effects of EDC exposure, including on reproductive health (which, by the way, has been amply documented in epidemiological studies of *human* exposures to EDCs, both at work and at home, obviating the need for frog-to-human extrapolation[90]). What I am suggesting is that focusing on proxies of reproductive fitness, which are themselves based on Eurocentric, human-centric, and (tacitly) eugenicist ideologies about natural law, biological rules, or physiological normalcy, will not bring about the political revolutions so necessary to reining in chemical corporate power and mitigating global crises of biodiversity.[91] Nor will this feminist critique of toxicology, I will be the first to admit. My concluding chapter sketches the contours of more radical shifts that both ecotoxicology and ecofeminism might embrace for environmental justice.

Journal Club Triage

I would be remiss in neglecting to note how generous the lab members were in their responses to the paper overall, and for inviting me to speak on it, including Ben. I also do not mean to single Ben out for his critical commentary and aggressive affect (in my experience). I certainly do not want to deter this exceptionally open-minded practitioner of dominant science from welcoming future feminist critics into his laboratory community. I hold Ben in high esteem and respect that he was freely expressing himself in a space where he feels perfectly entitled and entirely safe to do so: at a meeting of the students, postdocs, and staff whom he employs and mentors. His students, moreover, confided in me, with gratitude, that he tends to cultivate a lab discussion space where they feel comfortable expressing themselves even when in disagreement.[92] What is more, to my knowledge, Ben is not trained in critical race feminist and queer theory, nor is anyone else in the lab, and I cannot expect them to demonstrate a level of expertise in these fields on par with what I have earned any more than they might expect me to demonstrate their high levels of training in toxicology.

It was rather Ben's argumentative, somewhat defensive, and mildly aggressive—in a word: masculinist—affect that I hope to constructively criticize here. Notably, Ben was the only member who spoke argumentatively, and I wondered how the conversation might have proceeded differently if he were not present, or if he had more mindfully taken up less space. Would the junior (and more senior) lab members have felt freer to speak in support of the article's position? Was Ben worried that his students *would* be swayed by the article's queer feminist STS position had he not stepped in to strongly disagree? (He remarked to me later that he suspected his students were on the quieter side because they had not read the article, but he nevertheless was genuinely concerned that they would mistakenly accept my work's "serious errors that were thinly but attractively cloaked in the language of progressivism."[93]) While several of Ben's lab members openly expressed their difficulty with the article, in terms of feeling defensive while reading it, they remained willing to be reflexive and think differently about their own research and writing going forward.

I even sensed, at some moments, that lab members were trying to silently come to my defense, to communicate to me in some subtle way, without explicitly contradicting their PI, that they were sympathetic to the paper's position and did not fully agree with Ben's criticisms. Bruno vocally concurred, for example, with the article's claim that descriptions like "transgender frogs" should be rejected because they are *both* offensive *and* incorrect. Another more senior member, Upton, was so moved by the quote our article included from disability rights activist and scholar Sunaura Taylor that he reread it aloud to the group: "Researchers and advocates must 'criticize the systems that often lead to disability while simultaneously allowing disabled people to experience their bodies in empowered ways—or at least in ways that are not defined by oppression, discrimination and the able-bodied world.'"[94] If the meeting had been in person (as opposed to via Zoom), these other lab members and I might have exchanged quick, furtive glances, silent signals of support while Ben was excitedly protesting. And while the more junior lab members mostly echoed Ben's objections, perhaps, in part, because of the power dynamic therein, they did not also imitate his masculinist affect. The other lab members all spoke calmly and quietly, encouragingly, waiting their turns to speak and sharing their criticisms with care. I also noted that Kelly, the senior member who had expressed concern about being untrained for conversations about the racist and sexist history of dominant science, and Olivia, the student who had taken the seminar in feminist STS and presented her coursework back to an equally excitable and critical PI, remained conspicuously silent throughout most of the two-hour-plus discussion. I can only speculate as to why these two women refrained from joining the conversation as frequently as the others, but I suspect their relative silence stemmed from some amount of disagreement with Ben or me, some amount of discomfort in challenging Ben or me publicly, and some amount of concern that they are not well-versed enough in critical STS to effectively contribute. (The latter of which I would disagree but can empathize with.)[95]

Immediately after the two-hour, fifteen-minute session—we ran well over time—I emailed Ben to thank him and asked him to encourage lab members to contact me with any additional comments and critiques. To my surprise, Ben emailed me back immediately, cc'ing the entire lab, to publicly commend me on how well I received and responded to criticism, adding that I was a model of professional integrity and grace under fire. *Was it a hazing?* I asked myself. *Did I pass some sort of test?* Here again, a conversation that I experienced as uncomfortably aggressive and masculinist was experienced by Ben, and presumably the other members of his lab, as perfectly acceptable, even normative, for a scientific journal club. Ben subsequently confirmed that he is, in fact, care-fully committed to my more accurate understanding of ecotoxicology and evolutionary biology, and hence expressed so much frustration because he believes I (at times willfully) still misunderstand these scientific fields. Which leads me to wonder whether his mentees' relatively calmer responses, then, are indicative of their less extensive knowledge of the field, and hence greater openness to my (mis)understandings of it? Or whether their calmer responses reveal that they are less invested in ecotoxicology-as-we-know-it, and hence more open to outsider critique of it, because they are not yet well-established ecotoxicologists who have built their careers around this dominant form of the discipline? A bit of both, I imagine.

Two other possibilities also occurred to me. The first was that I was being commended for correctly playing my part in a heteropatriarchal play: the gentle, pliable female who accommodates everyone else's concerns and takes care of everyone else's feelings above her own.[96] I distinctly remember a moment during my master's program when one of my advisors, an older man and full professor, stopped himself midcritique of my thesis to remark "You take criticism *really* well" (his emphasis) and that this (feminized) receptivity would serve me greatly throughout graduate school. He meant the remark as a compliment, I am sure, but I cringed internally. The exchange felt icky, to use the technical term, and part of me felt similarly after receiving Ben's praise, like being patted on top of the head for being a good girl. Would Ben have been less complimentary, less impressed, if I had instead mirrored his argumentative affect? This recollection and questioning led me to the second possibility: that I had in fact left a genuinely positive and meaningfully different impression because I had indeed modeled an alternative way to conduct journal club. Perhaps my intentional decision to refuse a debate-like, binary structure—even within one—and to welcome critique and listen actively, to gently push back without digging in, cultivated a critical feminist rhizome that will continue to spread. Encouragingly, Olivia and Kelly did later share with me how much they enjoyed my presence in lab meetings over those twenty weeks and regretted that once I left, feminist STS never came up again in lab until that journal club gathering approximately one year later.[97] Ben later pressed me to consider a third possibility: that I felt threatened or embarrassed by my lack of scientific knowledge, and was thus defensive because I did not understand his valid criticisms.[98] I will return to my apparent misunderstandings of the science at the close of this chapter.

Metaphors and Materials

Having run out of time, Olivia did not make it to the "mind-blowing" part of her presentation described earlier, which she alluded to with great excitement when she began: "Metaphors have material consequences!" The point of feminist STS critique of dominant scientific language is not to police language, but rather to illuminate, and interrupt, the direct connections between harmful language and harmful acts. As Toni Morrison stated in her 1993 Nobel Prize acceptance speech, "Oppressive language does more than represent violence; it is violence; does more than represent the limits of knowledge; it limits knowledge."[99] As I finalize this chapter, legislators in Texas and Alabama have criminalized gender-affirming care for trans children.[100] Legislators in Florida have banned public school districts from teaching about sexual orientation, in a law dubbed the "Don't Say Gay" bill by its critics.[101] Similar bills are popping up in left-leaning states such as Rhode Island (where I myself was a queer school child), to say nothing of the proliferation of state-level bans on critical race theory or the US Supreme Court's regressive decision to overturn *Roe v. Wade*, deposing pregnant people's rights of bodily autonomy in a major blow to reproductive freedom.[102] I am not blaming EDC toxicologists for such reactionary policies. Nor does my analysis mean to "conflate the identification of biological/reproductive impacts with the human rights abuses of historically marginalized folks," as Ben remarked.[103] Rather, I am drawing from feminist STS and critical race theory more broadly to emphasize how the scientific perpetuation of heterosexist ideology, hiding in plain sight as natural biology and normal behavior, does nothing to uproot nor burn down these "deeply penetrating lies," to borrow Ben's turn of phrase.

Perhaps this PI, had we more time to discuss metaphors' material consequences, would ultimately agree. During a previous conversation on structural racism in higher education, for instance, Ben reflected again on intentionality (just as he had during Olivia's lesson on so-called invasive species, described earlier):

> What role, if any, does intentionality play here? Clearly there are forms of intentional violence, but you tend to think of pollution as unintentional. *Using language associated with violence implies intent—part of me wants to push back, but another part of me acknowledges being part of a system that benefits from this—their disadvantage is indirectly your advantage—then that is a form of violence* [emphasis added]. I'm thinking about this in terms of [Black Lives Matter] in the last year. It's no longer good enough to say, "*I'm* not shooting Black people; *I'm* not *not* hiring people because they're Black." That's not good enough because we all benefit from this system [his emphasis].[104]

Environmental justice scholars and activists can certainly cite many examples of *intentional* pollution, another point which Ben would not disagree with, but I highlight his reflection here to show the work that committed scientists are doing, many of whom became motivated by the most recent social movements for Black lives and environmental justice. These scientists' reflections, alongside my mixed experiences as the lab's temporary, resident critical feminist STS scholar, also reveal what work remains to be done. The deep, structural demands of the global movement for Black lives, for instance, are in danger of being reduced to institutionalized forms of DEI that start and stop at hiring more Black people. Representation is undeniably important, but merely hiring more Black professionals or enrolling more Black students, to extend this same example, without simultaneously pursuing longer-term, institutional and cultural changes that would more firmly support a true diversity of *ideas*, as well as people, returning to Bruno's words quoted at the beginning of this chapter, comes nowhere near close enough to burning it down and building something better. As Black feminist STS scholar Ruha Benjamin cautions, "Changing individual sentiment from animus to tolerance, or even affection, will not transform the status quo so long as the underlying design of our socio-technical world is left in place."[105]

Overall, this lab's warm welcome, productively imperfect conversations, and possibly continued efforts to integrate critical theory into their regular scientific work is encouraging for a feminist STS scholar such as myself, and hopefully not too discouraging for ecotoxicologists such as these. Centuries of indoctrination into the dominant scientific worldview will not be un-learned in a handful of seminar discussions or lab meetings. Welcoming a critical feminist STS presence, whether materially or theoretically, in a traditional scientific laboratory creates openings and catalyzes conversations nevertheless. As Ben wrote in his response to my draft chapter, "I think that we can do two things at once: Identify and raise alarm over the violence caused by environmental pollution, and at the same time care for those folks that are affected by those exposures. In fact, it is critically important that we do both."[106]

Ben, I could not agree more.

Seeking Sea Change

I draw on the concept of a sea change, meaning a material and irreversible transformation (and drawn from Shakespeare's *The Tempest*[107]) with caution, as it has apparently been reduced to a corporate buzzword, much like sustainability or DEI.[108] I cautiously reclaim sea change here for it is a particularly apt metaphor in the context of marine-focused toxicology. The ethnographic observations detailed in this chapter, following my analyses in chapters 1 through 3, evidence a normalization, and hence tacit acceptance, of the masculinism and eugenicism permeating dominant toxicology (in "intra-action," to borrow feminist physicist

Karen Barad's term), with the broader society from which toxicology emerges[109], such that even practitioners committed to environmental justice unwittingly reentrench ableism, queer- and transphobia, patriarchy, and white supremacy in their analyses and praxes—and moreover reject the suggestion that their work may be doing so. I am sympathetic to scientists' defensiveness and indignance—"Why is the pressure on *us* to be so careful with our language?"—given industry's concerted and continuous attacks on environmental and climate scientists. I draw again from Ben's care-full critiques of my first draft of this chapter: "[Your] curt treatment of [Guillette's] statements [that US Congressmen are half the men their grandfathers were] . . . and whether his statements 'worked' is missing an opportunity to make a better case, lest readers respond simply by thinking . . . 'of course the testimony of one scientist is no match for the hegemonic power of big chem and political corruption.'"[110] Making a better case, in my view, would involve less dependence on and prioritization of the unavoidably uncertain findings of ecotoxicology—remember, toxicology is both a science and an art, and biology breaks rules all the time—turning instead to a greater reliance on and valuing of the lived experiences of overexposed communities (but more on this radical pivot in my concluding chapter).

Notably, Ben's tenacity extends in caring ways too. I admired his righteous indignation, for example, when an oil industry representative disrupted one of his student's academic conference presentations on the adverse effects of oil exposure on marine life:

> [Industry-consulting scientists] are paid to go to [scholarly association] meetings by BP [British Petroleum, an oil corporation responsible for numerous exposure disasters] and harass your grad students and try to heckle them if they give a presentation and try to embarrass them in front of the [scientific] poster—like, this is next-level, this is not—this is no longer respectful. This is, clearly you have an agenda. And I'm not going to engage with that, you know, I'm not going to engage in discussion with you [as an oil industry consultant]. You're heckling my students. I'm going to tell you to fuck off. And if you ask me a ridiculous question in front of an audience, I might not say "fuck off" but I'm going to communicate that, right? And I'm going to tell everyone who you are, and I'm going to embarrass the shit out of you. You know, I think that that's—just that

dishonesty and those kinds of agendas, I just—like I have a hard time just ignoring that then, so it gets under my skin as something that's wrong.[111]

While demonstrating Ben's care for his students, this anecdote also underscores the dependencies created by the hierarchical academic system: without tenure, emerging scholars remain precariously dependent on the benevolence of their tenured mentors—and I think it's fair to say Ben is an unusually kind and supportive R1 PI—to defend them against such nefarious attempts to discredit their scientific results.[112] This anecdote also illustrates that scientists *are* careful with their language when reasons for doing so matter enough to them.

During one of the first lab meetings I attended, to offer another example, I observed with admiration how lab members spent considerable time thoughtfully reworking a graphic to display on their website.[113] Kyle, a senior member, had worked up a variation of the "science is real" posters, buttons, bumper stickers, and lawn signs that became popular (in certain quarters) during the Trump administration. He sought his lab mates' and Ben's approval of the final design—clearly the sentiment was not up for debate—before uploading the image to the lab's website. Kyle's version read "Science is progress," so naturally I asked why he had chosen "progress" instead of the more typical "real." This little question from the critical feminist STS peanut gallery prompted an extended, care-full discussion, during which I remained mostly silent, about the connotations of such terms and which words might better convey the meaning they hoped this image would project. Lab members reflected, for example, that "progress" may not be the best term because it implies that other fields or disciplines are somehow backward. As Upton observed, "Science is not the only way of understanding the world"—and this discussion occurred well before my mini-presentation on the field of critical feminist STS. They eventually dropped "progress" and put two suggested replacements to a vote, resulting in a tie between "important" and "valuable." (I had thoughts on these two options as well, but I held my tongue.) Ben then directed Kyle, as designer of the graphic, to choose his preference between the two alternates, marking the end of the approximately twenty-minute discussion.

I share this vignette to underscore that practitioners of dominant science are perfectly capable and willing to "be so careful with [their] language" when the validity and status of Science seems to be on the line. "Real" was the established term, but someone thought "progress" might work better, and all it took was one gentle inquiry to open up a productive conversation about the connotations and implications of word choices. What makes such care-full intellectuals resistant to reconsidering established terms in the EDC literature like feminizing and demasculinizing? Or resistant to the suggestion that evolutionary theories regarding the centrality of procreation and a purely genetic basis for animal behavior are human constructions from the dominant culture? In this apparently antiscience or posttruth historical moment, are environmental health advocates so fearful, and exhausted, that any questioning of the status quo is perceived as illegitimate and dangerously unscientific?

Through my partial vision as a critical feminist STS scholar, I observed multiple moments of lab work as care work, or fuzzy family feelings. Sharing my research on the militarist and masculinist history of US toxicology, and on the tacit eugenicism of contemporary ecotoxicology, sparked uncomfortable yet generative conversations, compelling this group of renowned toxicology researchers to think more deeply and expansively about what diversity, equity, inclusion, and justice truly means, and might look and feel like, within educational institutions and scientific spaces. I also found it telling that even a lab self-selected into my ethnographic study, being already committed to environmental and racial justice, is not immune to the hegemonic influences of patriarchal hierarchy and masculinist affect, as evidenced by the intralab dynamics under an exceedingly benevolent PI who nevertheless functions as head of household.

The fact that Ben does mentor his students so well, even paternally, may make it *more* difficult for them to bite the hand that feeds, as it were. It is generally easier to rebel against a lousy authority figure than an excellent one. Nevertheless, in my observations, any and all uncomfortable conversations, whether prompted by my mere presence, my verbal provocations, or my written scholarship, spurred acts of care. My presentation on the limits of representation, or the need for a diversity of scholarship as well as scholars, inspired lab members to voice their frustrations with their institution's disingenuous and surface-level attempts at cultivating DEI, including the lack of structured education about dominant science's prejudicial histories and ongoing inequities.[114] Ben's mildly aggressive, argumentative manner of speaking, during two different lab discussions explicitly about critical feminist STS, elicited caring words, gestures, and glances from senior to junior members and back, while the hierarchical and gendered norms we all performed may have suppressed more overt resistance. At times Ben's paternal affect served as a caring act, as when he protected his students from oil industry consultants' heckling at professional conferences. What is more, Ben generously opened his lab to a feminist STS critic such as myself, creating space and time for what the lab labeled as nonscience conversations, modeling to his students that social justice and scientific inquiry need not be separate endeavors.

Perhaps Tironi's concept of a hypo-intervention is the best I can make of my short stint as a critical feminist interlocuter within this reflexive yet traditional toxicology lab.[115] The hierarchical structure of a US R1 university scientific laboratory provided several openings for care between and across lab members—sometimes in response to hierarchy under their PIs, sometimes while navigating the hierarchies of the larger institution and the political economy of pollution science more broadly. Offering and receiving care within a particular set of restraints not only supports critical thinkers in their efforts to survive a stratified system, but also exposes the failures of said system, unsettling established terms, practices, and theories in generative if unfinished ways.

There is another hierarchy that is more difficult to dismantle, however. Here I return to Ben's repeated insistence that I simply do not understand evolutionary biology and ecotoxicology and, moreover, that it is my feelings getting in the way of my understanding. As Carol Cohn found in her ethnographic research with nuclear defense intellectuals, when she intentionally avoided using their highly specialized terminology, they dismissed her as unknowledgeable. When she then tried to speak to defense intellectuals using their language, she found she could no longer articulate her own feminist and antinuclear position: "The better I got at engaging in this discourse, the more impossible it became for me to express my own ideas, my own values. I could adopt the language and gain a wealth of new concepts and reasoning strategies—but at the same time as the language gave me access to things I had been unable to speak about before, it radically excluded others. I could not use the language to express my concerns because it was physically impossible. This language does not allow certain questions to be asked or certain values to be expressed."[116]

It may be that Ben and I continue to misunderstand each other, no matter how much we each try to clarify and reclarify, because the language of evolutionary biology and ecotoxicology does not allow certain feminist questions to be asked or certain feminist values to be expressed. I cannot say what I want to say in the language of evolutionary biology and ecotoxicology (and maybe Ben cannot say what he wants to say in the language of critical feminist STS).[117] But arguably this observation amounts to a cop-out. Max and I wrote two articles together, after all, and I continue to collaborate with other biological scientists, such as Ambika Kamath, who are no less intelligent and well-meaning than Ben. And of course I am not the only critical feminist STS scholar who collaborates with natural scientists. We humans do share a language, even if our intellectual and lived experiences are widely divergent, and we also share a planet. Therefore we must continue to try, however uncomfortable such efforts might make us, to dismantle the walls and build bridges instead between practices of science and social studies of science.

The next chapter traces another promising crack in the hegemonic structure, analyzing how these biological scientists grapple with the pollution-related harm that has been inflicted on the species and ecologies they care for and hence research—including the chemical exposures these scientists themselves produce in their efforts to better understand and communicate more precisely how damaging toxicants are to the world.

5

Fishy Exceptionalism

The feminist care tradition in animal ethics urges us to attend to other animals in all of their difference, including differences in power within systems of human dominance in which other animals are seen and used as resources or tools. So another way that the [feminist] care tradition differs from traditional [ethical] approaches is through its analysis of the economic, political, racial, gendered, and cultural underpinnings of systems of animal exploitation, commodification, and cruelty.
—Lori Gruen[1]

An Unfeeling for the Animal

As part of my ethnographic research for this project, I enrolled in a graduate-level toxicology course. One of my most vivid memories from that semester, which I recall with a strange mixture of bemusement and disappointment, occurred not during official coursework or lecturing but rather during a brief flicker of my attention. Because the course met midday, students often brought their lunches and ate at their desks during class. An equally common practice of these industrious students was to keep their laptops open when the instructor was speaking, maintaining the appearance of typing notes while in actuality working on other assignments (or doing something unrelated to schoolwork altogether). This particular afternoon, I happened to glance over at the open laptop of the toxicology PhD student sitting next to me, who was happily crunching away at her lunch while finishing up a presentation that was clearly for another course, or perhaps for a professional conference. I became distracted by her screen because she was rapidly browsing through internet image search results of experimental mice in an assortment of situations I can only describe as sadist. Some mice appeared alive, with bits of plastic and metal laboratory equipment puncturing different orifices, veins, and skins of their bodies, presumably to administer toxicants. Some were pictured at various stages of vivisection and dissection, having either died from the administered toxicant, or, more likely, having been "sacrificed" by the scientist to determine the effects of the substance under study.[2]

My eyes were unhappily glued to her computer screen, as when one struggles to turn from an accident scene on the highway. I felt nauseated and saddened by what I saw as imprisoned, tortured, and mutilated animals—poked and prodded and poisoned in cold, clinical cages for the duration of their unlucky lives, only to have their hides splayed and internal organs removed and systematically sliced into sections.[3] The PhD student worked rapidly, expertly, selecting and placing these gory scenes of everyday toxicological torture into her presentation slides, seemingly so unperturbed by the visual content that she could simultaneously enjoy her delicious lunch.

There was nothing atypical about this PhD student in general, and I encountered this same casual attitude toward toxicology's use of experimental rodents consistently throughout this project. As science and technology studies (STS) scholar Tora Holmberg notes in her article "A Feeling for the Animal," the title of which I borrow for this section, "[Laboratory] animals are standardized through, for example, breeding, keeping, and experimental design . . . *the experimentalists too become standardized* . . . through [Institutional Animal Care and Use Committees] and curricula."[4] The historically contingent practice of using mice and rats,[5] among other "model organisms,"[6] for biomedical and scientific research has become so normalized that people who *protest* such practices are regarded warily, if not angrily dismissed, by scientists thus standardized.[7] While studying alcohol addiction researchers and their experiments on mice, for instance, STS researcher Nicole Nelson found herself pretending she was *not* a vegetarian, so as to build trust with her interlocuters, who remained outraged by what they perceived as animal rights activists' irrational, emotional, and thoroughly antiscientific stance against the use of animals for research.[8] (She conspicuously ordered a burger for lunch, at one point, so that the scientists she was observing would not suspect her to be an undercover animal rights extremist.)

Animal rights advocates are of course not alone in their concerns over the (a)morality of scientific and militaristic experimentation on more-than-human animals, including chimpanzees, rabbits, cats, dogs, dolphins, and other creatures humans tend to view particularly fondly or as more charismatic.[9] (As a recent profile of a primate-researcher-turned-PETA-activist in the *Guardian* put it, "Few people care what researchers do to insects or other invertebrates."[10]) Several proposals have been submitted by scientists themselves for the phasing-out, if not eventual end, of the practice of killing more-than-human animals for research purposes.[11] Without digressing into an important but unwieldy discussion of animal ethics vis-à-vis dominant science's taxonomies, in what follows I critically analyze my ecotoxicologist interlocuters' deliberate choices to study, and hence conduct experiments on, fishes rather than furry beasts.[12] While exhibiting touching (pun intended) moments of tenderness and care for the animals they affectionately if possessively called "their" fish, these scientists nevertheless subjected these fish to toxic exposures, viral exposures, water temperature and salinity stressors, and certain death. Here, I attempt to explicate yet another fractal of contradictions inherent to (eco)toxicology: the systematic harm of animals for the intertwined goals of environmental and human health. Ultimately, I suggest that these deeply caring toxicologists intentionally turn to fish in order to avoid—in vain—the messy, uncomfortable, and undeniably human politics of pollution.[13]

As mentioned in my introduction to this book, I did not expect to end chapter 5, and this monograph, with a call for laboratory animal liberation. However, after working through and against the binary hierarchies reproduced by dominant science—Man over Animal, Woman, Other; Culture over Nature, Mind over Body—I found no other place to land.[14] Only within the worldview of dominant, US toxicology does it make sense that an environmental-health-leaning toxicologist would "develop a model for juvenile warfare exposure," as I discuss in chapter 1; or assume that a toxic substance that kills insects, rodents, or fungi will not also be harmful to so-called nontarget organisms and ecosystems, as I critique in chapter 2; or systematically, irrevocably pollute the environment for the sake of feeding the world, as analyzed in chapter 3; or steal fish from the wild, expose them to toxicants, and then kill them, all in the name of environmental justice, as I shall examine in this chapter.

Overall, I do *not* suggest that the toxicological knowledge that has been amassed thus far is worthless. Quite the contrary, as nearly everything known about toxicants has come at the expense of an othered body.[15]

I do, however, assert that toxicological exposure experiments on animals should be swiftly phased out. I take this stance not only because experimenting on animals is part of the same hegemonic worldview that environmental justice movements seek liberation from,[16] but also because status quo toxicology has always been deeply uncertain and has not sufficiently protected human and environmental health from "some unforeseen toxic catastrophe," as Harold C. Hodge, one of toxicology's founding fathers, assured us it would half a century ago.[17] *Toxicology cannot tell us what we need to know about toxicants* both because its quantitative methods are inherently flawed, and because it deliberately separates the toxicant from its sociopolitical preconditions, or the poison from the poisoner.

"You Can't Use Tongs on Mice"

The ecotoxicologists I observed for twenty weeks conducted their exposure experiments on different species of fish, as opposed to human cell lines or other officially recognized model organisms. (The vast majority of toxicology experiments are performed on rodents, which is in itself no accident.[18]) For many lab members, the choice to intentionally expose this particular type of organism to toxic harm was not one taken lightly, nor was it arbitrary. Several admitted to me during our one-on-one interviews that they would, or have had, a much harder time experimenting on mice or other mammals, particularly when it came time to sacrifice—their term, meaning *kill*—the animal, either for the purposes of the experiment itself or once the experiment was completed.[19] Upton recalled in horror a previous job he had held at another laboratory, where he was assigned the unlucky task of sacrificing thousands of mice, and quickly: "I had to 'sac'—sacrifice—something like 1,800 mice within three days, and that took a *toll* [*emphasized heavily*] on me, killing that many animals. I was killing, you know, zebrafish left and right, and they're one thing, but then moving up the taxonomy of complex organisms, something more furry like this; it really took a toll on me, and I was like, I don't want to do that anymore, and I got a job as a lab tech in a lab that worked on cancer, childhood leukemias."[20]

Silently noting that killing that many mice was so traumatizing to this PhD candidate that researching childhood leukemia felt like a relief in comparison, I cautiously asked him to reflect more on the difference between sacrificing zebrafish versus mice, for science's sake. Haltingly, he explained:

> Yeah, this is something that I thought, I thought about before, and a lot of it is the difference between the zebrafish and a mouse. Well, fish—they can feel pain. And as far as emotions, I don't know if they have emotions, but I—yeah, I think, I think I know [fish] can feel pain and I know they can, they can—probably have a sense of suffering that's somewhat similar to ours, so they do have somewhat of a memory. It was . . . [*pauses thoughtfully*] The difference between killing all those mice and killing maybe an equal number of fish was the shortened period of time I had to do it in. We had to have all those mice sac'd within like three working days, and they require handling, right? So *fish don't require handling*, you just transfer them with a net to another tank or you transfer tanks to tanks, and it's not that—*it's very impersonal*. Whereas with the rodents, mice and rats, it's—you have to pick them up, right? And so you're handling a lot of animals, and this is, I think, the kind of interface that—kind of—I don't know, *that kind of closeness that you have with the animal*. Just as a practical measure, just because of the way you have to handle—you can't, like, use tongs on mice, or—You have to actually pick them up by their scruff and put them in the gas—you know, the CO_2 chamber, you know, one by one . . . [*trails off*] And so it's just, *it really kind of hits home. You don't—you're just much closer to the animal that way*. I don't think I'm cut out to dispatch animals on a mass scale like that. I certainly have, you know, I—probably when I die and I go, you know, to the pearly gates it seems like, "Well, let's look at how many animals you've sacrificed, let's add it all up," right? [*laughs*] To me a lot of fish I've killed throughout my—mostly for research, pretty much all for research purposes. That's not to justify it, but it's more like—it's not, it wasn't—*there's at least a means to an end, not just for sport*. I think if done right CO_2 is a humane way to euthanize a mouse as long as you nail—get the dosing correct,

right? And they just like, kind of lose consciousness. Or if—you can over-dose them and they start gasping for air and that's a form of suffering and distress, and you're just basically suffocating them while they're still awake. Not cool. I think if done correctly it's like going to sleep. I think. Not everyone—everyone has different—thinks differently about that, but that's my impression.[21]

"That kind of closeness that you have with the animal" (emphasis added) that Upton repeatedly expressed in the interview excerpt above, is one that troubles many an animal researcher, despite decades-old offi-cial protocol calling for the "three Rs": "refinement of treatment, replace-ment with in silica or in vitro or other alternatives where possible, and reduction of numbers of animals used."[22] Holmberg similarly found, in her ethnographic research on animal handling training courses for sci-entists, that "a gentle and humane death for the [experimental] animals also includes the experimentalists' feelings."[23] And as psychologist John Gluck argues in his book *Voracious Science and Vulnerable Animals*, "That observation—*they're just like us*—is . . . the paradox at the heart of the debate about primates in research. . . . when researchers want to extrapolate their animal results to humans, they emphasize the simi-larities between animals and humans. . . . But when they want to justify research that causes pain, fear, or death—protocols that would never be approved for humans—they emphasize the differences. In other words, we can learn from them because they're just like us; we can experiment on them because they're not like us."[24] Rather than grapple with this unsettling paradox head-on, or refuse it by declining to conduct animal experimentation in general (more on the impossibilities of such refusals below), several of the toxicologists in this particular lab opted to study fish and marine invertebrates instead of mammals—and definitely not primates—because working with these other species is "very imper-sonal."[25] *"Fish don't require handling*, you just transfer them with a net to another tank or you transfer tanks to tanks . . . , *it's very impersonal*," but "you can't use tongs on mice, you have to actually pick them up by their scruff and put them in the gas [chamber]."

Later, I learned about research demonstrating that fish do indeed feel and express pain, as Upton himself noted, however our human sensi-bilities are so different from those of fish that we don't know how to see or otherwise comprehend their fishy expressions of pain.[26] As Upton observed, handling fish feels "very impersonal" as compared to mice. Ethologist Jonathan Balcombe reports that humans cannot hear fishes' pain vocalizations because such sounds may only be heard underwater (presumably diving so as to be underwater with fish still doesn't allow us humans to hear their pain). As Balcombe writes in his book *What a Fish Knows*, "We hear no screams and see no tears when their mouths are impaled and their bodies pulled from the water. Their unblinking eyes— constantly bathed in water and thus in no need of lids—amplify the illusion that they feel nothing."[27] Just as early toxicologists interpreted no observable toxic effect as harmless (see chapter 2), no observable pain response is all too easily interpreted as painless.

"Charismatic Little Species"

The impersonality of fish is a matter of degree, and perspective, however, and these fish-focused toxicologists also opted to study sea-dwellers precisely because certain fishes *are* more charismatic, to use their word, and in some ways similar to humans.[28] Kyle, for instance, taught me that 80 percent of human and fish genes are orthologous, meaning genes of different species that evolved from a common ancestral gene. Humans and fish also share vulnerability, differently and similarly, from exposures to the same toxic substances and environmental disturbances, including everything from crude oil explosions and pharmaceutical residues in the water to global warming and drought. Writing primarily about animal experimentation for human health, as opposed to ecological health, feminist STS scholar Charis Thompson explains in her book *Good Science* that "the logic of animal experimentation in bioethics is sequential, and the epistemology and the ethics reinforce each other. Two things follow from this. First, the substitution of animals for humans makes a fundamental if implicit ethical *distinction* between humans and other animals. Second, the sequential logic makes a fundamental if implicit *connection* between animals and humans: animals must continue to be good (enough) models for humans in whatever system is being investigated, or the sequential epistemological purpose would not be served."[29] While my toxicologist interlocutors were not necessarily *substituting* more-than-human animals for humans, the shared vulnerabilities and other affinities between fishes and humans remain important. For some lab members the extrapolation from animal or ecological health to human health is built-in, for others, their experiments are purely for more-than-human animal and ecological health—more on this tenuous distinction to come.

Kyle, for example, told me how excited he was as a graduate student, and now a postdoc, to transition from fruit flies to mice to fish. He felt particularly excited about the species of fish he was currently working on precisely because of this fish's importance to human communities and economies.

> I switched from drosophila [fruit flies] to fish because I was rotating in a lab that I was really interested in that did drosophila work. And then I rotated in another lab and realized that I kind of liked that system better—*It's a little more exciting to work with vertebrates*, and some of the questions that I was interested in one can really only ask with that type of system . . . [and] I was really excited to work in a system where *other people cared about the fish*! Mice, the species I worked with in grad school, were pretty nice and only one other group [had] fish in that lab at all. So *the idea that my science was contributing to questions that a larger community cared about was really exciting.*[30]

I asked Kyle to elaborate further on why he felt more excited to study fish than fruit flies or mice. He expressed both his commitments to informing environmental policy and having an affinity with the animal:

> KYLE: I kind of viewed my efforts in grad school as really just learning a bunch of methods and learning how to think critically. And as I was coming out the other side, my [mentor] had moved from [university A] to [university B], so I was working remote the last year, and kind of had a lot of time to think about what I wanted to use this skill set for. And I was thinking that *the most obvious way that my skill set could be useful is in informing [fisheries] management and policy decisions.* So, if we can find out something interesting about these fish populations, then maybe that'll affect some type of legislation that influences how humans interact with that population.

MELINA: I love what you shared about finding fish more interesting than fruit flies. So can you tell me—let's talk a little bit more about that. I mean, I know you said certain [scientific] questions you can only ask with vertebrates, but what was it about studying fish and working with fish that captivates you, do you think?

KYLE: Yeah, *it was just a really charismatic system.* So the fish species that I worked with, they—well, I can give you the whole spiel that I normally give in the intro to a talk . . ."[31]

Kyle then proceeded to tell me an evolutionary history of this "really charismatic system" ("system" as in species of fish). In brief, a single population diverged thousands of years ago because of a geographic barrier, eventually producing spatially separate populations that are now phenotypically quite different because of their respective populations' adaptations to differing environmental factors, and yet still share the same genetic material with their ancestral population. Kyle finished, "I just think that story is so much cooler than any [fictional] story you can tell."[32]

His fascination with certain fishes' charisma, and his commitments to fishing communities and sustainable management policies, do not preclude hierarchical relations however. He continued to express his enthusiasm for recent technological advances in genome editing, such as CRISPR, that allow him to manipulate this fish species in the lab in order to better understand which genes are behind which phenotypes.[33]

KYLE: One of the other things that had me really excited about joining this [fish] lab over a fruit fly lab is gene editing experiments are kind of old hat [with fruit flies]. . . . They had a lot of really nice, you know, the tools to be able to do that type of stuff where *you can grow legs where they're not intended to be* and a whole bunch of different stuff, but in nonmodel systems, we're just beginning to use, like, CRISPR-Cas9 tools *to be able to disrupt function.* So I was really keen on trying to use CRISPR to like swap those genetic changes between species and then look at the offspring and see if I could see any differences in . . . phenotype.

MELINA: I want to ask—this is just something that comes up for me and I think it betrays the differences in our training, but to me it always seems like a contradiction—and I'd love to hear your thoughts on this: On the one hand, clearly you are like, really fascinated by and even sort of impressed by these fish, you know, the way that they change [phenotypically] and, you know, it is really neat. But then, on the other hand, you're manipulating them in a lab environment, almost like they're objects, right? So I wonder how, how that—I don't know. Is that a contradiction for you as well? Or is that just part of the work of... [*trails off*]? I'm just curious, what do you think?

Kyle's response was telling, revealing again Gluck's voracious science and vulnerable animals paradox: we can learn from them because they're like us, we can experiment on them because they're not like us. In response to my questions, this senior lab member reflected that fish are genetically similar and culturally important enough to humans to feel an affinity with, and learn something from, yet not so close as to prohibit laboratory manipulation or extraction from their wild habitats.

> So whenever we were out, collecting fish, we would use these really gi-ant seine nets which are like these twelve-foot long things that you have two people just drag across the ground and then pull it up on shore and you have hundreds of fish there. . . . We always made an effort to make sure that the net was all clear of [unwanted] fish, and that any stragglers were thrown back into the water, *lest we upset the [fish] gods.* So I think . . . there is this appreciation for the species and what they could teach us. . . . And *if these charismatic little species could teach us something that was new or provide some insight . . . as long as we are following protocols to make sure that no fish are unnecessarily suffering, then it would be worth it. Even if you're creating, like, these Frankenstein monsters in the lab* where you're trying to just manipulate genes that might influence their . . . development, maybe influences a whole bunch of other different things—*It does make you feel like kind of a, a cruel person to potentially be creating these deformities that are affecting fish in a negative way, but at the same time I would be so excited if one of my genetic constructs*—what, like I swapped those things between species, and then one of their offspring had really big [phenotype A] or really tiny [phenotype B] or . . . Um, but yeah *it is a strange balance where we have a lot of respect for this species and what they can teach us, but that*

comes at the cost of needing a system where we can do this manipulation.
Which is why I found fish a good place to start because it's a vertebrate still
so it shares—like, 80 percent of its genes are orthologous to our own, but it
is a step away from mice, or anything furry and cuddly.[34]

His joke about "upsetting the [fish] gods" suggested to me that I was
not the first colleague to raise questions about how experiments for the
sake of scientific progress can cause harm to the animals used as re-
source or substrate—"it does make you feel like kind of a cruel person
to potentially be creating these deformities" (never mind removing fish
from their natural habitats, though this latter concern did not come up
in this discussion).

Moral arguments about sacrificing animals for science are as old
as science itself, and I will not rehash this protracted debate here.[35]
Yet these care-full ecotoxicologists' somewhat paradoxical practices
and reflections led me to wonder whether a truly feminist toxicology is ever possible. The description "charismatic little species" may
be interpreted as more condescending than complimentary. The critical strands of feminism that I subscribe to—Black, Indigenous, queer,
socialist and Marxist, postcolonial, ecological—are ultimately about
unsettling and refusing the binary hierarchies that position Man over
Woman, Human over Animal, Culture over Nature, White over Black,
Brown, Yellow, Red.[36] How, then, could an ecofeminist toxicologist,
let's say—meaning one who is committed to environmental justice and
so works to generate the socially legible, dominant-culture-revered
scientific data that might hold polluters accountable precisely because
she is ideologically opposed to the uneven and unethical poisoning of
peoples and ecologies—reconcile her acts of taking fish from the wild
(or breeding fish in the lab), deliberately and systematically exposing
said fish to toxicants and other stressors, and then eventually killing
the fish, as also, somehow, about environmental justice? And what are
the alternatives?

For Donna Haraway, whose academic career began in biology and
who suggests there may always be a justifiable need for experimental
animals, feminist lab practices might include recognizing the experimental animals as workers alongside the scientists; she calls this practice
"response-ability." In *When Species Meet*, for instance, Haraway writes:

It is important that the "shared conditions of work" in an experimental lab make us understand that entities with fully secured boundaries called possessive individuals (imagined as human or animal) are the wrong units for considering what is going on. That means not that a particular animal does not matter but that mattering is always inside connections that demand and enable response, not bare calculations or ranking. Response, of course, grows with the capacity to respond, that is, responsibility. . . . Calculation, such as a risk-benefit comparison weighted by taxonomic rank, suffices within relations of bounded self-similarity, such as humanism and its offspring. Answering to no checklist, response is always riskier than that. If an experimental lab becomes a scene only of calculation in relation to animals or people, that lab should be shut down. Minimizing cruelty, while necessary, is not enough; responsibility demands more than that.[37]

However, Haraway continues, "real pain, physical and mental, including a great deal of killing, is often directly caused by the instrumental apparatus, and the pain is not borne symmetrically. Neither *can* the suffering and dying be borne symmetrically, in most cases, no matter how hard the people work to respond. To me that does not mean people cannot ever engage in experimental animal lab practices, including causing pain and killing. It does mean that these practices should never leave their practitioners in moral comfort, sure of their righteousness. Neither does the category of 'guilty' apply."[38]

All of the lab members I spoke with about experimenting on animals, whether furry or fishy, felt conflicted about instrumentalizing organisms. They recognized that "the pain is not borne symmetrically" no matter how hard they might "work to respond." As revealed through our interviews, lab members also expressed uneasiness; they certainly were not "in moral comfort, sure of their righteousness." Nevertheless, the relative ease of falling back on dominant science's taxonomical hierarchies and standardizations of experimental animal use was difficult for these care-full practitioners to resist.[39] Katie, the lab manager, poignantly reflected:

I'm always recognizing and grateful that we get to work with organisms and that we're sacrificing them to try to help, you know, answer greater questions, *but those are individual lives* [emphasis added] that most of the—oftentimes we're taking from the wild and bringing back [to the lab] and doing research on, or sacrificing right there [in the wild], you know, and so *I don't want that to be in vain and I don't ever want anybody in our lab to take that lightly* [emphasis added]. And that's something that [Ben] and I—I think everybody in our lab gets it. You know, we've had a couple of times where we've been housing fish, and sometimes things get sloppy and there's some issues that come up and we address that extremely quickly because it's like, *from an undergraduate helping to all the way up to the PI, every single one of us is responsible for those animals,* [emphasis added] and we don't—these are not just research organisms. *These are organisms* [her emphasis].[40]

Here again, Holmberg's observation that both the experimental animals and the experimentalists become standardized, if unevenly, rings true.[41] Fulfilling a somewhat maternal role on how to handle with care, while expressing an anti-Cartesian enchantment with the natural world, Katie as lab manager, alongside her husband Ben as PI, models to students how to become care-full toxicologists: "From an undergraduate helping to all the way up to the PI, every single one of us is responsible for those animals . . . these are not just research organisms. *These are organisms*" (original emphasis). She also reflected critically on the irony of an environmental-health-focused toxicology laboratory creating its own not insignificant share of toxic waste, and the limits of a regulatory structure that produces such paradoxes:

We're very aware of—Sometimes we have to work with nasty chemicals to get to the question, you know, like to actually, like, get to the DNA or the RNA that we need to address these questions. We're also producing plastic waste, we're using some nasty compounds. And *we have long conversations about how, as scientists, we grapple with these issues,* that *we really are trying to help species, the environment. Yet as scientists we also are contributing to the problem.* So you have to truly believe that what you're doing is really going to make a difference. And that—you have to address the questions in such a way that they will, you know, and it's hard in science not to get burned out sometimes, you know, about—everybody makes mistakes. And so sometimes that costs, unfortunately, animals' lives that you're researching, or sometimes costs like a field season of research, and you just have to be okay. You just have to forgive yourself and forgive others that make those mistakes. Because, you know, people that genuinely—I mean, I don't think I've ever met anybody that, you know, obviously was making—you know was being callous about things, because clearly then they need to be leaving [science]. . . . They don't belong in this sector. But everybody makes mistakes, and you just have to be able to forgive ourselves and forgive them and know that *what we're doing is ultimately really trying to help address these questions so that we can be better in the future*, you know. But it is also super frustrating that—how much more science do we need to . . . [*trails off*]? It is frustrating that everything is so data-driven in our policies now, that you have to have a scientific study for species A when species B is very similar and why do we need to have the same question in species A when we know that they should be having the same response to say, for instance, for example, like for different pesticides, you know? I mean, it, it's frustrating that the policy is so, so slow to catch up to what the science is saying, you know?[42]

Just as feminist critiques of scientific language can sometimes seem misplaced (see this book's chapter 4 and outro), I also wondered whether Katie's expressions of guilt—"You just have to forgive yourself"—over producing toxic waste and sacrificing animals for the purposes of reducing toxic waste and saving animals were similarly misdirected, in the sense that the military-industrial complex clearly deserves more of the condemnation for today's pollution-related crises than environmental health scientists. As Ben felt compelled to underscore, after reading my first draft of this chapter, "Chemical pollution contributes to the biodiversity crisis and lab research does not."[43] Chemical pollution and lab research are not unrelated, however. Registering *a single pesticide* in the United States leads to the death of 10,000–15,000 experimental animals, to say nothing of the lives harmed and lost because of that pesticide's eventual dissemination out into the world. More alarmingly, this estimate only includes laboratory animals killed for human health assessments, not for ecological health, and also "does not include 'non-guideline' studies (e.g., mode of action studies)" nor "[reproductive toxicity] and carcinogenicity tests," which "consume a particularly large number of animals to fulfill regulatory requirements

(for [ecological] and human [health])"; in other words this 10,000–
15,000 laboratory animal deaths per registered pesticide estimate does
not include the sort of experiments my interlocuters might conduct on
the same toxicant.[44]

STS scholar Shiv Visvanathan powerfully wrote, in 1987, "Vivisection,
which has acquired a central and permanent status within science, has
now become totally banal. The pervasive everydayness of it masks the
metaphysical shock one would otherwise have experienced. Today, over a
hundred million animals are used up in the pursuit of research, in experiments ranging from hair dyes to cancer research. . . . One can add to it now
a roll call of patients, prisoners, the poor, inmates of old people's homes,
and name-less peasants in the third world."[45] Perhaps my toxicologist colleagues' expressions of guilt carry more weight after all, and later in this
chapter I offer some suggestions, drawing heavily from Thompson's work
in *Good Science*, on how said guilt might be more productively channeled.

The "strange balance," as Kyle put it, between revering and objectify-
ing a given species and the "long conversations about how, as scientists, we grapple with these issues" of producing toxic waste and killing
animals in the name of environmental health and justice, as Katie described, led these particular scientists to deliberately take a "step away
from mice, or anything furry and cuddly"—a move that arguably helps
allay any guilt. "Everybody makes mistakes, and you just have to be able
to forgive ourselves and forgive them and know that what we're doing
is ultimately really trying to help address these questions so that we can
be better in the future." Experimenting on animals who are more furry
and cuddly, in other words, might have made confronting these ethico-
onto-epistemological questions, to borrow Karen Barad's term, that
much more unsettling.[46] At one point during our conversation, I asked
Katie to elaborate on why she decided against an earlier career choice, to
become a veterinarian. She frankly admitted:

> KATIE: I knew that *there was no way I could ever work in a lab that*
> *worked on mammals*, because, you know, I mean, *fish are hard*
> *enough, and abalone are hard enough*, you know? But for whatever
> reason, for me, you know, I can't work with—I can't sacrifice a furry
> animal. No thank you. And I can't know that I'm working on tissue
> that came from a furry animal, you know, that kind of thing, so . . .

MELINA: I've actually heard this a lot, people sort of draw the line—
KATIE: That's sad! [*laughs ironically*]
MELINA: —between fish and mammals.
KATIE: Yeah, I know, and I do feel bad because I think fish are amazing, you know? And it is weird. It's a weird thing that we have that, right? Is it just because we can't, like, hold the little fish and, you know, pet it? [*mimes gently stroking a small animal in her cupped hands*][47]

The strange balance swung the other direction as well, as when members of this same caring, reflexive group of ecotoxicologists spoke quite casually about killing and dissecting their experimental animals. In nearly the same breath, for instance, Olivia spoke with concern for her fishes' stress levels and then pragmatically discussed her timing and rationale for dissecting them: "We want them [the experimental fish] happy and eating and getting fed and not being stressed in order to spawn well, so not tagging individual fish is better. . . . Once I'm done spawning these fish I don't see any reason not to dissect them and take tissue samples. . . . For my [qualifying exams] I had to think a lot about [statistics] and replication and so I want to make sure I get something out of these data because it's going to be a lot of work."[48]

It's worth quoting Visvanathan once again: "The pervasive everyday-ness of [scientific vivisection] masks the metaphysical shock one would otherwise have experienced."[49] These fishes' happiness and low stress levels (assuming we could gauge their emotional states) were merely for the sake of a sound experiment—"I want to make sure I get something out of these data because it's going to be a lot of work"—and perhaps also for the experimentalists' conscience; certainly not for the fishes well-being overall, as they were sure to be exposed to toxicants, killed, and then dissected. To draw from Holmberg once again: "This mutual figure (happy [experimental animals] and good science) has become rather dominating and is constantly rehearsed in legislation, ethics-committee guidelines, and scientific publications."[50] Revealing the darker side of care,[51] then, like the PhD student described in this chapter's opening vignette, these toxicologists become standardized alongside the experimental animals, learning to handle with care the animals they are nevertheless poised to kill, for respectable science and to be a respectable scientist.[52]

Importantly, however, Olivia's response to my first draft of this chapter pressed me to complicate my initial assessment. She admitted that at first, she turned to "the in vitro world" and fish after a challenging experience in a lab that experimented on species she happened to love, namely alligators and turtles, because sacrificing and dissecting these more charismatic creatures was too disturbing for her.[53] After working in that reptile lab, "the ethics of the in vitro world appealed to me, not having to do animal research." And yet, as she shared with me, she soon discovered that "even with fish, many dissections every day didn't feel good either. . . . Animal use could definitely be reduced and done better. . . . I'm not one to talk because *how many fish did I have to euthanize for my project? But at least it's not easy for me. It's hard to imagine that some scientists are completely unfazed by it.*[54] Olivia also remarked on how sad she felt to break down the fish experiment she had built over a multistep, multirelational process of two years, noting all the memories and collaborations and work in which these fish were active participants. "It was the culmination of a long study, multiple lab members helped me take care of these fish, I had very mixed feelings. I was excited to be done with experiment but having to break it down after two years felt wrong."[55] Her newfound feelings for fish must also extend to cell cultures, Olivia further reflected, as "a lot of in vitro work still uses animals—those cells are from rats; *in vitro work still means animal lives,*" and deaths.[56] I will return to in vitro and in silico alternatives later in this chapter. Overall, Olivia's responses to my first draft helped me see that her efforts to keep experimental fish "happy and eating and getting fed and not being stressed in order to spawn well" were not simply part of some cold, self-serving calculation that merely prioritizes her experimental results. Rather, her efforts were part of her desire to take response-ability for the fish unwillingly enrolled in an experiment that harms them as individuals but also aims to improve lives for their future fish relatives and other, more distantly related organisms.

These care-full ecotoxicologists' practices in "culturing a radical ability to remember and feel what is going on and performing the epistemological, emotional, and technical work to respond practically in the face of the permanent complexity not resolved by taxonomic hierarchies"[57] were important to them; during our interviews, each lab member eventually circled back to justifying experimental animal sacrifice for the

greater cause of environmental health science—thus still seeking reso-
lution in taxonomic hierarchies—but not without conflict. Kelly, who
works with a highly endangered species of fish, spoke of her struggles
sacrificing *any* living entity for science, not to mention those nearly ex-
tinct already:

> KELLY: The first experiment I did [in graduate school], I had all these
> really beautiful corals that I had been looking after and growing for,
> like, months. And I had to kill them and sacrifice them at the end,
> and I hope that they're like—*you know, they don't think, they're in-*
> *vertebrates, I don't think they feel pain the same way we do, but it was*
> *like, I was a little sad to have to kill them. But I think maybe, it sounds*
> *really bad, you just do it enough that you kind of become immune to*
> *it*, like, I don't know. Yeah. I think a lot about the number of animals
> killed for science.
>
> MELINA: Do you think it's possible to do science without that kind of
> sacrificing?
>
> KELLY: Um, yeah, it just depends what the end goal is. I do a lot of
> genomics work and so kind of have to sacrifice the animal to get
> DNA out of it. And one of the questions I did have about work-
> ing with [X fish] is that they're an endangered species and so you
> obviously don't want to be taking from the population if it's going
> to significantly affect their population size in the wild. And so I was
> concerned, when I started the [X fish] project like, is there going to
> be enough species for me to really answer these questions and not
> significantly affect the population? I don't want to be the cause of an
> animal going extinct, clearly. But because there's the hatchery there
> is a lot of fish to work with and so that made me feel better. I could
> still do a project out of it and not feel guilty. But you know I did feel
> really guilty when last summer—I don't know how much you heard
> but, like, things did not go well and there was just—fish were not
> kept at the temperatures they're meant to be and there was a lot of,
> like, tension over that between me and the hatchery and, like, whose
> fault it was and so that did make—I don't know, I felt like a—maybe
> I ruined a few relationships. I have to repeat [the entire experiment]
> basically and I was—that was so many fish that I just felt got wasted
> because people were not properly looking after the fish. . . . I have a

lot of guilt about that. . . . . I was able to repeat a little bit of the experiment towards the end of the summer but there just weren't that many fish left in my experiment because I'd already sacrificed like 3,000 of them. So, when I did it the second time there was only 1,000 left, so I got something out of it which is good because it was just, like, a lot of money and resources and fish.[58]

Kelly's observation that "I think, maybe, it sounds really bad, you just do it enough that you kind of become immune to it," well-encapsulates my unease over the ways that environmental-health-motivated toxicology too somewhat rationalizes, and thus normalizes, toxic pollution. Kelly clearly felt uneasy as well, repeatedly expressing feelings of guilt and potential regret. The best-intentioned ecotoxicologists, in other words, are often still limited to "playing the industry's game,"[59] as one of my advocacy interviewees bitterly reflected. Does a pollution scientist lose her moral standing over a polluting corporation if she also kills animals and spreads toxicants in an effort to hold that polluter accountable? Or, to ask a different but related question, returning to my book's core argument (that dominant toxicology is inherently white supremacist and masculinist), what openings might occur if toxicologists and other biological scientists *refused* to "become immune to it," and in the process both refused to normalize vivisection for the sake of scientific discovery and refused to emulate or embody the masculinist and white supremacist norm of the clinical and superior scientist?

The notion that in order to be a true, proper and rational scientist one must steel oneself against feeling emotional attachment to experimental organisms is also as old as dominant science itself. Writing of antivivisectionist movements in nineteenth century Britain, for example, historian Paul S. White notes how scientists navigated public outcry about their experiments on dogs: "That experimenters were dog owners and dog lovers, *that they possessed sympathy and tenderness and yet were able, on entering the laboratory, to mobilize their curiosity, stem the tide of sentiment, and perform like well-tuned instruments for the pursuit of truth and medical mercy was a crucial part of their self-legitimization*; it asserted their preeminent position on the physiological and moral scale of being, ahead of their critics, who, like the lower creatures they advocated, were slaves to their sentimental affections."[60]

I would hope for a feminist toxicology that would not "stem the tide of sentiment" but rather allow our emotions to inform our ethics, practicing what animal ethicist Lori Gruen terms "entangled empathy," an explicitly feminist blend of *both* cognition *and* affect.[61]

Chasing the Holy Grail of Pure Pollution

My analysis suggests that these particular ecotoxicologists navigated these challenges and tensions by attempting to distance themselves from explicitly human-related research questions. Seeking a sort of *pure pollution*, or the transcendent scientific aesthetic raised in chapter 4, my interlocutors repeatedly admitted their preference for more abstract data. Bruno noted the irony of having to make his research about humans in order to generate funding, when his true interests lie in marine ecologies—a tacit separation of these interconnected worlds.[62] Olivia expressed her preference for studying, in the hopes of ultimately improving, fish and amphibian life rather than human life because she was dismayed by what she described as human-centric science and polluters:

> I never was someone who wanted to do strictly human health research, because I've always—I don't know, I mean, like, it's hard to put words to it but, you know, there's— *We tend to be very human-centric [pauses to think]* . . . that we're the most important. But we're just one species and having the earth—and *our habitation of the earth causes a lot of issues for many, many issues for other species*, as you know. And so I never—*for me the motivation was never simply human health research. I wanted it to always have, like, an environmental component. And that's more important to me honestly, but then I realized, I mean it is linked* and it's easier to relate to as a human and also to, to make other humans care, when it's something that, okay it doesn't just, you know, impact these alligators or these turtles, like, it can also have an impact on me and on my children, and *I think it just, yeah, it makes it easier to get people to care.*[63]

While remaining cognizant of the obvious links between human-generated pollution and polluted ecologies and remaining aware of the need to "make other humans care" (and hence receive project funding and inform policy) by linking ecological health issues to human health issues, these ecotoxicologists prioritized nonhuman life. In the process, they somewhat fetishized cold, dead data—not furry, not cuddly, not personal—as a means of avoiding the paradoxes canvassed in this chapter. As Upton explained to me, with intentional irony, "By the time we get them they're—We don't get any live fish, these are all samples now, been reduced to their DNA and RNA. There's no IACUC [Institutional Animal Care and Use Committee] oversight for that."[64] Upton also explained his attraction to the newer field of toxicogenomics, self-deprecatingly sharing a mildly masculinist fixation on big, giant, tons of huge data and "the bright, shiny, new instrument to play with":

I like the idea of the bright, shiny, new instrument to play with, and the new analysis to do. . . . When I read science literature . . . I always stick with genomics and genetics . . . the idea of, you know, heredity and genes being passed, you know mutations and variants being passed down from parent to offspring and the different things, environmental interactions that can affect those mutations. . . . I find this super awesome and really complicated and really interesting, it's always been a kind of puzzle. It's kind of like engineering . . . it's like a puzzle I can solve. That's why, like, *molecular data—it's a lot of ones and zeros, lot of binary stuff and it's not, it's not so descriptive.* And so I think, in my mind, *I like the rigor that it provides, it might be a little false rigor because, you know, the [statistics] can tell you anything* [unclear] *the numbers give this false sense of like,* [emphasis added] *"Oh yeah, I'm doing, like,* real *science,"* [his emphasis on *real*] but, um, yeah it's big data too, so it's *a ton of data,* a ton of ton of ton of [*his emphasis*] data to analyze and to sort through, so I think if you can find a creative way to take all that giant chunk—I'm looking at a giant data set right now. You know, 450 fish, 30,000 genes for each fish— [*questions himself*] 30,000, right? 30,000 genes for each transcriptome, 450 transcriptomes, right? Analyze all that data to tell a very concise, basic, kind of funnel of, like, huge data, down to, like, a small little thing. And I like that. I like the challenge of doing that.[65]

Gently mocking his own desires for bright shiny new scientific toys and the "false rigor" of binary ones and zeros—"Oh yeah, I'm doing *real* science"—Upton also laughed about how such molecular data displeased the EPA lawyers trying to leverage his scientific findings, on the adverse effects of crude oil exposure, against an oil corporation in court. Again, the contradictions of animal charisma arose:

> Kind of an eye-opening experience for me, while I was working on [oil exposure] stuff, we were trying to generate data, get data that would, could be used in the courts by government, EPA lawyers, as part of their case against [X oil company], right? . . . And I was working on molecular phenotypes, right? *We were working with fish, for one, not with oil and birds, which was really flashy, or mammals, right? Nothing charismatic like that,* working with—but *not only working with fish, working with, like, molecular phenotypes—that doesn't translate well into an image that the public can wrap their heads around.* And so the lawyers were really not interested in what we were doing. . . . "It's not going to sway a judge or a jury, looking at some sort of, you know, plotted data. *We want pictures of, of like bleeding fish, or oil-covered fish, give us those.*" And so a lot of it, you know, we did a lot of imaging and showing these little embryos with their oil and they're all deformed, that would—*that's what they [the EPA lawyers] want, right? That, like, really gross kind of, like, anatomy . . . the most interesting stuff, the sub-lethal doses, the stuff that doesn't kill [the fish] outright but impacts them long-term, that's what we [scientists] are really interested in, but it's hard to get people on board to care about that kind of stuff.* . . . The lawyers have been, and the government policy officials have been, "No, we don't want anything to do with this molecular data, that's working with mumbo jumbo stuff," right? "*We want to see oil on animals,* that's the only thing that's going to convince anyone." So it's been an uphill battle [getting lawyers and the public to care about molecular data] since then. So it's a weird situation, yeah.[66]

In this case, literally, the very distance between charismatic fish and humans (as opposed to charismatic mammals and humans or charismatic birds and humans) that these toxicologists preferred, comprised a charismatic *lack* for a judge, jury, or the (imagined) general public: "We were working with fish, for one, not with oil and birds, which was really flashy, or mammals, right? Nothing charismatic like that." Making matters worse for the EPA lawyers, Upton's scientific team was working with, and more interested in, the "mumbo jumbo stuff" of molecular data: "[We were] not only working with fish, [but also] working with, like, molecular phenotypes—that doesn't translate well into an image that the public can wrap their heads around. And so the lawyers were really not interested in what we were doing. . . . 'It's not going to sway a judge or a jury, looking at some sort of, you know, plotted data. We want pictures of, of like bleeding fish, or oil-covered fish, give us those.'" In other words, the lawyers sought similarities and shared vulnerabilities between fish and humans, such as sympathy-generating images of "bleeding fish," whereas the scientists sought "the most interesting stuff, the sub-lethal doses, the stuff that doesn't kill [fish] outright but impacts them long-term," or the intellectual puzzle produced by a giant chunk of binary data, fish "reduced to their DNA and RNA." Charisma cuts both ways, it would seem. My toxicologist interlocutors swam uneasily between "that, like, really gross kind of, like, anatomy" and a transcendent aesthetic of *pure pollution*, free of messy, contradictory human politics and human-centric environmental concerns.

Exxon Babies

Another recurring tension throughout these toxicologists' work was the fact that their very lab's existence depended on the same industry they are ostensibly working against. Nina, one of the junior PhD students in the lab, observed sardonically that the ubiquity of chemical pollution is "job security."[67] Upton also recalled how his mentors are known in the field as "Exxon babies," referring to the 1989 *Exxon Valdez* oil tanker disaster out of which their research careers grew. Lab members remained well aware of this tension but were perhaps less troubled by it than I was. Ben explained to me, for instance, also in the context of oil tanker explosions he had researched, in terms of how crude oil exposure causes long-term, adverse effects on sea life:

> I think terrible things happen. And people should be studying them. And we have no shortage of terrible things happening. It's not like I'm elbowing other scientists in the face to go and study, you know, terrible things. There's plenty to go around. [*Laughs*] If it was like, really sort of much more cut-throat in that way, and very, like, competitive, then that might be a little bit weirder. But I guess my opinion is these things happen. And

I think our lab had—takes a slightly different angle than a lot of research groups and their approach to studying these problems that I think is—adds something to what is, sort of [the] standard science that's done. And so *I think we bring something unique. And I think that's useful.* I hope it's useful. I think it is. *So yeah, I'm not—I'm not terribly conflicted about that.*[68]

In the same interview, Ben summed up this seeming contradiction of environmentally focused toxicology when describing how a prior lab of his took advantage of a crude oil tanker disaster geographically close to his research institution at the time. Because they knew the oil was headed to the coastline, he and his fellow lab members were able to take baseline measurements immediately before the oil arrived, to which they could then compare the same measurements after the oil had wreaked its havoc on the ecosystem. In short, because of "terrible things happening," his lab was able to create the conditions of a controlled laboratory experiment out in the field. The situation was, as he memorably put it, "a toxicologist's dream-slash-nightmare." Clearly an individual as enchanted by the natural world as he did not desire such an ecological disaster, but as an ecotoxicologist, the event presented ideal research conditions: a dream-slash-nightmare.

Upton interpreted the fact that oil companies were forced to fund his research demonstrating that oil exposure harms marine life as "poetic justice":

I'm working on money from a corporation that has been forced to—has been sued by the government, and it's been forced to give up this money. So in that sense, you know, it gives you kind of this, kind of, um, [*pauses thoughtfully*]. . . . Yeah, I guess the feeling I have from that is it's pretty cool that I'm working on basically stolen—not stolen money, but like money that wasn't willingly offered to me. But I got it anyways and I'm doing hopefully something that that company, a corporation should have done before they started drilling or before they started moving oil across open ocean. And that is doing due diligence, with their—they're making a lot of money off oil and they should see what the environmental impacts of this, the profit are. . . . Here [in the US] it's all after the fact. . . . There's no money for oil spill research unless there's an oil spill. No one wants to fund it. No one will fund it. So you have to actually pull the money out of the corporations, by suing them to get the money to research it. So it's kind of a weird—it's definitely messed up. So the fact that we get to work on it at all, and get to work on it after the fact, it's still sad but also kind of, you know, poetic justice a little bit.[69]

Unlike the stem cell research that comprises the focus of Thompson's *Good Science*, wherein animals are *substituted* for human research subjects, these good scientists intentionally expose the very same species of fish to oil, for example, for the purposes of arguing that this specific species of fish that was accidentally (or inevitably, depending on who you ask[70]) exposed to oil is indeed dying because of said oil exposure—"[Oil corporations are] making a lot of money off oil and they should see what the environmental impacts of [their profits] are." Thus, while Thompson makes a strong case for why "systematic efforts should be made to improve in vitro human models in such a way as to make them more in vivo-like, rather than putting resources and energy into humanizing non-human animal models,"[71] it seems an equally strong case still has to be made for why even biological experimental models that are *not* substitutive, such as those conducted by these toxicologists, may not constitute "good science" in its ethical sense. Put another way, is the claim that "we really are trying to help species, the environment" enough to absolve scientists of the guilt of also "contributing to the problem" of toxic waste production and animal suffering? What is more, to what extent does *researching* the ubiquity of chemical contamination *normalize* the ubiquity of chemical contamination? Are ecotoxicologists inadvertently condoning the same "there is no alternative" and "exposure is inevitable" mindset as the proindustry, pesticide-happy toxicologists I described in chapters 1, 2, and 3? Alternatively, to what extent might all the small yet significant acts of care work that take place in an ecotoxicology lab—caring for fish, caring for corals, caring for mice, caring for one another—hold more radical potential?

Toward an Ecotoxicology with Ecofeminist Ethics; Or, Telling Different Stories

In her analysis of "sciences with ethics," such as human stem cell research, and to which I would add toxicology, Thompson claims that a high level of political attention to the ethics of the life sciences . . . is a good thing for science and democracy. This argument is counter-intuitive to many, who fear . . . that non-scientific attention imposes unrealistic regulatory burdens on researchers, is anti-science (or criti-cal of scientists), interferes with the relation of trust underlying the public funding of science, is a distraction to scientists and an invasion of research autonomy, stokes false hopes and fears about the field, mis-understands the role of science in stimulating the economy, and/or is under-informed about science. If attention from non-scientists in fact slowed down research aimed at finding cures [or reducing pollution] and undermined freedom of inquiry and the public understanding of science, such attention could hardly claim to serve democracy or science. . . . Sci-ences with ethics, because of the attention given to their conduct, offer an unprecedented opportunity to reset how science as usual is carried out.[72]

The environmental and ecotoxicologists I had the privilege of ob-serving, learning from, and gently challenging from 2020 to 2022 were unquestionably committed to improving environmental conditions for all life and to holding polluting perpetrators accountable via their lab's scientific findings. They therefore rationalized even the gory and cruel practices of their laboratory- and field-based research, including the theft of animals from the wild, the production of toxic waste, and the systematic killing of "amazing," "charismatic" species, while nevertheless openly struggling with these asymmetrical relationships. Although the scale and scope of these particular ecotoxicologists' experiments rep-resent a mere fraction of the millions of animals sacrificed for science, not to mention the unfathomable quantity and quality of lives lost due to toxic pollution, such practices still emerge from the same European Enlightenment-derived dominant science, wherein Man is entitled to mastery over Nature, Animal, Other. Just as appeals to purity and nor-malcy in endocrine-disrupting chemical science and advocacy reinforce the very same eugenicist logics that positioned some people and places as more pollutable than others to begin with, claims of serving environ-mental health and justice through a reliance on (less) theft, death, and contamination rest on questionable ethical grounds.[73]

What, then, are viable alternatives to animal experimentation? Highly distinguished scientists and longtime anti-toxics advocates decried the

Trump-era EPA move to phase out chemical testing on animal models as a backdoor maneuver to deregulate toxic substances. The prestigious science journal *Nature* reported, for instance,

> The move represents an "unholy alliance" between the chemical industry and animal-rights groups that are pushing to halt animal tests, says Jennifer Sass, a senior scientist at the Natural Resources Defense Council, an environmental advocacy group in New York City. Sass says that the EPA has reduced its reliance on animal testing in certain areas. For instance, tests to see whether a chemical is corrosive to the skin can now be done on skin that is grown in a Petri dish. But without tests on animals such as mice or rabbits, the only way for companies to study chemical interactions in the body is to use computer models, she says. And those models are often proprietary, which makes it hard to assess their accuracy.[74]

While recent history confirms that chemical corporations must be eyed with suspicion and regulated more stringently,[75] I am less convinced that toxicological studies conducted on animals are somehow more accurate than computer models, for some of the reasons elaborated in chapter 2, and even less sure that said studies ultimately result in environmental health, given today's highly toxicologically studied and yet "permanently polluted" world. To be sure, the toxicology laboratory I worked with has successfully leveraged their scientific findings against polluting corporations, and there are numerous, righteous stories of environmental justice activists teaming up with scientists to help hold polluters accountable.[76] Nevertheless, I remain unconvinced that these occasionally positive ends justify what ought to be more metaphysically shocking means. The financial settlement Exxon was forced to pay after their 1989 *Exxon Valdez* disaster, to cite an unusually successful example, totaled $100 million "for the injuries caused to the fish, wildlife, and lands of the spill region," a number that pales in comparison to the record profits Exxon Mobil continues to rake in almost forty warmer years later—$36 billion in 2023 alone—to say nothing of the irremediable damages done.[77] Instead, I agree with Thompson's take on human stem cell research, wherein she compellingly argues that it takes work to make *any* model system stand in for any target group; there is no mimesis or self-evidently self-same model system. . . . if a research subject is being tested on for the benefit of someone else, there are likely to be limits to how good a model the research subject is for those for whom the subject stands in. The more we conceptualize health in terms of genetic and epigenetic and environmental specificity, the less compelling the idea of allowing some to be researched upon for the benefits of others becomes. . . . We need to begin to work as hard and with as much ingenuity to make life-like in vitro human [and animal] models as scientists and others have worked over the last 60 years to establish the current standards of animal care and use and the extraordinarily refined animal tools and animal-model systems.[78]

Again, adapting Thompson's analysis of animals as *substitutes* for humans, to these ecotoxicologists' work on captives of the *same* species, whether taken from the wild or bred in the lab, I submit that stealing and killing living organisms for the sake of environmental health and justice is untenable and unethical. In other words, I have found that toxicology cannot be ecofeminist unless and until it helps dismantle heteropatriarchy *and* anthroparchy, working toward sociological *and* ecological justice.

Readers might argue that I, too, am pursuing an impossibly pure politics, a criticism to which I am open. None of us are innocent. Just this week I deliberately killed some ants tracking tiny morsels across my kitchen floor; I drive my gas-guzzling old car almost every day. I am not suggesting that environmental toxicologists immediately stop doing their good science because it cannot be done without animal death and dismemberment. Perfection is the enemy of the good. At any rate, industry-employed toxicologists are certainly not going to stop producing their "bad science," and for government-required risk assessments at that. I would, however, respectfully challenge environmental toxicologists to start telling different "cool stories," as Kyle put it, to themselves, to their colleagues, and to the general public. Like all researchers, my ecotoxicologist interlocuters' have a personal stake in their science; some were drawn to certain charismatic little species, others were motivated by a long-standing enchantment with the natural world, still others relish the challenge of an engineering-like puzzle, or selflessly seek to improve public health, clean up contaminated ecologies, and punish polluters—or some combination of all these interests. Taken together, my social location, critical feminist training, and ethnographic research leads me to the position that environmental health toxicologists and environmental justice advocates are making a categorical, ethico-onto-epistemological error by turning to "the basic science of poisons" to provide answers to the problems produced by powerful poisoners' synthetic poisons.[79]

As I (and others[80]) have argued, US toxicology was designed by and for the military-industrial complex, based on its founding fathers' thoroughly interested premise that toxicants could, and should, be made safe. Some may recall the old Monsanto Company tagline: "Serving industry, which serves mankind."[81] Even if today's environmental and ecotoxicologists recognize the myopia of their field's founders and predecessors, their laboratory practices and experimental methods continue to rely on and reinforce the same hierarchical logic of what Black feminist theorist Alexander Weheliye calls the "Western Liberal Man Master Subject."[82] A science that rationalizes and normalizes the systematic death of millions of organisms for the sake of (other) organisms' lives cannot claim to be a science for justice. In Haraway's analysis, "The animals in the labs . . . they are somebody as well as something, just as we humans are both subject and object all the time. To be in response to that is to recognize copresence in relations of use and therefore to remember that no balance sheet of benefit and cost will suffice. I may (or may not) have good reasons to kill . . . but I do not have the majesty of Reason and the solace of Sacrifice."[83] As I hope this and the previous chapter have effectively demonstrated, these ecotoxicologists are exceptionally care-full and reflexive scientists. Having been trained in the dominant tradition, however, their caring and reflexivity, in terms of whether and how to use experimental animals, still tended toward the "balance sheet of benefit and cost" or relied on the "majesty of Reason and the solace of Sacrifice."

What if contemporary ecotoxicologists were motivated by and passed along different stories? Chris, a federally employed ecotoxicologist PI who frequently collaborates with this academic lab, candidly questioned the good his ecological research does for the world, as a sort of environmental civil service:

[Environmental civil service] has always been in the background in my family. It's a pretty politically engaged family. My dad was teaching at a public university, my mom worked at the university. I think they both took pretty seriously that that they worked for the taxpayers of the state. . . . My dad's research was almost always, like everybody's, federal or state funded, and he really felt like "I have been paid to do this, and I have to deliver a product for the taxpayers" like that, you know—he would actually literally talk about that sort of stuff. So I think, you know, I had that kind of influence, and we were always a family that, you know, talked about politics, voted, talked about the environment. . . . in the last, you know, [Trump] administration, I just felt like it consumed every part of life, that you needed—It was kind of an "all hands on deck" moment, and I was, I was never going to go disappear and become an environmental lawyer, or, or human rights lawyer—I mean honestly, I will say that the one thing I do think about when I talk about this is it is a little ridiculous, that—*if I really want to do the most to help, there are a lot of other things that—"Oh yeah I'm gonna be a civil servant helping to protect minnows," [gently mocks himself] or things like that. You know, like, in the environmental field, it's really climate change. I mean, like, the—almost nothing matters if we don't deal with climate change.* So there's a part of me that's like . . . *you know, if I really was, really really really putting my money where my mouth is I'd probably be stopping doing, you know, some noodley academic research* that, you know, can take a long time in a lot of ways to pay off. . . . I really am particularly concerned with wild populations and I'm in an [ecological] program and that sort of stuff. But—*I certainly think that that is an important, you know, preserving the ecosystems around us that may or may not have what people see as direct benefit to people's, you know, everyday life and especially when you're talking about people who are just trying to get by. I mean they don't give a spit about, you know, populations of small fish. If they're not eating them. So, you know, some of the public probably doesn't think I serve much purpose. Even the ones who agree with the need to control environmental chemicals.*[84]

Anthropological research and activist movements alike suggest that "people who are just trying to get by" do in fact "give a spit" about "populations of small fish," whether or not they depend on them for sustenance, but Chris's overarching sentiment is well-understood: "noodley academic research" (mine included) is unlikely to serve justice at the speed current crises demand. And the public's dissatisfaction with the EPA's ecological research programs is not necessarily because said public does not care about toxic environmental exposures, but rather because government research divisions appear to be prioritizing the wrong questions and methods. Environmental scientists know all too well the exigencies of climate emergency and related human and ecological violations. Rather than feeling guilty for killing corals, or like a cruel (or powerful?) person for making Frankenstein fish, rather than rising above the fray to immerse oneself in the transcendent aesthetic of genetic code, toxicologists committed to environmental justice might instead reroute their genuine care for charismatic marine life, and enduring passions for preserving ecosystems, into stories and practices that refuse the dominion of Man, that place greater value in nonscientific forms of expertise, disabled and neuro-atypical experiences, and critical feminist and animal perspectives and positions.[85]

I imagine my interlocuters and other constructive critics protesting that I am asking for too much, erecting all the obstacles in Thompson's summary; imposing unrealistic burdens on researchers; being anti-science; interfering with the public funding of science; distracting scientists; invading research autonomy; stoking false hopes and fears; misunderstanding the role of science in the economy; being underinformed. As an outsider to the discipline, many of these criticisms hold some truth. However, my outside perspective also affords me a partial vision that has arguably been trained out of toxicological insiders—"You just kind of become immune to [laboratory organism death]." Moreover, as animal ethicist Brian Luke notes, ending our violent reliance on experimental animals creates far more possibilities than it eliminates: "Animal liberation does not limit action through control of self and others, it develops the individual's capacity for a broader range of action. It is creative, not restrictive."[86] After twenty plus weeks with such diligent environmental scientists, I could not help but notice, and was moreover repeatedly struck by, how the material realities of sacrificing animals deeply troubles these practitioners, evidencing these toxicologists' ethics of care for more-than-human organisms. Which is to say that they are *already* doing the good work; they already recognize that "instead of being pure objects for scientific inquiry . . . animals constitute parts of significant relationships."[87] Olivia, for example, felt sad and wrong breaking down her fish experiments after two years of significant relationships, and furthermore quite frustrated that IACUC rules require her to kill *all* fish (nonconsensually) enrolled in the experiment, even if Olivia didn't need their specific deaths for her scientific analyses. (IACUC regulations prohibit scientists from releasing live, used-and-no-longer-needed experimental animals into the wild, for fear of disease spreading to endemic species and other forms of potential contamination.) And as Katie so poignantly observed, "How much more science do we need . . . ? It is frustrating that everything is so data-driven in our policies now, that you have to have a scientific study for species A when species B is very similar. . . . Why do we need to have the same question in species A when we know that they should be having the same response to . . . different pesticides, you know?"

While open, if skeptical, to the idea that animals might eventually (need to) be phased out of research, Kelly was still unsatisfied after reading my first draft of this chapter:

> I think a lot of us in the lab are all for this and do want to be ethically better with our science, but if there's one thing grad school taught me is to be humble and admit the things that I don't know. . . . I admit that I don't know the best way forward and I can't help but think when reading this sentence ["Toxicologists committed to environmental justice might instead reroute their genuine care for charismatic marine life."] that it doesn't really answer my question. But how do I do this? . . . This all seems well and good to make these improvements, but how do we do this while still doing rigorous science that we've been trained in?[88]

My response to Kelly's excellent, heartfelt question, will likely still leave her unsatisfied, but I will venture out on this limb, by her side, all the same: making these improvements means changing what "rigorous science" looks and feels and sounds like, radical changes which require significant amounts of untraining and what Black feminist geographer Katherine McKittrick calls "non-hierarchical collaboration."[89] Rather than play the chemical "industry's game of catch-up," as one of my public health interviewees bitterly remarked, while using the industry's tools,[90]

I humbly yet boldly challenge ecotoxicologists (and government regulators) to rapidly phase out animal experimental models and redouble their efforts to strengthen in silico, high-throughput toxicant screenings instead, while engaging in a frequent, regular practice of examining the unquestioned tenets of their scientific disciplines—many of us trained in critical feminist STS are eager to collaborate on these efforts![91] An organization called "Free Radicals," for example, has developed a "research justice worksheet" that includes generative questions traditionally trained scientists (of both natural and social persuasions) can ask themselves.[92]

In his own care-full response to the first draft of this chapter, Ben reminded me that in silico modeling does not preclude the lives and deaths of experimental animals.

> In silico models require extensive validation for them to have any worth, and that validation is going to come from nothing other than animal research. You can't have one without the other. We, and many of our colleagues, are big advocates for in silico prediction/modeling that may reduce and perhaps eventually replace our need for animal models, and for many folks, including us, this is a big focus of their research programs. But we aren't there yet, and to suggest otherwise is either ill-informed or disingenuous, and making that switch prematurely will do nothing other than let polluters off the hook because the modeling results would not be defensible in court.[93]

I agree with Ben that "we aren't there yet," and would not wish for toxicology to make this move prematurely. But making moves in this direction will seem premature as long as the belief persists that standard(ized) toxicological experiments on animals can actually tell us what we need to know about toxic chemicals, or that animal model validation will always be necessary, in terms of holding polluting corporations and complicit regulators accountable. The research I compiled into this book shows that status quo toxicology does not do the work that environmental justice demands, in large part due to its founding fathers and their enduring, hierarchical perspectives and concomitant presumptions. These include better living through chemistry, serving industry serves mankind, exposure is inevitable, the dose makes the poison, chemicals can be made safe, certain beings are pollutable, quantitative data are more valid than qualitative, and so on.

Many of my interviewees readily acknowledged that the US chemical regulatory system is fundamentally flawed, only to hastily add that "it's the system we've got" and we cannot afford to lose any more ground to industry—a complaint plus compliance that has existed since the first toxicant-related acts became law.[94] What if those of us who wish to repair ecosystems, and make polluters pay, broke free from this fatalistic and, frankly, "boys will be boys" narrative? Results from in silico modeling are only indefensible in court if the court believes that animal models are somehow superior to computer models, which renders even more bizarre the fact that lived, human experience, such as that testified to by overexposed individuals, is deemed *less reliable* than toxicology's animal models. Admittedly, in the historical moment during which I type these pages, I have less and less faith every passing moment that there is any hope of US judges and juries holding oil corporations meaningfully accountable for the environmental destruction they've wrought.[95] Let us not forget Upton's illuminating story about the EPA lawyers: "We want pictures of, of, like, *bleeding fish*, or *oil-covered fish*, give us those." All this is to say that my suggestions are not disingenuous, even if my informedness is necessarily limited, and I recognize and appreciate how difficult doing toxicology differently will be. The next and final chapter offers some "otherwise" stories we feminist scientists and scientist feminists might tell, about toxicity, charisma, science, and justice.[96]

Outro

Purity and Drag

This is just what queer critique must do: use our historically
and presently quite creative work with pleasure, sex, and
bodies to jam whatever looks like the inevitable.
—Elizabeth Freeman[1]

The title of this brief conclusion, "Purity and Drag," purposefully references several somewhat contradictory notions.[2] Ideals of purity are inextricable from eugenic ideologies, which is why contemporary environmental health advocates' nostalgia for some imagined, prepolluted body or nature gives me pause.[3] The concept of drag is likewise central to eugenics. The expression "the drag of the race," which today is primarily used in the context of animal breeding, refers to the notion that without selective breeding of, for example, purebred dogs, all dogs would eventually devolve into some sort of awkward, homely, and not particularly intelligent mutt or mongrel.[4] The human-related eugenic anxiety behind this idea, what former US president Theodore Roosevelt referred to as "race suicide," is that supposedly superior humans interbreeding with supposedly inferior humans will *drag* down the quality, and hence threaten the survival, of the so-called white race.[5]

My chapter title deliberately evokes more playful yet no less political uses of the term drag in response. For drag also refers to how queer folks dress and perform to unsettle gender norms and underscore cultural constructions of binary sex and other limitations of heteronormativity.[6] Additionally, drag performance may be understood as a refusal of linear time.[7] Here I draw from Elizabeth Freeman's concept of "temporal drag," which understands drag performance "as the act of plastering the body with *outdated* rather than just cross-gendered accessories, whose resurrection seems to exceed the axis of gender and begins to talk about, indeed talk back to, history."[8] Given temporal drag's insistence on exceeding the gender axis *and* talking back to history, endocrine-disrupting chemicals (EDCs) are perhaps best reviewed through this lens of queer theory. EDCs exceed the axis of gender by revealing how malleable sexed traits and characteristics can be, even on a biological—as opposed to "merely cultural"[9]—level. Moreover, via their transgenerational and low-dose effects, EDCs begin to talk about and talk back to colonial and capitalist, masculinist and militarist histories, through what queer theorist Eva Hayward calls "intoxifornication . . . a kind of queer sexual becoming that is shot through with toxins—the toxins of endocrine disruption, of poisonous working conditions, of the uncertain ecstasy of hormone replacement therapy or gender realignment."[10] Put another way, the unruly movements and unrelenting residues of EDCs thwart dominant understandings of linear time and mathematics, including scientific beliefs that the dose makes the poison or that organisms exist solely to reproduce and maximize fitness, as well as capitalist (and eugenic) commitments to maintaining the ever-onward, forward march of better living through chemistry.

What is more, within Freeman's queer theorization of temporal drag, truly queer approaches do not simply "dissolve forms, disintegrate identities, level taxonomies, scorn the social."[11] Freeman speculates, rather, that "the point may be to trail *behind* actually existing social possibilities: to be interested in the tail end of things, willing to be bathed in the fading light of whatever has been declared useless" (emphasis added).[12] A queer ecofeminist study of toxicity, then, might talk back to history—directly confronting the power asymmetries that lead to the overproduction and uneven dissemination of toxic chemicals—while simultaneously offering radical care for, and being willing to be bathed in the fading light of, all the organisms and ecosystems that dominant toxicology and powerful social actors have either directly or indirectly declared useless—whether before, during, or after toxic exposure. As Freeman righteously yet tenderly argues. "Queers have, it is fair to say, fabricated, confabulated, told fables, and done so fabulously . . . in the face of great pain. This is the legacy I wish to honor here, that of queers as close enough readers of one another and of dominant culture to gather up, literally, life's outtakes and waste products and bind them into fictitious but beautiful (w)holes. Because in taking care of our own we have also been forced to stay close, to wash one another's sweat-soaked sheets in Fab when no one else would."[13]

Queer reclamations of drag, in other words, might help environmental toxicologists turn against purity[14]—of nature, of bodies, of scientific aesthetics—without downplaying the injustices of and illnesses produced by differently distributed toxic exposures. In this speculative epilogue, then, I summarize the overarching argument of *Toxic Sexual Politics* and suggest ways that queer ecofeminist practices might open up otherwise possibilities for justice-centered studies of toxicants, in part by urging scientists to see outside the waters they/we are swimming in.

Reckoning with Toxicological Eugenics

Toxicology research on EDCs provides a good illustration of the unarticulated eugenicist assumptions limiting toxicological studies and subsequent chemical regulations. Toxicology, as a scientific practice, defines purity and hence impurity, normal and hence abnormal, desirable and hence undesirable. These are value-laden, culturally derived decisions located in particular social, political, and historical contexts. If, as discussed in chapter 1, a founding toxicologist like Harold C. Hodge is *defining* "the requisite purity" then we ought to be concerned about his enthusiasm for synthetic pesticides, not to mention his unethical yet government-funded experiments on uninformed human subjects. If a textbook-authoring toxicologist like Michael A. Gallo receives a prestigious award from the Society of Toxicology in 2021, then we ought to be concerned about his praise for the Manhattan Project and DDT in 2013. The message that influential practitioners such as these are imparting on toxicologists-in-training is that certain people and places are more pure, valuable, and worth protecting from pollution, whereas other(ed) peoples and places are impure, less valuable, and more pollutable. Toxicology's eugenic thinking has likewise permeated the subfield within toxicology that focuses on EDCs.

Authors of a 2006 review of the scientific literature on EDCs, evolution, and disease, for instance, ominously warned, "In nature, individuals (particularly females) actively discriminate and choose among potential mates; successful mating requires a reciprocal synchronicity in behavior and physiology among males and females. We know that EDCs influence the behavior of animals both in nature and in the lab; might they also influence the embryo's developing nervous system such that, in adulthood, the individual's ability to discriminate and choose between possible mates is compromised? Extrapolating from altered behaviors to evolutionary significance is straightforward."[15] As stressed in chapter 4, I do not wish to suggest that the ways in which EDCs might influence behavior (sexual or not) and affect development (sexual or not) are either nonexistent or nonconcerning. Rather, I wish to emphasize that the primary lens through which such outcomes are interpreted—part and parcel of the dominant culture that rationalizes economic poisons—occludes broader, more justice-centered understandings of the harmful effects (and causes!) of EDCs. What might this focus on "mate choice"—assuming scientists thoroughly know all the complexities of such behaviors—be blurring in the background? Who gets to decide what makes for properly "discriminating" behavior or choosing the "right" mate? None of these supposedly rational biological questions address, moreover, why or how EDCs have become so ubiquitous, legal, profitable, and unevenly deployed in the first place.

In ideological alignment with chemical corporations, the US military, and industry-friendly government regulators of their times, toxicologists such as Hodge and Gallo embraced the widespread yet uneven dissemination of chemical weapons and synthetic pesticides, among other economic poisons. This ideological position forms the foundation of the objective, quantitative science of toxicology, practice of weed science, and regulatory process of chemical risk assessment, which taken together, effectively *rationalize* toxic exposures for certain communities and ecologies, allowing and approving the use of purportedly safe amounts of toxicants. Put another way, making value judgements about which communities and landscapes were pollutable, influential US toxicologists and chemical regulators reinforced the dominant race-, sex-, and class-based hierarchies of the day, contributing to the plethora of environmental injustices that marginalized communities continue to struggle against.

So when well-intentioned environmental health scientists and advocates sound the alarm over EDCs "shrinking penises," "plummeting" sperm counts, and "threatening" intelligence, I hear some alarm bells of my own.[16] Put simply, this is the very same eugenicist thinking that entered the planet into this toxic mess to begin with. The ideology of eugenics is what drives claims that people with so-called deviant sexualities, neuro-atypical or differently abled people, working-class people, and people of color are somehow less evolutionarily fit, less intelligent, less desirable members of society.[17] Environmental advocates' use, and I choose that verb intentionally, of people with disabilities, people with lowered IQs, and intersex folks (or frogs, as the case may be) as examples of everything that does and could go wrong because of EDC exposure is an approach that reinforces eugenic thinking—and eugenic thinking is what reproduces environmental injustice.

To be sure, today's toxicologists have come a long way from their industrial chemical-enthusiast predecessors of the 1970s, and perhaps especially those in the subfields of environmental and ecotoxicology. As exemplified by the toxicology PhD student working on "a model for juvenile exposure to chemical warfare," discussed in chapter 1, contemporary environmental toxicologists work diligently to measure and predict the harmful health effects of toxic chemicals. Even weed scientists, who admit their discipline may be more accurately named "herbicide science,"[18] are increasingly seeking alternatives to the masculinist myth of chemical control, as I mentioned in chapter 3.[19] Still, I found implicit biases in toxicological premises that deserve critical attention. Importantly, I bring these critiques to the fore in an effort to help create better, more stringent chemical policy, certainly not to add fuel to the fire of industry-led attacks on the environmental health sciences and overburdened communities.

Toward Scientifically Honest Politics

Admittedly, while pursuing this project I became increasingly uncomfortable with queer feminist critiques, including my own, of integrative biologist Tyrone Hayes's research findings specifically, given how he had already been viciously singled out by Syngenta Corporation for being an uppity African American scientist who dared to report the harmful effects of exposure to Syngenta's agrochemical atrazine.[20] Scientists can and ought to do better than "chemical castration,"[21] but Hayes is not alone in the field of endocrine disruption in compounding what Giovanna Di Chiro termed "heteronormative sex panic."[22] But of all EDC researchers invoking offensive, or, at best, unthoughtfully chosen, words to describe EDCs' adverse effects on reproductive and developmental biology, why does Hayes continue to receive so much negative attention, from both the chemical industry and queer feminist critics of the chemical industry? Is this yet another example of the general tendency of the Left to endlessly critique and hold its (Black, Indigenous, and other people of color) comrades to the highest, impossibly perfect standards while the Right grows ever more bonded, empowered, and solidified in their crystal-clear, oversimplified demands?[23]

Alongside my uneasy critiques of Hayes, I also frequently found myself in the uncomfortable position of justifying my queer feminist science and technology studies (STS) critiques of such luminaries as biologist Theo Colborn. For example, one highly accomplished public health practitioner respectfully yet quizzically noted, after a research talk I gave in 2021, "I did not quite get your critique of Theo Colborn. She's one of my heroes!" Dr. Theo Colborn, lead author of the popular 1996 book *Our Stolen Future: Are We Threatening Our Fertility, Intelligence, and Survival?: A Scientific Detective Story*,[24] is regarded by many in the environmental advocacy world as a hero for standing up to chemical gaslighting and for inspiring scientists to venture outside their laboratories and get explicitly political. I too applaud environmental health researchers for sticking their necks out and taking a public stance, especially against the powerful influences of Big Ag and Big Chem (which are increasingly indistinguishable), industry blocs that can easily destroy an academic career, as Syngenta attempted in the case of Hayes, among many others.[25]

What is more, as one of my undergraduate students so plainly and plaintively put it (see chapter 4), frogs—and people!—overexposed to EDCs like atrazine *are* harmed. EDCs undoubtedly cause harm, though not necessarily in ways related to sexual reproduction, gonadal development, or sexual behaviors. While I and other critical STS scholars would firmly agree with Robbins and Moore's call for more politically honest science,[26] I have come to believe that left-leaning critics of science also need to cultivate a more *scientifically honest politics*. We must do our best to root out the heterosexism, racism, and ableism that permeates scientific knowledge production on chemical pollution (among other phenomena), and we must simultaneously be "unflinchingly pessimistic" about the bodily harms wrought by EDC exposures and manufacturers, as well as name and undermine the "interlocking systems of oppression" that reproduce such "unevenly distributed vulnerabilities to premature death."[27]

Moreover, as feminists have long argued, those of us acting in solidarity with environmental justice struggles would do well to avoid fetishizing care work. Some of us are "forced to care," to borrow feminist sociologist Evelyn Nakano Glenn's turn of phrase, while the "care chains" of reproductive labor, as conceived by feminist sociologist Rhacel Salazar Parreñas, reinforce race-, class-, and gender-based hierarchies.[28] Women do not equally bear the heavy burdens of care work; socially and economically marginalized women of color are disproportionately more saddled with this load. Because of these power asymmetries, care work has limited capacity to stop the poisoner from drawing his bow; care is a necessary response, a necessary antidote, but can care work halt the production of poisons to begin with? Given persistent gendered and racialized disparities in social, economic, and political power, perhaps the question is rather about *who* needs to care for the sake of environmental justice. While I would not separate an essentialized "women's" ethics of care from an essentialized "men's" ethics of justice, as psychologist Carol Gilligan proposes, I do suggest that centering care work—by focusing *both* on its gendered devaluing *and* on its gendered fetishization—is fundamental for justice.[29] Sexually and racially marginalized people cannot, should not, be the only ones caring.[30]

Overall, my ethnographic research compelled and inspired me to offer a bit of recuperative and bridge-building work in this epilogue. The ecotoxicologists I engaged for twenty-plus weeks, for instance, are highly attuned to chemical corporations' outsized influence on research and policy. They have been taught, however, that expressing their personal and political positions delegitimizes their science, and, in turn, their authority to speak as scientists. In response to a question I posed about how toxicologists might become more explicitly political in their publications, Ben explained that not only will the chemical industry use environmental toxicologists' advocacy against them—"You're not objective, you have an agenda. Look it's right here in your [scientific] paper"[31]—but scientific publications themselves, no matter how "woke," are unlikely to inspire social movements or policy changes on their own.

I mean, they [chemical corporations] are going to use whatever tactic they can to discredit you. . . . If you don't have [explicit political standpoints] in your science paper they try to discredit you in other ways. . . . So I think there's some pretty hard inertia there because really, honestly, when it comes down to it, *the vast majority of people that read primary research articles are other scientists, and you're preaching to the choir.* Right? And maybe a journalist picks it up and actually reads your article. But they're in—and if a journalist picks it up, then I'm more than happy for them to write about it because they are . . . probably more qualified than I am to communicate this in efficient ways. Sometimes. [*Laughs*] They're definitely more qualified, whether they always do a good job of it. They don't always do a good job of it. But yeah, I think, I sort of *stick to the science.* . . . I'm just not sure that, you know, "we should do this, we should write these laws this way, we should . . ." [*trails off*]—*not sure you're speaking to the right audience by doing that in your scientific article.* And I don't think that that's just a cop-out, I think it's wasted words. And probably not only wasted words but deleterious words because you're going to get this pushback on it from colleagues.[32]

If ecotoxicologists will face censure from both colleagues and adversaries by "taking sides"[33] in their scientific journal articles, then it's no wonder so few of them do. Of course, easily the core contribution of STS is that "sticking to the science" is not in fact an apolitical position. Toxicologists would have had to have encountered STS, however, or have been consciously marginalized in some way by dominant toxicology, to recognize that science is always already political. Some recent and increasing efforts to bring critical theory and political history into scientific training early on provide some hope on this account.[34] I tend to agree with Ben's point that criticizing the chemical industry in toxicology journals often (but not always) amounts to preaching to the choir. However, the notion that scientific papers are *not* political simply because authors do not make their political positions explicit in them seems to me to be where the "pretty hard inertia" lies.

Ben went on to share a story about his own choice to be more explicitly political in a scientific journal. Two research papers he published received multiple rebuttals from a toxicological consultant paid by the very same industry whose toxic substance caused serious ecological damages, according to Ben's research.

> So, the second time, our second [toxicant] paper, when [the manufacturing corporation] hired another consultant, again—now, this, this started to really piss me off. And, you know, when they write a letter to the editor that the journal thinks has value, you as the author of the original paper that's been criticized have an opportunity to respond. And they usually publish both together. And so we're like, you know, we always respond because we don't want them to just publish the critique without our response. Sometimes we think it doesn't warrant a response, but they're going to publish [the critique] anyway even if we don't respond. And so we respond very carefully, point by point and—but by the second one I'm like, you know, people should see this for for for [stuttering with frustration] what it is. And it wasn't a terribly bold or brave thing to do but at the end of that letter to the editor, the response to [the industry consultant's] letter to the editor I'm like, I'm calling them out, like, this— you need to call them out, like that this is—I forget what we actually said but it's definitely something that I would never say in a paper. [*Laughs*] And it's just saying like, "Look, your industry has a responsibility in managing public resources for the public good. And this is clearly a violation, that we need to hold them responsible, and them hiring consultants to try to discredit the work is—Everyone should see this for what it is. And it's, and it's not okay." So, you know, it wasn't a particularly brave place to say it, in a response to a letter to the editor. I don't know how many people read that, but that seemed like an appropriate place to do that. The research article didn't seem like the appropriate place to do that.[35]

It is hard to convey in writing the intensity of Ben's aural delivery of this particular anecdote, which is why I left all the repeated phrases and stuttering of his mildly agitated speech in the interview transcript excerpted above. He may be correct that the "research article didn't seem like the appropriate place" to call out chemical manufacturers, and not because research articles are supposed to be free of politics, but because research articles do not necessarily reach the right audiences—audiences that have the collective strength and will to rein in chemical industry power.

As discussed in chapters 4 and 5, these particular ecotoxicologists care deeply about environmental health and justice and are tremendously proud, as they should be, that their toxicological studies have helped hold polluting industries to account. Going against the scientific grain in this way, prompting pushback from well-resourced industry consultants on top of pushback from their well-intentioned (but perhaps less brave) colleagues, is not a welcome task for those who would prefer to stick to the science. I began to wonder whether queer feminist STS critiques of EDC research and advocacy, in their worthy efforts to counter stigmatization and discrimination, are too frequently (mis)interpreted as trivializing the adverse, physiological effects of toxic exposures, while putting would-be scientist allies on the defensive. Thinking with reflexive ecotoxicologists, as chronicled in chapters 4 and 5, not to mention my weed scientist accomplice who plays a leading role in chapter 3, leaves me in search of a middle path, wherein harmful outcomes of chemical pollution are taken seriously and yet not at the expense of overexposed and racialized communities, people living with disabilities, and queer, trans, and gender-non-conforming communities, and not in ways that counterproductively leave would-be scientist allies (or accomplices) playing defense.

I am also left wondering how a queer scientist feminist study of toxicants might approach the physiological harms caused by EDC exposures that are *not* related to animal sex or behavior, and moreover *do* generate serious bodily harms, in contrast to the imagined harms of gayness. And what about those synthetic hormones that are not so easily maligned? Environmental health advocates, myself included, love to hate pesticides and chemical weapons, but the synthetic estrogens of hormonal birth control comprise another ubiquitous EDC causing widespread harm to more-than-human and human animals.[36] Certainly defenders of environmental and social justice cannot and would not support the banning of hormonal birth control, or wish to prevent the conscious ingestion of synthetic hormones as part of gender-affirming care.[37] Without having definitively answered such questions, I am confident that approaches informed by critical feminist STS, namely those that take a principled stance against purity while radically caring for whomever and whatever has been declared useless, help scholars and activists generatively grapple with such nuance and complexity. The need for hormonal birth control is not the same as the need for chemical control of weeds. Killing animals for environmental health research is not the same as killing animals for chemical industry profit. But it is the historical, political, social, and cultural data—exceeding the axis of gender and talking back to history—that elucidates the crucial distinctions between these qualitatively different desires.

What I hope *Toxic Sexual Politics* has illustrated is that environmental health advocates and critical feminists alike want healthy, happy families and thriving ecosystems, however they may be conceived. I further hope that this critical feminist intervention helps turn efforts away from such a heavy reliance on, and privileging of, the highly uncertain results of conventional toxicology. Queer feminism-trained practitioners of a newly critical toxicology might instead turn toward the indisputable historical-material facts of unchecked corporate power, veraciously connecting those two most common collocates of *toxic*: "chemical" and "masculinity." An explicitly politicized study of toxicants will argue that it is not the dose that makes the poison, nor is it the timing that makes the poison, it is rather the poisoner who makes the poison—the *toxikon*, not the *pharmakon*. For it is critical feminist studies of toxic pollution that reveal how the transnational chemical industry's undue power to poison the planet with practical impunity is what most demonstrably, and most certainly, threatens the livability of all life on earth. Put simply, power is far more accurately measured than poison.

ACKNOWLEDGMENTS

I am most indebted to the animals, peoples, plants, and other organisms whose bodies unwillingly generated everything we think we know about toxicants. I also wish to thank the toxicology practitioners, researchers, environmental advocates, chemical and public health regulators, journalists, activists, and other experts who generously shared their time and knowledge with me, even if, and perhaps especially because, we experience and interpret the world quite differently.

For turning my food systems research toward the politics of toxic exposures, I thank Phil Brown, whose qualitative methods course in environmental sociology, on the ancestral homelands of the Narragansett Indian Tribe (Brown University), quite literally changed my life. I am likewise grateful to Mercedes Lyson and Meghan Kallman for noticing that I "think like a sociologist" and modeling how to have fun and look great while doing so. Kerry Smith, Kathy Spicer, and Ross Cheit also propelled me on to a PhD through their material, institutional, and philosophical support.

My time on the unceded territories of the Chochenyo speaking Ohlone people (at the University of California, Berkeley) profoundly shaped both my politics and my intellect. I give thanks to Louise Fortmann and her "lady lab," including Carolina Prado, Laura Dev, Margot Higgins, Juliet Lu, Christine Wilkinson, and Margiana Petersen-Rockney. My thinking and writing also owe a tremendous debt to Ashton Wesner—my first critical race feminist science studies role model—who ingeniously assembled the Queer Ecologies | Feminist Biologies working group that subsequently pollinated fruitful collaborations between me and Max Lambert, Ambika Kamath, and Beans Velocci. Thanks are likewise due to the many PhD peers who sharpened my analyses while softening the edges and brightening the depths of an unavoidably anxiety-producing doctoral program: Matt Libassi, Brian Klein, Vera Chang, Julie Gorecki, Sebastián Rubiano-Galvis, Julie

Pyatt, C. N. E. Corbin, Frances Roberts-Gregory, Laura Ward, Jim La-Chance, Adam Calo, Guillermo Douglass-Jaimes, Hossein Ayazi, Patrick Baur, Hekia Bodwitch, Maywa Montenegro, Jane Flegal, Lisa Kelley, Ted Grudin, Jennie Durant, Robert Parks, Akos Kokai, Sarick Matzen, Cleo Woelfle-Hazard, Jesse Williamson, Katie Wolf, Mindy Price, and Ataya Cesspooch. I am equally grateful to and ever-inspired by the insurgent scholar-activists (formerly) of the UC Berkeley Center for Race and Gender, especially Maria Faini, Desiree Valadares, John Mundell, Alisa Bierria, Pam Matsuoka, Rachel Lim, and Evelyn Nakano Glenn. The Food, Identity, and Representation reading group, summoned by Rosalie Z. Fanshel and graced by the presence of Lila Sharif and Marilisa Navarro, played a pivotal role in my political and intellectual journey as well, as did Kara Young and Hortencia Rodríguez, and my Science and Technology Studies comrades at Berkeley, particularly Santiago Molina, Morgan Ames, and Julia Lewandowski. I must thank the various toxicity scholar-activists scattered across campus too, particularly Mackenzie Feldman, Annie Shattuck, Mauricio Najarro, Ailén Vega, and Natalia Duong, alongside my sociology interlocutors Tara Gonsalves and Caleb Scoville, and cultural geography and anthropology accomplices Meredith Palmer and Julia Sizek, respectively. My fellow participants in "STS camp," or the 2019 annual California STS summer retreat on Coast Miwok territory (also known as the Marin Headlands), provided much intellectual and natural rejuvenation. I appreciate all my undergraduate and master's students at UC Berkeley, Mills College, and Middlebury College, whose endearing enthusiasm and unique insights helped me realize how healing teaching can be.

In addition to learning from my esteemed peers and students, I enjoyed the great privilege of receiving intellectual training from such scholarly giants as Charis Thompson, Alastair Iles, Trinh T. Minh-ha, Carolyn Merchant, Nancy Peluso, Leslie Salzinger, Minoo Moallem, and Cori Hayden. I was most fortunate to participate in a seminar with the unmatched Carolyn Finney during her last year at UC Berkeley, and I am also forever changed, in a good way, because of Julie Guthman's STS and food seminar at UC Santa Cruz—through which I reconnected with Charlotte Biltekoff and met the fantastic Stephanie Maroney, Andy Murray, and Emily Reisman—not to mention an innovative quad-seminar on the "alterlife" of chemicals cotaught by Michelle Murphy, Joe Masco,

Tim Choi, and Jake Kosek. UC Berkeley bioscience librarian Becky Miller was always exceedingly helpful, as was faculty graduate advisor Damian Elias and departmental administrators Bianca Victoria and Althea Grannum-Cummings. Many, many thanks are of course due to my all-star dissertation committee: Jake Kosek, Michael Mascarenhas, Rachel Morello-Frosch, and Raka Ray.

Luxuriating in the abundance of two postdocs, I could not have produced this work were it not for the intellectual, material, and moral support variously provided by Jade Sasser, Chikako Takeshita, Juliann Allison, Traci Brynne Voyles, David Pellow, Liz Carlisle, Lisa Materson, Lawrence Cohen, Julie Sze, Liza Grandia, Rebecca Herzig, Banu Subramaniam, Jenny Reardon, Jane Ward, and Ambika Kamath. Additional highlights from my (remote) time with the University of California, Riverside, and the University of Colorado, Boulder, include my stellar writing group with Natalia Duong, Heidi Amin-Hong, Reena Shadaan, and C. N. E. Corbin; the public health disparities writing group convened by Tanya Nieri; as well as critical conversations with Asa Bradman, Steven Haring, Emily Lim Rogers, Tamara Pico, Nadia Gaber, Yogi Hendlin, Anila Daulatzai, S. Chava Contreras, Sarah McCullough, Kalindi Vora, Salvador Zárate, and Stephen Molldrem.

I presented a version of chapter 2 at the UC Berkeley Center for Science, Technology, Medicine, and Society, and versions of chapter 3 at the Science and Justice Research Center at UC Santa Cruz as well as the Center for Ideas and Society at UC Riverside; I thank those hosts and audiences for their insightful questions and comments. I am especially grateful to the brilliant members of Ambika Kamath's Feminist Lenses for Animal Interaction Research (F.L.A.I.R.) Lab too. Last, I am delighted to be building my newest intellectual and political home alongside the critically engaged faculty, staff, and students at the University of Wisconsin–La Crosse, on Ho-Chunk Nation land. My colleagues in the Department of Race, Gender, and Sexuality Studies, namely Richard Breaux, Andrea Hansen, Sana Illahe, Shuma Iwai, Sona Kazemi, Alec Lass, and Terry Lilley, are truly enjoyable to work and think with. At UW–La Crosse, I am also buoyed by the friendly yet cunning mentorship of Kelly Sultzbach and Marie Moeller.

Elements of this research were funded by the UC Chancellor's Postdoctoral Fellowship Program; the UC Office of the President; the

Berkeley Food Institute; UC Berkeley Graduate Division; the UC Berkeley Department of Environmental Science, Policy, and Management; the UC Berkeley Department of Gender and Women's Studies; the UC Berkeley Center for Race and Gender; the UC Berkeley Center for Science, Technology, Medicine, and Society; the Great Lakes Scholar Program; and the P.E.O. Foundation.

I am deeply grateful to the executive social sciences editor at NYU Press, Ilene Kalish, and the Health, Society, and Inequality series editor Jennifer Reich, for their enthusiastic support of this project, as well as Yasemin Torfilli and Priyanka Ray for their manuscript shepherding skills. The constructive criticisms generously offered by anonymous peer reviewers significantly improved this book, as did the scrupulous editing of Valerie Zaborski and Annie Boisvert; I take full responsibility for any remaining mistakes.

There is of course a vast and enchanting world beyond the towers and moats of academia. Nic and Dewi randomly affirmed and inspired me in ways they likely and charmingly remain unaware of. Annie: thank you for being the best radical fairy goddessmother a girl could dream up. B: you will always be my favorite apothecary. Unpayable debts are due to Lilli, Allie, Pepper, Bowie, Iman, and Rex, for incessantly and adorably pulling me outside of my brain and pushing me back into my body. Brett, Julie W., Mom, Winona, Zack, Langhorne, all my aunts on both sides, and the entire Nahid family extended the kind of unconditional love and indispensable distractions that only kindred spirits and (chosen) relatives can. Somehow the stubborn ghost of my father silently, steadfastly, held my heart the entire way. And S. L. A.: who knew we would be the antidote?

APPENDIX

Queer Feminist Methods

Sociologist Jane Ward beautifully summarizes queer feminist methods as follows:

1. intersectional (queer projects are designed to investigate the ways that imperialism, settler colonialism, white supremacy, poverty, misogyny, and/or cissexism give shape to queer lives and queer resistance) (Nash and Browne 2010);
2. intimate, reflexive, and/or collaborative, often anchored within the extant subcultural and political affiliations of the researcher (Ward 2008);
3. infused with the erotic, or marked by a conscious recognition of sex practices, bodies, and desires and their place within the presumably asexual realm of research (Newton 2000);
4. interdisciplinary, or comprised of humanistic approaches concerned with the particularities of cultural representation and discourse, social science approaches concerned with behavioral patterns, and hybrid methodologies (Nash and Browne 2010);
5. focused on fluid or "messy" categories, shifting classifications, and people and practices often illegible within prevailing disciplinary schemas (Ahmed 2006).[1]

I was especially pleased to come across this list because I did so *after* completing the research for this book project, in a telling example of queer time,[2] and hence appreciated the affirmation that my unconventional methodological approach is no less rigorous than standard(ized) sociology or anthropology. Even antiassimilationist queers want to fit in sometimes. At the risk of limiting queer feminist methods to this numbered list, I check these boxes somewhat cheekily, recognizing that queer methods are not set in stone (pun intended). I have already described the intersectional feminist genealogies that inform my reading, thinking, and writing (list item number 1) in the introduction.

Regarding number 2, my choice to study up, meaning study scientists rather than activists, was intentional, heeding the sage advice of not only anthropologist Laura Nader, who coined the term "studying up," but also cultural theorists Eve Tuck and K. Wayne Yang, who caution well-intentioned liberal scholars against "damage narratives"—those serious yet myopic studies of disadvantaged peoples, often conducted by advantaged academics, that dwell on said communities' so-called damages so much so that the seemingly sympathetic studies themselves become yet another medium of damage.[3] I decided to pursue ethnographic research with relatively powerful figures in certain subfields of toxicology, rather than, say, fence-line environmental justice (EJ) activists, because I am not an EJ activist. While I support the work of EJ activism, I felt that given my particular social location and background, my scholarly intervention would be better directed toward the highly trained, US-based researchers and professional advocacy organization and government agency staff with whom I appear, on the surface, to have a greater affinity. Overall, my interlocutors and I shared environmental, if not political, commitments, and I conducted my ethnographic research as reflexively, ethically, and collaboratively as possible, sharing drafts with and incorporating feedback from my ecotoxicologist interlocuters before any other readers, for example.

Both my discursive and ethnographic analyses are "infused with the erotic," referring to list item number 3, as I underscore the implicit and explicit sexual politics that permeate toxicology textbooks, classrooms, laboratories, and field sites, differently detailed in each of this book's chapters. This mentioning of research materials and sites leads me to queer methods clue number 4: by critically analyzing scientific texts as cultural texts, and by observing, interviewing, and collaborating with ecotoxicologists, I draw from humanistic and social science disciplines, namely critical theory and the environmental humanities, as well as environmental sociology and medical anthropology. The scientific texts of my queer feminist archive include classic and contemporary

US toxicology textbooks, scientific papers on EDC toxicology more specifically, federal chemical risk assessment manuals, and, to a lesser extent, toxic tort transcripts and US congressional testimony.

My ethnographic research took me from graduate-level toxicology classrooms and professional toxicology conferences to outdoor toxicological experimental field sites and indoor toxicological research laboratories. I also interviewed twenty-four experts who regularly interface with toxicology for some core aspect of their careers—ranging from fresh young US activist to seasoned supranational health agency director—as well as nine members of the toxicology laboratory I embedded myself within for the second part of this project.[4] Throughout the book, I cite the first twenty-four interviewees as "expert interviews" and the second nine interviewees as "lab interviews," though the laboratory scientists are of course experts as well.

The arguments in chapters 1–3 are based primarily on my textual analyses, twenty-four expert interview transcripts, and participant observation of toxicology classrooms, conferences, and outdoor experimental field sites. Chapters 4 and 5 draw almost entirely from my ethnographic research with the aforementioned toxicology lab, which consisted of twenty weeks of participant observation and nine lab member interviews. The thirty-three interviews I conducted in total lasted anywhere from fifteen minutes to ninety minutes, with the majority averaging about one hour in length. I audio-recorded ten of these thirty-three interviews, which I then transcribed word-for-word. For the other twenty-three interviews I took copious, hand-written notes while listening (table A.1). I coded all texts (inclusive of scientific and regulatory texts and my field notes and interview transcripts) with the help of MaxQDA software, versions 2018 and 2020.

Last, my queer feminist methodological approach dwells in fluid, messy categories, not the least of which are endocrine-disrupting chemicals themselves, discussed in more depth in chapter 2, and including everything from what "sex" means in different contexts to what "safe" means to different actors. As chapters 4 and 5 demonstrate most explicitly, queer people and queer ecologies generally remain illegible in mainstream ecotoxicology, as does the agency and desire of disabled peoples and experimental animals alike. A proudly queer ecofeminist practice of ecotoxicology just might change that, reclaiming science for justice.

TABLE A.1 Interviews

Count	Sector	In person, phone, or Zoom	Transcribed recording (R) or handwritten notes (N)
Expert Interviews (conducted spring and summer 2019)			
1.	Research	Phone	N
2.	Regulatory Policy	Phone	N
3.	Advocacy	Phone	N
4.	Regulatory Policy	Phone	N
5.	Advocacy	Phone	N
6–7.	Multiple (toxicology conference)	In person	N
8.	Advocacy	Phone	N
9.	Advocacy	Phone	N
10.	Advocacy	Phone	N
11.	Regulatory Policy	Phone	N
12.	Research	In person	N
13.	Research	Phone	N
14.	Research	Phone	N
15.	Journalism	Phone	N
16.	Research	Phone	N
17.	Research	Phone	N
18.	Regulatory Policy	Phone	N
19–22.	Multiple (weed science conference)	In person	N
23.	Industry	Phone	N
24.*	Research	Zoom	R
Lab Interviews (conducted spring and summer 2021)			
25.	Research	Zoom	R
26.	Research	Zoom	R
27.	Research	Zoom	R
28.	Research	Zoom	R
29.	Research	Zoom	R
30.	Research	Zoom	R
31.	Research	Zoom	R
32.	Research	Zoom	R
33.	Research	Zoom	R

*conducted spring 2021

NOTES

PREFACE
1 Nixon, *Slow Violence and the Environmentalism of the Poor.*
2 Hendlin, "Surveying the Chemical Anthropocene."

INTRODUCTION
1 Brown, "Finding the Man in the State," 14.
2 Boast, "Theorizing the Gay Frog."
3 For scientific reports on EDCs, see Colborn and Clement, "Chemically-Induced Alterations in Sexual and Functional Development"; Bergman et al., *State of the Science of Endocrine Disrupting Chemicals—2012.* For queer feminist critiques of such reports, see Di Chiro, "Polluted Politics?"
4 Swan and Colino, *Count Down.*
5 Guerre, *Disappearing Male*; Brockovich, "Plummeting Sperm Counts, Shrinking Penises."
6 White, "Experimental Animal in Victorian Britain."
7 Laskow, "Sad Sex Lives of Suburban Frogs."
8 Lambert and Packer, "How Gendered Language Leads Scientists Astray."
9 Fausto-Sterling, *Sexing the Body*; Davis, *Contesting Intersex*; Human Rights Campaign, "Attacks on Gender Affirming Care by State Map," Human Rights Campaign, last updated November 13, 2023, https://www.hrc.org.
10 Bagemihl, *Biological Exuberance.*
11 Lambert et al., "Molecular Evidence for Sex Reversal."
12 Packer and Lambert, "What's Gender Got to Do with It?"
13 *Wikipedia*, "American Chemistry Council," accessed May 18, 2022, https://en .wikipedia.org.
14 I dwell in toxicant science and its applications for this book. For critical studies of toxicant regulation, see Boudia and Jas, *Powerless Science?*
15 Board of Governors of the Federal Reserve System, "Celebrating 100 Years of the Industrial Production Index," The Fed—Industrial Production and Capacity Utilization—G.17, January 18, 2019. https://www.federalreserve.gov.
16 Environmental Protection Agency, "CDR Data Limitations Summary," Chemical Data Reporting, September 20, 2022, https://www.epa.gov.
17 Environmental Protection Agency, "Summary of the Toxic Substances Control Act," Laws and Regulations, last updated September 29, 2023, https://www.epa.gov.

18 Environmental Protection Agency, "Chemical Production Data," Chemical Data Reporting, September 20, 2022, https://www.epa.gov.

19 Gross and Birnbaum, "Regulating Toxic Chemicals for Public and Environmental Health"; ChemicalSafetyFacts.org, "Debunking the Myths."

20 Moore et al., "2023 Guide to the Business of Chemistry."

21 Adams, *Glyphosate and the Swirl*, 10.

22 For various political and chemical legacies of the insecticide DDT, see Grier, "Ban of DDT and Subsequent Recovery of Reproduction in Bald Eagles"; Davis, *Banned*; Conis, "DDT Disbelievers."

23 Cone, *Silent Snow*; Petryna, *Life Exposed*; Boudia et al., "Residues: Rethinking Chemical Environments."

24 Masri et al., "Toxicant-Induced Loss of Tolerance for Chemicals, Foods, and Drugs."

25 Landecker, "Antibiotic Resistance and the Biology of History"; Blum et al., "Mercury Isotopes Identify Near-Surface Marine Mercury in Deep-Sea Trench Biota."

26 Liboiron, Tironi, and Calvillo, "Toxic Politics."

27 Oxford University Press, "Oxford Word of the Year 2018," Oxford Languages, 2018, https://languages.oup.com.

28 Oxford University Press.

29 It remains politically important to distinguish *toxins*, which are naturally occurring in certain plants and animals, from *toxicants*, which chemical companies invent and synthesize. See Liboiron, "Toxins or Toxicants?"

30 Oxford University Press, "Oxford Word of the Year 2018."

31 For a more thorough review of the literature, in which I rehearse a similar argument regarding what's missing from "deceit and denial" explanations, see Packer, "Chemical Agents."

32 Markowitz and Rosner, *Deceit and Denial*.

33 For example, see Ross and Amter, *Polluters*; Oreskes and Conway, *Merchants of Doubt*; Michaels, *Doubt Is Their Product*; Markowitz and Rosner, *Deceit and Denial*; Proctor, *Cancer Wars*; Krimsky and Gillam, "Roundup Litigation Discovery Documents."

34 Michaels, *Doubt Is Their Product*.

35 To offer only a small handful of examples, see Pellow, *Resisting Global Toxics*; Lerner, *Sacrifice Zones*; Bullard, *Dumping in Dixie*; Brown, *Toxic Exposures*.

36 Notable exceptions to the tendency to take toxicological findings at face value include Murphy, *Sick Building Syndrome and the Problem of Uncertainty*; Chen, "Toxic Animacies, Inanimate Affections"; Wiebe, *Everyday Exposure*; Shapiro, Zakariya, and Roberts, "Wary Alliance"; Liboiron, *Pollution Is Colonialism*.

37 United Church of Christ Commission for Racial Justice, *Toxic Wastes and Race in the United States*; Bullard, *Dumping in Dixie*; Taylor, *Toxic Communities*.

38 For excellent histories and more recent analyses of the US environmental justice movement, see Taylor, "Rise of the Environmental Justice Paradigm"; Kojola and Pellow, "New Directions in Environmental Justice Studies."

39 For other EJ-supportive critics of environmental health science, see Shapiro, Zakariya, and Roberts, "Wary Alliance"; Adams, *Glyphosate and the Swirl*. Adams also cautions STS critics of toxic exposures, reminding us that "the science of chemical toxicity frequently lets us down in efforts to source accountability and redress. So too does the analytical toolkit of science studies scholarship when it comes to aligning activism with science. We cannot use the scientific facts when they go our way but dismiss them when they align with a consensus we disagree with" (8).

40 On science as disinterested, see Merton, *Sociology of Science*.

41 Gallo, "History and Scope of Toxicology," 8th ed.

42 "DuPont Song."

43 Casarett and Doull, *Toxicology*.

44 Davis, *Banned*.

45 For more on (white and male) epistemic entitlement, see Manne, *Down Girl*; Prescod-Weinstein, "Making Black Women Scientists under White Empiricism." The sociocultural meaning of the term "gaslighting" is fairly well defined by the *Encyclopedia Britannica*:

> The term is derived from the title of a 1938 British stage play, *Gas Light*, which was subsequently produced as a film, *Gaslight*, in the United Kingdom (1940) and the United States (1944). Those dramas vividly, if somewhat simplistically, depicted some of the basic elements of the technique. These may include attempting to convince the victim of the truth of something intuitively bizarre or outrageous by forcefully insisting on it or by marshaling superficial evidence; flatly denying that one has said or done something that one has obviously said or done; dismissing the victim's contrary perceptions or feelings as invalid or pathological; questioning the knowledge and impugning the motives of persons who contradict the viewpoint of the gaslighter; gradually isolating the victim from independent sources of information and validation, including other people; and manipulating the physical environment to encourage the victim to doubt the veracity of his [*sic*] memories or perception. (Brian Duignan, "Gaslighting," in *Britannica*, last updated March 25, 2024, https://www.britannica.com.)

Feminist philosopher Kate Manne elaborates on the inherent misogyny of the practice, a topic I return to in chapter 3, see Manne, *Down Girl*. See also Sweet, "Sociology of Gaslighting."

46 Throughout this book, I use "environmental toxicology" when I am referring to toxicology conducted for human health, and "ecotoxicology" for toxicology conducted for ecosystems and more-than-human animals.

47 Bergman et al., *State of the Science of Endocrine Disrupting Chemicals—2012*.

48 A couple good places to start include Crenshaw et al., *Critical Race Theory*; Scott, "Gender."

49 Crenshaw, "Mapping the Margins."

50 Crenshaw, "Demarginalizing the Intersection of Race and Sex."

51 Cho, Crenshaw, and McCall, "Toward a Field of Intersectionality Studies." See also Nash, *Black Feminism Reimagined*.

52 Brown, "Finding the Man in the State," 14.

53 On the politics of inclusion more broadly, see Ahmed, *On Being Included*.

54 Schor, *Overworked American*.

55 Bhattacharya, *Social Reproduction Theory*.

56 Glenn, "From Servitude to Service Work"; Parreñas, "Reproductive Labour of Migrant Workers"; Bhattacharya, *Social Reproduction Theory*.

57 Hochschild, *Second Shift*; Matchar, *Homeward Bound*; Kasymova et al., "Impacts of the COVID-19 Pandemic on the Productivity of Academics Who Mother"; Kreeger et al., "Ten Simple Rules for Women Principal Investigators During a Pandemic."

58 Even "hard science" struggles against chemical regulation, for instance, when the rules around toxic exposures have not yet been updated to accommodate the latest advances in scientific measurements of toxicity. See Shostak, "Environmental Justice and Genomics."

59 Wiebe, *Everyday Exposure*, 147.

60 See also Cordner's work on "strategic science translation" in Cordner, *Toxic Safety*.

61 The postcolonial and feminist STS literature is rich and vast; here I list but a few resources: Bordo, "Cartesian Masculinization of Thought"; Smith, *Decolonizing Methodologies*; Schiebinger, *Nature's Body*; Anderson, *Race and the Crisis of Humanism*; Keel, *Divine Variations*; Subramaniam, *Ghost Stories for Darwin*; Harding, *Postcolonial Science and Technology Studies Reader*; Tilley, *Africa as a Living Laboratory*.

62 Kim, *Dangerous Crossings*; Ko, *Racism as Zoological Witchcraft*; Jackson, *Becoming Human*; Miller, *Why Fish Don't Exist*.

63 For instance, see Pratt, *Imperial Eyes*; Polcha, "Breeding Insects and Reproducing White Supremacy in Maria Sibylla Merian's Ecology of Dispossession."

64 Pratt, *Imperial Eyes*.

65 Kim, *Dangerous Crossings*; Keel, *Divine Variations*; Jackson, *Becoming Human*; Wynter, "Unsettling the Coloniality of Being/Power/Truth/Freedom."

66 Visvanathan, "From the Annals of the Laboratory State"; Messing and Mergler, "Rat Couldn't Speak, But We Can"; Ahuja, *Bioinsecurities*; Grimm, "How Many Mice and Rats Are Used in U.S. Labs?"

67 Markowitz, "Pelvic Politics"; Schiebinger, *Nature's Body*; Russett, *Sexual Science*; Oyěwùmí, *Invention of Women*.

68 Aph Ko offers "multidimensional feminism" as a way of capturing the coconstitution of gender, race, sex, and species. See Ko, *Racism as Zoological Witchcraft*.

69 Somerville, "Scientific Racism and the Emergence of the Homosexual Body"; Ferguson, "Of Our Normative Strivings"; Lugones, "Coloniality of Gender."

70 Patil, "Heterosexual Matrix as Imperial Effect."

71 Brown, "Finding the Man in the State."

72 I did not know what Casarett meant by "the distaff set" so I had to look it up. This phrase was used to refer to women because women were typically assigned the work of weaving; a distaff is part of the apparatus of a weaver's loom. Casarett, "Origin and Scope of Toxicology," 6.

73 For a classic essay on how European and Euro-American women's contributions to science have been dismissed and omitted, see Rossiter, "Matthew Matilda Effect in Science."

74 Thus named in reference to the French Enlightenment-era philosopher René Descartes who (in)famously separated thought from sense, mind from body, and culture from nature (and whose followers hence justified, among other horrid practices, the live dissection of animals because, in their worldview, nonhuman animals and "lesser humans" cannot experience suffering). Descartes, *Descartes*. Descartes did not, apparently, dissect live animals himself, but practitioners who did so cited his philosophies as justification. See Riskin, *Restless Clock*. See also the harrowing accounts of public surgeries performed without anesthesia, repeatedly, on African American women in particular, a heinous practice which brought us today's gynecology. Washington, *Medical Apartheid*. Tu's history of dermatology also documents how imprisoned men in the United States, most of whom were African American, were experimented on without adequate pain medication because researchers considered them to be more animal-like and hence more tolerant of, if not impervious to, pain, as compared to their white counterparts. Tu, *Experiments in Skin*.

75 For a variety of historical examples of non-Cartesian modes of thought and being, see Irigaray, *This Sex Which Is Not One*; Taylor, *Sources of the Self*; Cajete, *Native Science*; Federici, *Caliban and the Witch*; Wynter and McKittrick, "Unparalleled Catastrophe for Our Species?"; Povinelli, *Geontologies*; Rusert, *Fugitive Science*; Kimmerer, "Covenant of Reciprocity."

76 Rachel Carson famously critiqued this idea in *Silent Spring*. Or as one of my interviewees, a toxicologist at a national environmental nonprofit, scoffed, "[Industry toxicologists] overcomplicate models to make data work in their favor; they create a certain model of how [they] think the body acts when you get exposed to a chemical—and people wanted really complicated models—you could put so many parameters into a model and still make it replicate the data you want . . . to get from point A to point B you don't need a Maserati . . . What a ridiculous idea [that a pharmaceutical] 'target' is the brain [for example]! It could go anywhere!" Expert interview no. 17, 2019.

77 Liboiron, *Pollution Is Colonialism*.

78 Porter, *Trust in Numbers*.

79 Taylor, *Rise of the American Conservation Movement*; Cronon, "Uses of Environmental History"; Zimring, *Clean and White*.

80 Haraway, "Teddy Bear Patriarchy"; Bederman, *Manliness & Civilization*; Stern, *Eugenic Nation*.

81 Colborn, Dumanoski, and Myers, *Our Stolen Future*; Swan and Colino, *Count Down*; Brockovich, "Plummeting Sperm Counts, Shrinking Penises."

82 Frickel, *Chemical Consequences*, 86.

83 Merchant, *Death of Nature*; Plumwood, *Feminism and the Mastery of Nature*; Ray, *Ecological Other*; Voyles, "Toxic Masculinity."

84 See, for example Ah-King and Hayward, "Toxic Sexes"; Agard-Jones, "Bodies in the System"; Pollock, "Queering Endocrine Disruption"; Shotwell, *Against Purity*.

85 Bagemihl, *Biological Exuberance*; Terry, "'Unnatural Acts' in Nature"; Monk et al., "Alternative Hypothesis for the Evolution of Same-Sex Sexual Behaviour in Animals."

86 Packer and Lambert, "What's Gender Got to Do with It?"

87 Packer and Lambert.

88 Roy, "Asking Different Questions."

89 Hird, "Naturally Queer."

90 I borrow the term "scientist feminist" from Roy, *Molecular Feminisms*.

91 Colborn, Dumanoski, and Myers, *Our Stolen Future*.

92 Stern, *Eugenic Nation*; Clare, *Brilliant Imperfection*; Schuller, *Biopolitics of Feeling*.

93 I borrow the phrasing "live, learn, work, play, pray, and eat" from environmental and food justice movements. For example, see Gottlieb, "Where We Live, Work, Play . . . and Eat"; Greenaction for Health and Environmental Justice, "Environmental Justice & Environmental Racism," accessed May 31, 2023. http://greenaction.org. See also Voyles, *Wastelanding*; Lerner, *Sacrifice Zones*.

94 Diamanti-Kandarakis et al., "Endocrine-Disrupting Chemicals"; Merrill et al., "Consensus on the Key Characteristics of Endocrine-Disrupting Chemicals as a Basis for Hazard Identification."

95 Krimsky, "Essay"; Benbrook et al., "Commentary."

96 Expert interview no. 11, 2019.

97 Expert interview no. 17, 2019.

98 I use "critical feminist" as shorthand for the numerous critical approaches I embrace throughout this book, including critical race theory, queer theory, feminist theory, postcolonial theory, and disability theory.

99 As cited in Ray and Sibara, introduction to *Disability Studies and the Environmental Humanities*, 10–11.

100 Packer and Lambert, "What's Gender Got to Do with It?"

101 Perret, "Chemical Castration."

102 Davis, *Contesting Intersex*; Viloria and Nieto, *Spectrum of Sex*; Barba, "Keeping Them Down."

103 A mere handful of examples include: Lancaster, *Trouble with Nature*; Richardson et al., "Focus on Preclinical Sex Differences Will Not Address Women's and Men's Health Disparities"; Clare, *Brilliant Imperfection*; Johnson, "Bringing Together Feminist Disability Studies and Environmental Justice"; Velocci, "Battle Over Trans Rights Is About Power, Not Science"; Karkazis, "Misuses of 'Biological Sex'"; Egede and Walker, "Structural Racism, Social Risk Factors, and Covid-19."

104 I thank Beans Velocci for pushing me to make this crucial distinction.

105 Seymour, *Strange Natures*, 180.

106 Shadaan and Murphy, "EDCs as Industrial Chemicals and Settler Colonial Structures."

107 Sustainable Pulse, "Glyphosate Herbicides Now Banned or Restricted in 20 Countries Worldwide," Sustainable Pulse, May 28, 2019, https://sustainablepulse.com.

108 Székács and Darvas, "Forty Years with Glyphosate," 248.

109 For specific, deliberate attempts to export US toxicological theory and method, see Frickel, *Chemical Consequences*; Zimdahl, *History of Weed Science in the United States*.

110 Haraway, "Situated Knowledges," 581.

111 Roberts, *Messengers of Sex*, 57. See also Martin, "Egg and the Sperm"; Spanier, *Im/Partial Science*.

112 Gallo, "History and Scope of Toxicology," 8th ed.

113 Expert interview no. 13, 2019.

114 Shostak, *Exposed Science*.

115 Akaba, "Science as a Double-Edged Sword"; Shapiro, Zakariya, and Roberts, "Wary Alliance."

116 For relatively early work on the masculinism of dominant science, see Bordo, "Cartesian Masculinization of Thought."

117 Casarett and Doull, *Toxicology*.

118 Linda Nash has argued that environmental toxicologists simply transferred occupational health toxicology, formerly known as "industrial hygiene," from the indoor conditions of the factory (and laboratory) to the outdoor conditions of the agricultural field, without making the necessary (if impossibly so) adjustments for the vagaries of wind (causing "pesticide drift" onto other plants, animals, and human agricultural laborers), soil and riparian ecologies (wherein agricultural chemicals leach into the soil and enter waterways), or biomagnification (wherein small amounts of pesticide ingested by smaller organisms become larger and larger amounts of poison for their predators, who inevitably consume greater quantities of poison by virtue of eating multiple, poisoned prey), among other differences between indoor and outdoor exposure settings. Nash, "Purity and Danger." See also Sellers, *Hazards of the Job*.

119 Food and Agriculture Organization of the United Nations, "Pesticides Use."

120 Seymour, *Strange Natures*, 27.

121 Seymour, 184.

122 Horkeimer and Adorno, "Concept of Enlightenment."

123 For more on biological science's use of the term "sacrifice," when it comes to experimental animal death, see Lynch, "Sacrifice and the Transformation of the Animal Body into a Scientific Object."

124 Lab interview no. 5, 2021.

125 For more on the history, politics, and ethics of substituting animals for humans in biomedical research, see Thompson, *Good Science*.

126 Herzig, *Suffering for Science*; Daston and Galison, *Objectivity*.

127 See also O'Brien, "Being a Scientist Means Taking Sides."

128 I thank Jake Kosek and Natalia Duong, respectively, for these excellent turns of phrase.
129 Murphy, "Alterlife and Decolonial Chemical Relations."
130 Murphy, "Alterlife and Decolonial Chemical Relations." I paraphrase the notion widely attributed to Antonio Gramsci, "pessimism of the intellect; optimism of the will." For recent reflections on this approach, see Antonini, "Pessimism of the Intellect, Optimism of the Will."

1. THE DEVIL TRICK

1 Cohn, "Sex and Death in the Rational World of Defense Intellectuals," 711.
2 Brown et al., "Gulf of Difference"; Masco, "Mutant Ecologies"; Lyons, "Chemical Warfare in Colombia"; Tu, *Experiments in Skin*.
3 *Casarett & Doull's* has remained one of Doody's Core Titles—"a book or software title that represents essential knowledge needed by professionals or students in a given discipline and is highly recommended for the collection of a library that serves health sciences specialists"—for as long as this honor has been bestowed, or since 2004. See Doody Enterprises, Inc., "Core Title Selection Process," Doody's Core Titles, last updated 2018, https://www.doody.com. The predecessor to Doody's Core Titles was the "Brandon-Hill list," on which *Casarett & Doull's* also made regular appearances.
4 See Sellers, *Hazards of the Job*; Frickel, *Chemical Consequences*; Murphy, *Sick Building Syndrome and the Problem of Uncertainty*; Shostak, *Exposed Science*; Davis, *Banned*; Conis, "DDT Disbelievers"; Cordner, *Toxic Safety*.
5 Frickel, *Chemical Consequences*, 63. Frickel characterizes the vein of genetic toxicology that emerged in the 1960s and '70s US as a "scientist social movement," though he concedes that these scientist-activists tended toward reform rather than revolution.
6 C. Wright Mills, "The Professional Ideology of Social Pathologists," (1943), *Power, Politics and People* (Oxford University Press, 1963, 525), as cited in Millett, *Sexual Politics*, 299.
7 Hodge, foreword to *Toxicology*.
8 Wexler and Hayes, "Evolving Journey of Toxicology."
9 Haraway appears to have been explicitly critiquing Thomas Nagel's claim that dominant science can adopt a view from nowhere. Haraway, "Situated Knowledges"; Nagel, *View from Nowhere*.
10 Wexler and Hayes, "Evolving Journey of Toxicology," 3.
11 Liboiron, "There's No Such Thing as 'We.'"
12 To name but a few: Bullard, *Dumping in Dixie*; Stein et al., *New Perspectives on Environmental Justice*; Pellow, *Resisting Global Toxics*; Taylor, *Toxic Communities*; Scott, *Our Chemical Selves*; Wiebe, *Everyday Exposure*.
13 Benbrook, "Trends in Glyphosate Herbicide Use."
14 Ryerson, "Blended Bifurcation."

15 Frickel, *Chemical Consequences*; Shostak, *Exposed Science*; Davis, *Banned*; Cordner, *Toxic Safety*.

16 Much feminist scholarship has identified how military cultures are particularly masculinist, so I will not repeat those arguments here but rather take it as a given that the military is necessarily also masculinist. For instance, see Cohn, "Sex and Death in the Rational World of Defense Intellectuals"; Enloe, *Bananas, Beaches and Bases*.

17 Expert interview no. 2, 2019.

18 Expert interview no. 3, 2019.

19 Expert interview no. 18, 2019.

20 Expert interview no. 10, 2019.

21 Welsome, *Plutonium Files*.

22 University of California Academic Senate, *University of California*.

23 Morrow, Bruce, and Doull, "Louis James Casarett (1927–1972)"; Klaassen, dedication in *Casarett & Doull's Toxicology*; Davis, *Banned*.

24 Morrow, Bruce, and Doull, "Louis James Casarett (1927–1972)."

25 Davis, *Banned*, 76. Given that Geiling's first graduate student, Frances Oldham Kelsey (PhD 1938), was a woman, one might be tempted to think he was refreshingly ahead of his social time. However, it was subsequently revealed that when Geiling accepted Kelsey he thought, based on her paper application, that she was a man. To his credit he did not withdraw his offer once she arrived, and Kelsey apparently thrived in the lab as a student and eventual colleague (73). The name Frances Kelsey may be familiar to readers for other reasons; she received the President's Award for Distinguished Federal Civilian Service from President Kennedy for rejecting the thalidomide pharmaceutical application during her time at the Food and Drug Administration (FDA). Chemical corporations sought to market thalidomide as a sedative for pregnant women, despite "a complete lack of studies to consider thalidomide's fetal effects" (175). Even as reports of severe birth defects emerged, from European women who had taken thalidomide while pregnant, the chemical manufacturers heavily pressured the FDA and Kelsey to approve their application. Nevertheless she persisted. See Davis, *Banned*.

26 Omenn, "Report on the Accomplishments of the Commission."

27 Casarett and Doull, preface to *Toxicology*, vii.

28 Casarett, "Origin and Scope of Toxicology," 9.

29 For more on the politics of "safe use," see Shattuck, "Risky Subjects."

30 Casarett, "Origin and Scope of Toxicology," 9–10. Emphasis added.

31 Thanks are due to Matt Libassi for this important observation.

32 Nixon, *Slow Violence and the Environmentalism of the Poor*.

33 Daston and Galison, *Objectivity*.

34 Latour, *Science in Action*.

35 Hodge, foreword to *Toxicology*, v.

36 Casarett, "Toxicologic Evaluation," 11.

37 Packer, "Becoming with Toxicity," 12.

38 Thomas, "Toxic Responses of the Reproductive System," 547.

39 Thomas, 547.

40 Drugs.com, "Thalidomide (Monograph) for Professionals"; *Wikipedia*, s.v. "Thalidomide," accessed May 29, 2021, https://en.wikipedia.org.

41 Dally, "Thalidomide."

42 Winerip, "Death and Afterlife of Thalidomide." This is indeed the same Dr. Kelsey who also happened to be E. M. K. Geiling's first graduate student, whom he had accepted under the mistaken impression that she was a man. Ah, the ways in which women have to twist patriarchy to their advantage. See Davis, *Banned*.

43 Thomas, "Toxic Responses of the Reproductive System," 547.

44 Gallo, "History and Scope of Toxicology," 4th ed., 3–11; Gallo, "History and Scope of Toxicology," 8th ed.

45 Gallo, "History and Scope of Toxicology," 8th ed.

46 Casarett, "Origin and Scope of Toxicology," 9.

47 Hodge, foreword to *Toxicology*, v.

48 Gallo, "History and Scope of Toxicology," 8th ed.

49 Gallo. Emphasis added.

50 Gallo. Emphasis added.

51 *Chemical & Engineering News* reports, "In what is being billed as progress toward a split-up next year, DowDuPont has named the three firms it intends to become. Two of the companies will retain the Dow and DuPont names. However, the third, an agricultural chemical and seed firm, will get a new identity: Corteva Agriscience. . . . Corteva, DowDuPont says, is taken from words meaning 'heart' and 'nature' in Latin and Hebrew, respectively." Tullo, "DowDuPont Names Its Three Planned Spin-Offs."

52 For example, see Markowitz and Rosner, *Deceit and Denial*; Ross and Amter, *Polluters*; Oreskes and Conway, *Merchants of Doubt*; Proctor, "Everyone Knew but No One Had Proof"; Gillam, *Whitewash*; Lerner, *Sacrifice Zones*.

53 Expert interview no. 13, 2019.

54 Murphy, *Sick Building Syndrome and the Problem of Uncertainty*; Cordner, *Toxic Safety*; Jill Lindsey Harrison, *From the Inside Out*.

55 Brian Cummings, "Michael Gallo Receives 2021 SOT Founders Award."

56 Gallo, "History and Scope of Toxicology," 8th ed.

57 Casarett, "Origin and Scope of Toxicology," 9.

58 For a variety of longer-term and widespread effects of nuclear production, see Masco, "Mutant Ecologies"; Voyles, *Wastelanding*; Cram, "Living in Dose"; Garcia, *Pastoral Clinic*; Petryna, *Life Exposed*.

59 Gallo, "History and Scope of Toxicology," 8th ed. Emphasis added.

60 For more on the abstract, distancing, and masculinist language of nuclear defense analysts, see Cohn, "Sex and Death in the Rational World of Defense Intellectuals."

61 Tu, *Experiments in Skin*. For additional examples of US military justifications for radioactive extraction and scientific experimentation, see Voyles, *Wastelanding*; De Chadarevian, *Heredity under the Microscope*.

62 "J. Robert Oppenheimer: 'I Am Become Death, the Destroyer of Worlds.'" 1965 television interview with J. Robert Oppenheimer. YouTube video, 0:00:53, August 6, 2011. https://www.youtube.com/watch?v=lb13ynu3Iac. Oppenheimer was head of the Los Alamos National Laboratory that developed the nuclear bomb under the directives of the Manhattan Project.

63 Wexler and Hayes, "Evolving Journey of Toxicology."

64 Wexler and Hayes, 3.

65 Nash, "Purity and Danger"; Davis, *Banned*.

66 Brown, "Finding the Man in the State."

67 Sellers, *Hazards of the Job*.

68 On the toxicity of newly industrializing capitalist economies, see Engels, *Origin of the Family, Private Property and the State*; Foster, *Marx's Ecology*.

69 Brown and Thornton, "Percivall Pott (1714–1788)," 69.

70 Rachel Morello-Frosch, personal communication, 2016.

71 The Global Movement for Black Lives being one prominent example, and also see Povinelli, "Windjarrameru, the Stealing C*nts,"; Roberts, "What Gets Inside."

72 Hacking, "Language, Truth, and Reason."

73 Keller, *Refiguring Life*, 35.

74 Thompson, "Critique in the Era of Trump."

75 For one such socio-chemical analysis, see Guthman, *Weighing In*.

76 Neil, Malmfors, and Slovic, "Intuitive Toxicology."

2. MAGICAL AUTHORITY

1 Manne, *Down Girl*, 140–41. Emphasis original.

2 Prescod-Weinstein, "Making Black Women Scientists under White Empiricism," 425.

3 Daniel Goldstein, *LinkedIn* profile, accessed August 6, 2020, https://www.linkedin.com/in/daniel-goldstein-76b06b9.

4 *Johnson v. Monsanto* involved a former landscaper, Dewayne "Lee" Johnson, who sued the US-based Monsanto Company following his diagnosis of the fatal blood cancer non-Hodgkin's lymphoma, because Monsanto advertises its flagship product, Roundup pesticide, as noncarcinogenic. A San Francisco County (California, US) superior court jury awarded Johnson $287 billion in damages, which the judge subsequently reduced to $78 million. Monsanto, which had recently been purchased by the German-based Bayer Corporation, appealed the verdict. For more on this protracted battle, see Gillam, *Monsanto Papers*.

5 The appropriation of ancient figures like Paracelsus is an old trick of conservative minds. As Martin Bernal's controversial work argues, beginning in the eighteenth century, dominant white culture reimagined Classical Greece as white, denying its African and Levantine roots, as a sort of intellectual justification for racism. See

Bernal, *Black Athena*; Bernal, "Race, Class and Gender." More recently, far-right supporters of former Brazilian President Jair Bolsonaro frequently used a Latin battle cry associated with the First Crusade—*Deus vult*, or "God wills it"—to legitimize their reactionary politics, "emphasizing a [fictionalized] historical continuity that casts white Brazilians as the true heirs to Europe." Pachá, "Why the Brazilian Far Right Loves the European Middle Ages."

Toxicology's founding fathers perhaps did not write in their textbooks and academic articles the sort of overtly racist pronouncements that eighteenth century intellectuals and twenty-first century neo-fascists have variously published. However, their reliance on selected practitioners and documents, from the (reimagined) European late Middle Ages and early Renaissance, to lend credence to a science devoted to the rationalization of twentieth century synthetic toxins demonstrates one of many ways that racial constructs remain central to the formation of modern institutions, from toxicology to Twitter. See also Morrison, "Academic Whispers [2004]"; Glenn, "Settler Colonialism as Structure."

6 Vogel, "From 'The Dose Makes the Poison' to 'The Timing Makes the Poison'"; Lanphear, "Low-Level Toxicity of Chemicals."

7 For instance, see Shapiro, "Attuning to the Chemosphere"; Wiebe, *Everyday Exposure*.

8 Levin, "Monsanto Trial."

9 For an excellent analysis of the ways measuring the "how much" happens at the expense of the "how," see Shapiro, Zakariya, and Roberts, "Wary Alliance." See also Akaba, "Science as a Double-Edged Sword."

10 I am indebted to B. Nahid for this observation.

11 Expert interview no. 13, 2019.

12 Casarett, "Origin and Scope of Toxicology," 3, 9. Emphasis added.

13 Casarett, 11.

14 Expert interview no. 13, 2019.

15 Hodge, foreword to *Toxicology*, v–vi.

16 Nash, "Purity and Danger"; Birnbaum, "When Environmental Chemicals Act like Uncontrolled Medicine"; Boudia, "Managing Scientific and Political"; Davis, *Banned*; Hepler-Smith, "Molecular Bureaucracy."

17 Gallo, "History and Scope of Toxicology," 8th ed.

18 Gallo.

19 Daston and Galison, *Objectivity*.

20 Daston and Galison, 325.

21 Thinking of the ways toxicology turns chemical uncertainty into neat and tidy mathematical graphs, apolitical diagrams, and all-too-real regulatory allowances, I was struck by another of Daston and Galison's analyses, quoted here at some length:

> The qualitative is not, by dint of being qualitative, indefinite. Again and again, one sees this cluster of terms now in the ascendant: what was needed is the subjective, the "trained eye," an "empirical art," and "intellectual"

approach, the identification of "patterns," the apperception of links "at a glance," the extraction of a "typical" subsequence within a wider variation. Reflections like these point to the complexity of judgement, to the variously intertwined criteria that group entities into larger categories that defy simplistic algorithms. *But . . . the complexity and nonmechanical nature of this identificatory process does not block the possibility of arriving at an appropriate and replicable set of discriminations.* It may take judgment to sort a B1 from a B2, but *such judgements can be nonmechanical and perfectly valid*: there is not a whiff of the arbitrary in . . . trained scientific judgements." (Daston and Galison, 333; emphasis added.)

22 On masculinist anxieties in the context of early science, see also Bordo, "Cartesian Masculinization of Thought."

23 Daston and Galison, *Objectivity*, 337.

24 Daston and Galison, 368.

25 Daston and Galison, 368.

26 Neil, Malmfors, and Slovic, "Intuitive Toxicology," 198.

27 A STS analysis of US chemical risk assessment processes would require its own book. Fortunately, scholars before me have completed such a worthy task. See Boudia and Jas, *Powerless Science?* See also Cordner, *Toxic Safety*.

28 Neil, Malmfors, and Slovic, "Intuitive Toxicology," 198. Emphasis added.

29 Neil, Malmfors, and Slovic, 199. Emphasis added.

30 Neil, Malmfors, and Slovic, 199.

31 Neil, Malmfors, and Slovic, 200.

32 Lanphear, "Low-Level Toxicity of Chemicals."

33 Faustman and Omenn, "Risk Assessment," 85–86. Emphasis added.

34 For example, see Bullard et al., "Toxic Wastes and Race at Twenty"; Peña, "Structural Violence, Historical Trauma, and Public Health."

35 Expert interview no. 3, 2019.

36 I work through different understandings of Charis Thompson's "good science" in chapter 5. Thompson, *Good Science*.

37 Prescod-Weinstein, "Making Black Women Scientists under White Empiricism." See also Mills, "White Supremacy."

38 Murphy has similarly theorized this depoliticized knowledge hierarchy as "chemicals in white space." "#AusSTS2021 Keynote Seminar: Prof Michelle Murphy," livestream recording, keynote seminar with Professor Michelle Murphy, YouTube video, 01:29:00, June 23, 2021, https://www.youtube.com/watch?v=4fTL-iRyM3U.

39 Flynn, Slovic, and Mertz, "Gender, Race, and Perception of Environmental Health Risks."

40 Flynn, Slovic, and Mertz, 1107.

41 Also criticized as the "mythical norm," "the West and the rest," "the Western Liberal Man Master-Subject," and "Reference Man"; see, respectively, Lorde, *Sister Outsider*; Hall, "West and the Rest"; Weheliye, *Habeas Viscus*; Olson, "Females

Exposed to Nuclear Radiation." bell hooks has also noted that the turn of phrase "women and nonwhite men" erases women of color, and Black women particularly. hooks, *Feminist Theory from Margin to Center*.

42 I paraphrase hooks, *Feminist Theory from Margin to Center*.

43 Flynn, Slovic, and Mertz, "Gender, Race, and Perception of Environmental Health Risks," 1107.

44 Neil, Malmfors, and Slovic, "Intuitive Toxicology," 200. Emphasis added.

45 Borzelleca, "Paracelsus"; Dominiczak, "International Year of Chemistry 2011."

46 Expert interview no. 24, 2021.

47 Lab interview no. 1, 2021.

48 Relatedly, see Pachá, "Why the Brazilian Far Right Loves the European Middle Ages."

49 Vogel, "From 'The Dose Makes the Poison' to 'The Timing Makes the Poison'"; Lanphear, "Low-Level Toxicity of Chemicals."

50 Langston, *Toxic Bodies*; Siegel, "Troubled Water."

51 Temkin, "Seven Defensiones."

52 Popper, review of *Paracelsus*.

53 Pagel, *Paracelsus*.

54 The old German reads "alle ding sind gift und nichts on gift; alien die dosis macht das ein ding kein gift ist." Webster, *Paracelsus*. See also Sigerist, *Four Treatises of Theophrastus von Hohenheim, Called Paracelsus*.

55 Temkin, "Seven Defensiones," 21.

56 Webster, *Paracelsus*, 150. Emphasis added.

57 Arguably, Rachel Carson sounded the alarm over hormone-interfering chemicals decades before, in her best-selling book *Silent Spring* (1962). See also Krimsky, "Epistemological Inquiry into the Endocrine Disruptor Thesis"; Vogel, "From 'The Dose Makes the Poison' to 'The Timing Makes the Poison.'"

58 Davis, *Banned*. See also Tu, *Experiments in Skin*.

59 Birnbaum, "When Environmental Chemicals Act like Uncontrolled Medicine"; Boudia and Jas, *Powerless Science?*

60 Casarett, "Toxicologic Evaluation," 17.

61 Wexler and Hayes, "Evolving Journey of Toxicology"; Aleksunes and Eaton, "Principles of Toxicology."

62 Wexler and Hayes, "Evolving Journey of Toxicology."

63 Franco and Olsson, "Scientists and the 3Rs."

64 Casarett, "Toxicologic Evaluation"; lab interview no. 10, 2021.

65 Casarett, 23.

66 Expert interview no. 2, 2019.

67 Casarett, "Toxicologic Evaluation," 24.

68 Casarett, 24.

69 Casarett, 24.

70 Webster, *Paracelsus*.

71 For a fascinating feminist discussion of thresholds via modern biomedicine, see Weir, *Pregnancy, Risk, and Biopolitics*.

72 *Oxford English Dictionary Online*, s.v. "Threshold, n.," accessed July 6, 2020, https://www.oed.com.

73 Faustman and Omenn, "Risk Assessment," 80.

74 Faustman and Omenn, 80.

75 Faustman, "Risk Assessment."

76 Faustman.

77 Casarett, "Toxicologic Evaluation," 24.

78 Casarett, 24. Emphasis added.

79 Casarett, 12.

80 Daston and Galison, *Objectivity*.

81 See Haraway, "Situated Knowledges," for a critique of Thomas Nagel's *View from Nowhere*.

82 Expert interview no. 9, 2019.

83 Casarett, "Toxicologic Evaluation," 22.

84 Nash, "Purity and Danger," 654.

85 Casarett, "Toxicologic Evaluation," 19. Emphasis added.

86 Frickel, *Chemical Consequences*; Landecker and Panofsky, "From Social Structure to Gene Regulation, and Back."

87 Vandenberg et al., "Hormones and Endocrine-Disrupting Chemicals"; Latham, "Unsafe at Any Dose?"; Lanphear, "Low-Level Toxicity of Chemicals."

88 Klaassen, *Casarett & Doull's Toxicology*.

89 Birnbaum, "When Environmental Chemicals Act like Uncontrolled Medicine."

90 For an environmental justice critique of "acceptable risk," see Peña, "Structural Violence, Historical Trauma, and Public Health."

91 Chen, "Monsanto and Growers Groups Sue California"; Environmental Protection Agency, "EPA Takes Next Step in Review Process for Herbicide Glyphosate, Reaffirms No Risk to Public Health," Pesticides, April 30, 2019, https://www.epa.gov.

92 Boudia et al., "Residues."

93 The US Hazardous Substances Act, first passed in 1960, includes household and consumer products only, not pharmaceuticals or pesticides. Pharmaceuticals are included in the Federal Food, Drug, and Cosmetic Act, first passed in 1906. Pesticides are regulated under the Federal Insecticide, Fungicide, and Rodenticide Act (FIFRA, first passed in 1910). The Toxic Substances Control Act (first passed in 1976) regulates newly synthesized chemicals as well as those excluded from the Hazardous Substances Act and FIFRA. See also Birnbaum, "When Environmental Chemicals Act like Uncontrolled Medicine."

94 Cordner provides a useful summary of the limitations of the Toxic Substances Control Act (TSCA), though her work was published before the most recent, 2016 amendments to the act:

> The EPA [US Environmental Protection Agency] has limited authority to impose regulations on the roughly 62,000 chemicals that were "grandfathered in" when TSCA was enacted, called "existing chemicals" in EPA parlance. As one EPA scientist explained to me during an informal meeting,

"TSCA is ineffective against old, nasty shit." Caught in a "data Catch-22," the agency cannot require further testing on a chemical or enact restrictions without data demonstrating that the chemical presents an unreasonable risk. . . . Manufacturers are not required to submit any toxicity or exposure data when requesting approval for new chemicals. According to EPA statistics, two-thirds of new chemicals are submitted with no measured data whatsoever. Only 15 percent are submitted with any data on health or toxicity, 10 percent with information in environmental fate or exposures, and only 4 percent with "repeated dose" studies, which track toxicity over a twenty-eight- to ninety-day period. Multigenerational, neurodevelopmental, or cancer studies in animals are almost nonexistent, despite the fact that these health outcomes are of significant concern for human health. (Cordner, *Toxic Safety*, 127–28.)

95 Nash, "Purity and Danger," 656.
96 Expert interview no. 1, 2019.
97 Expert interview no. 18, 2019.
98 Expert interview no. 17, 2019.
99 Expert interview no. 9, 2019.
100 Nash, "Purity and Danger," 656.
101 Wexler and Hayes, "Evolving Journey of Toxicology."
102 Hodge, foreword to *Toxicology*, vi.
103 Wexler and Hayes, "Evolving Journey of Toxicology."
104 Wexler and Hayes, 4. Emphasis original.
105 Wexler and Hayes.
106 Webster, *Paracelsus*.
107 Personal communication, 2021.
108 Webster, *Paracelsus*.
109 Hodge, foreword to *Toxicology*.
110 As science fiction author Octavia E. Butler writes, "There is nothing new under the sun, but there are new suns." Canavan, "There's Nothing New / Under the Sun, / But There Are New Suns"; brown and Imarisha, *Octavia's Brood*. I must credit B. Nahid for the turn of phrase "knowledge seeking is magic seeking."
111 Kaba, "Free Us All."

3. TOXICANT MASCULINITY

1 Ahmed, "Feminist Killjoys."
2 On hegemonic and other masculinities, see Connell, *Masculinities*.
3 G. Jervais, B. Luukinen, and D. Stone, "2,4-D General Fact Sheet," National Pesticide Information Center, Oregon State University Extension Services, 2009, http://npic.orst.edu. For more social history and commentary on the lingering toxic legacies of Agent Orange and other chemical weapons deployed in Vietnam, see Tu, *Experiments in Skin*; Duong, "Homing Toxicity."
4 Zimdahl, *History of Weed Science in the United States*, 44.

5   Zimdahl, 63.

6   Zimdahl, 71.

7   As with all interviewees, Tim is a pseudonym.

8   Personal communication, 2021.

9   On the sociocultural and economic context of defining agricultural "pests," see Morales and Perfecto, "Traditional Knowledge and Pest Management in the Guatemalan Highlands." See also Ritvo, *The Platypus and the Mermaid*; Brookshire, *Pests*.

10 "Mansplaining" is the vernacular term drawn from Solnit, *Men Explain Things to Me*; Manne, *Entitled*.

11 Pulido, *Environmentalism and Economic Justice*; Guthman and Brown, "Whose Life Counts"; Williams, "That We May Live."

12 Zimdahl, *History of Weed Science in the United States*, 2. Providing some such historical reflection, Scott Frickel, in his social study of genetic toxicology, likewise found that academic scientists welcomed their industry-employed counterparts from the outset: "Even though there were no for-profit genetic toxicology laboratories in the United States until the early 1970s and federal regulations would not require mutagenicity testing of new compounds until 1976, industrial laboratories contributed 16 percent of the EMS [Environmental Mutagenesis Society] membership in 1969. *Their presence was in part a reflection of an early decision by the charter members of EMS to actively recruit representatives from industry* and in part an acknowledgement by pharmaceutical or chemical laboratories that their economic and political interests would be best served by becoming involved in mutagenicity research." Frickel, *Chemical Consequences*, 75. Emphasis added.

13 Zimdahl, *History of Weed Science in the United States*, 88.

14 Guyton et al., "Key Characteristics Approach to Carcinogenic Hazard Identification."

15 For example, see Sze, "Boundaries and Border Wars"; Langston, *Toxic Bodies*; Mansfield, "Environmental Health as Biosecurity"; Richardson et al., "Society"; MacKendrick, *Better Safe than Sorry*; Scott, Haw, and Lee, "Wannabe Toxic-Free?"

16 As environmental health scientist James P. Keogh dryly remarked, "If you poison your boss a little each day it's called murder; if your boss poisons you a little each day it's called a Threshold Limit Value." Cited in Proctor, *Cancer Wars*.

17 Casarett, "Origin and Scope of Toxicology," 4.

18 Never mind that contemporary anthropologists and archaeologists believe, based on material evidence, that "harvesting wild plants and turning them into food, medicine and complex structures like baskets or clothing is almost everywhere a female activity, and may be gendered female even when practised by men. . . . where evidence exists, it points to strong associations between women and plant-based knowledge as far back as one can trace such things." Graeber and Wengrow, *Dawn of Everything*, 237.

19 For more on the biological and political differences between toxins and toxicants, see Liboiron, "Toxins or Toxicants?"

20 Millett, *Sexual Politics*, 300.

21 Casarett, "Origin and Scope of Toxicology," 4.

22 Millett, *Sexual Politics*, 310.

23 Parreñas, "Hunting," 167.

24 Casarett, "Origin and Scope of Toxicology," 5.

25 *Wikipedia*, s.v. "Sulla," accessed June 1, 2021, https://en.wikipedia.org.

26 Casarett, "Origin and Scope of Toxicology," 5.

27 Casarett, 6. Emphasis added.

28 Zimdahl, *History of Weed Science in the United States*, 20. Emphasis added.

29 Zimdahl, 31.

30 Zimdahl, 33. Emphasis added.

31 For example, see Hine, "Female Slave Resistance"; Davis, *Women, Race & Class*; Federici, *Caliban and the Witch*; Schiebinger, "Feminist History of Colonial Science."

32 Casarett, "Origin and Scope of Toxicology," 4.

33 Hodge, foreword to *Toxicology*, v.

34 Zimdahl, *History of Weed Science in the United States*, 146, 149. Emphasis added.

35 Thompson, "Dr. Charis Thompson."

36 Expert interview no. 13, 2019.

37 Proctor, "'Everyone Knew but No One Had Proof'"; Oreskes and Conway, *Merchants of Doubt*.

38 For two of thousands of papers on the unknown threats posed by thousands of toxicants, see Birnbaum, "When Environmental Chemicals Act like Uncontrolled Medicine"; Wiesinger, Wang, and Hellweg, "Deep Dive into Plastic Monomers, Additives, and Processing Aids."

39 Expert interview no. 13, 2019.

40 Author field notes, 2019.

41 Expert interview no. 17, 2019. Emphasis original.

42 Expert interview no. 2, 2019.

43 Benbrook, "How Did the US EPA and IARC Reach Diametrically Opposed Conclusions."

44 Prescod-Weinstein, "Making Black Women Scientists under White Empiricism," 425.

45 Manne, *Down Girl*.

46 Patel, "Long Green Revolution."

47 Expert interview no. 23, 2019.

48 Hodge, foreword to *Toxicology*, v.

49 Ward, *Tragedy of Heterosexuality*, 158.

50 Baltzell, *Protestant Establishment*; Hochschild, "Inside the Clockwork of Male Careers."

51 "Land-grant universities" refers to those created out of the 1862 and 1890 Morrill Land-Grant College Acts, which made federal lands available to states to sell for the specific purpose of establishing agricultural and applied science schools. As

historian Margaret A. Nash has written, such land sales depended on the dispossession and genocide of Native Americans. She also notes how the focus on agriculture and applied science was meant to counteract the "liberal elite" universities of the Northeastern United States. Nash, "Entangled Pasts."

52 Examples include Davis, "Pesticides and the Paradox of the Anthropocene"; Tu, *Experiments in Skin.*

53 Lorde, "Master's Tools Will Never Dismantle the Master's House."

54 I typically eschew the ethnographic term "informant," but in this particular instance it seemed more apt than research "participant."

55 Here is one poignant example: while conducting surveys with Cakchiquel Maya farmers in Patzún, Guatemala, in an effort to understand this indigenous community's "pest control" practices, agroecologists Helda Morales and Ivette Perfecto found that when they asked something akin to "What do you do about pests?," nobody seemed to understand the question—what is this "pest"? When the researchers rephrased, asking these farmers whether they saw specific insects in their fields, they received many more affirmative answers. They also found that they had to rephrase "*control* [insects]" to "*avoid* [insects]." Such differences in onto-epistemology, or ways of being and knowing, help explain how medicinal plants come to be known as "noxious pests" or "invasive weeds" that must be eradicated, justifying the production and deployment of highly toxic synthetic chemicals, endangering all our lives, some clearly more than others. Morales and Perfecto, "Traditional Knowledge and Pest Management in the Guatemalan Highlands."

56 McWilliams, *Factories in the Field*; Walker, *Conquest of Bread*; Guthman, *Agrarian Dreams*; Henke, *Cultivating Science, Harvesting Power.*

57 Zimdahl, *History of Weed Science in the United States*, 197. See also Jensen, "Amid Plenty"; Howard, "Myth of 'Feeding the World.'"

58 California Department of Food and Agriculture, "Encycloweedia: Data Sheets for California Noxious Weeds," CDFA: California Department of Food and Agriculture, last updated June 22, 2021, https://www.cdfa.ca.gov.

59 Dryly as ever, Zimdahl observes, "The methods of control have changed but as Appleby (1993, p. 147) points out 'many of the problems and thought processes have not changed since 1938.' His comment could be interpreted as praise for the strength and ubiquity of weeds or as an indictment of the thought processes of weed scientists." Zimdahl, *History of Weed Science in the United States*, 121.

60 Agency for Toxic Substances and Disease Registry (ATSDR), "Medical Management Guidelines for Methyl Bromide (Bromomethane)," Toxic Substances Portal, Medical Management Guidelines for Methyl Bromide, 2014, https://www.atsdr.cdc.gov.

61 Schubert, "US Pushes Limits on Ozone Destroyer."

62 "#AusSTS2021 Keynote Seminar: Prof Michelle Murphy," livestream recording, keynote seminar with Professor Michelle Murphy, YouTube video, 01:29:00, June 23, 2021, https://www.youtube.com/watch?v=4fTL-iRyM3U.

63 Kimbrell, *Fatal Harvest.*

64 Foster and Hobbs, *Field Guide to Western Medicinal Plants and Herbs*, 200.

65 Foster and Hobbs, 201.

66 Sosnoskie, "Biology of Field Bindweed."

67 Anker, *Imperial Ecology*; Banu Subramaniam, "Aliens Have Landed!"; Hayden, *When Nature Goes Public*; Kloppenburg, *First the Seed*; Schiebinger, *Colonial Botany*; Pratt, *Imperial Eyes*.

68 For feminist critique of the similarly problematic term "invasive species," see Subramaniam, "Aliens Have Landed!"

69 Native American nations past and present, as well as Euro-American herbalists, value this plant, known in English as "orchard morning glory," for several of its medicinal and edible properties. Orchard morning glory may be ingested as a laxative, purgative, antihemorrhagic, treatment for spider bites, intestinal stimulant, and "gynecological aid." Its flowers make a tea for reducing fevers and healing wounds, the leaves can be eaten as a vegetable or condiment, and the vines may be braided into ropes to tie and carry. What is more, the vine's binding properties reduce soil erosion and help stabilize steep hillsides. Mitich, "Intriguing World of Weeds"; Austin, "Bindweed (Convolvulus Arvensis, Convolvulaceae) in North America, from Medicine to Menace"; Goodrich and Lawson, *Kashaya Pomo Plants*.

70 The militarism and xenophobia of "invasive" species rhetoric (see Subramaniam, "Aliens Have Landed!") is especially overt in the US agricultural space. Consider this recent report from *Chemical and Engineering News*:

> North Dakota State University weed scientist Brian Jenks can tell you exactly when, where, and how Palmer amaranth first appeared in his state. In 2018, the noxious weed sneaked, via seed, across state lines using a variety of clever tactics, then sprouted in five locations. The crop saboteur was quickly detected by sharp-eyed farmers, who alerted the authorities. . . . the specimens that Jenks pounced on last year arrived already resistant to glyphosate—commonly known as Roundup—and were likely resistant to other chemicals as well. Palmer amaranth's ability to quickly develop resistance to herbicides is a major reason that the Weed Science Society of America voted it the country's most troublesome weed in 2017. . . . Weed scientists and agriculture chemical company experts describe the many ways that biology and growth habits make this king of weeds uniquely difficult to kill or contain. It will likely require brand-new technology—technology that does not yet exist—to regain the upper hand. It wasn't always this way. There was a time when Roundup could kill any Palmer amaranth plant. But populations resistant to glyphosate emerged in the southeastern US in 2006 and soon began to move about the country." (Bomgardner, "Palmer Amaranth, the King of Weeds, Cripples New Herbicides.")

71 Bederman, *Manliness & Civilization*. I borrow "United Statesean" from Halley, *Split Decisions*. On masculinities, see Connell, *Masculinities*.

72 For example, Fanon, "Colonial Violence and Mental Disorders"; McClintock, *Imperial Leather*; Stoler, *Carnal Knowledge and Imperial Power*; Anderson, *Cultivation of Whiteness*; Ahuja, *Bioinsecurities*. See also Pellegrini, *Performance Anxieties*.

73 See also Haraway, "Teddy Bear Patriarchy"; Herzig, *Suffering for Science*; Ray, *Ecological Other*; Stern, *Eugenic Nation*; Voyles, "Toxic Masculinity."

74 Tonn, "Evolutionary Brotherhood." See also Cronon, "Uses of Environmental History"; Wohlforth, "Conservation and Eugenics"; Pico, "Darker Side of John Wesley Powell."

75 See also Herzig, *Suffering for Science*.

76 For instance, Pico, "Darker Side of John Wesley Powell"; Prescod-Weinstein, "Making Black Women Scientists under White Empiricism."

77 Lab interview no. 4, 2021.

78 Ahmed, "Feminist Killjoys."

79 Personal communication, 2021.

80 "North Central Weed Science Society Student Weed Contest (2017)," NCWSS Collegiate Weed Contest Iowa State University at the Iowa State University Field Extension and Education Lab (FEEL) in Ames, IA on July 27, 2017, YouTube video, 00:01:24, January 4, 2018, https://www.youtube.com/watch?v=-5wufijco9g.

81 North Central Weed Science Society, "2021 NCWSS Weed Contest," 2021, https://ncwss.org.

82 North Central Weed Science Society. Sociologist Jill Harrison's critical work on pesticide drift comes to mind here as well. See Harrison, *Pesticide Drift and the Pursuit of Environmental Justice*.

83 North Central Weed Science Society, "2021 NCWSS Weed Contest."

84 "North Central Weed Science Society Student Weed Contest (2017)."

85 North Central Weed Science Society, "2021 NCWSS Weed Contest."

86 North Central Weed Science Society.

87 North Central Weed Science Society.

88 Personal communication, 2021.

89 Personal communication, 2021.

90 Benbrook, "Why Regulators Lost Track and Control of Pesticide Risks."

91 Zimdahl, *History of Weed Science in the United States*, 167, 171.

92 Zimdahl, 189.

93 Zimdahl, 194.

94 Zimdahl, 131.

95 Hodge, foreword to *Toxicology*, vi.

4. FUZZY FAMILY FEELINGS

1 Frickel, *Chemical Consequences*, 145.

2 Di Chiro, "Polluted Politics?"

3 In 2020 Professor Hayes published an open letter to his colleagues, signed by many supporters, describing the micro- and macro-aggressions he experiences as

a Black biologist at UC Berkeley. See Rothfels Lab, "Rothfels Lab Stands against Racism Everywhere."

4 "The Atrazine Rap," Dr. Tyrone Hayes performing, YouTube video, 00:01:57, March 21, 2008, https://www.youtube.com/watch?v=3MxrH4lNo-A.

5 See also Ah-King and Hayward, "Toxic Sexes"; Pollock, "Queering Endocrine Disruption"; Shotwell, *Against Purity*; Perret, "Chemical Castration."

6 For a brief history of the use of such terms in EDC research, see Packer and Lambert, "What's Gender Got to Do with It?"

7 For example, see Frederick and Jayasena, "Altered Pairing Behaviour and Reproductive Success."

8 Bagemihl, *Biological Exuberance*; Terry, "'Unnatural Acts' in Nature"; Lancaster, *Trouble with Nature*; Monk et al., "Alternative Hypothesis for the Evolution of Same-Sex Sexual Behaviour in Animals"; Packer and Lambert, "What's Gender Got to Do with It?"

9 I thank lab interviewee no. 8 for this reminder, personal communication 2022. See Erickson, "US EPA to Impose Atrazine Restrictions."

10 Branch et al., "Discussions of the 'Not So Fit.'"

11 Horkeimer and Adorno, "Concept of Enlightenment."

12 Lab interviewee no. 2, personal communication, 2022.

13 Robbins and Moore, "Ecological Anxiety Disorder."

14 See also Liboiron, "There's No Such Thing as 'We.'"

15 For example, see Federici, *Wages Against Housework*; DeVault, *Feeding the Family*; Glenn, "From Servitude to Service Work"; Hochschild, *Time Bind*; Glenn, *Forced to Care*; Manne, *Down Girl*.

16 Scott, *Our Chemical Selves*; Shapiro, "Attuning to the Chemosphere"; Zota and Shamasunder, "Environmental Injustice of Beauty." Pregnant women and mothers are also socially pressured to shelter their unborn infants, and children from toxic exposures, or to somehow *prevent* contamination. See Mansfield, "Environmental Health as Biosecurity."

17 See especially eco-feminist engagements with care work, such as Schroer et al., "Introduction: Multispecies Care in the Sixth Extinction."

18 Here I borrow Saidiya Hartman's wonderful turn of phrase, "care is the antidote to violence," from her interview with Kaba, "Free Us All."

19 Hobart and Kneese, "Radical Care," 2.

20 Piepzna-Samarasinha, *Care Work*.

21 Spade, "Solidarity Not Charity."

22 Hobart and Kneese, "Radical Care," 3.

23 Hobart and Kneese, 1.

24 Millett, *Sexual Politics*. I feature Millett so prominently with some misgivings. Like many white feminists of her day (and today), she perpetuates the persistent myth that sexism is somehow more fundamental than, or otherwise predates, racism, while also, contradictorily, arguing that US women's experience of sexism is comparable to African American people's experiences of racism (as singular

forms of oppression), thus erasing those who experience both sexism and racism (particularly African American women), never mind that the categories of sex and race are historically coconstitutive. Overall, her Euro-American-centeredness and sweeping generalizations regarding non-Western cultures are cringe worthy by today's standards. Nevertheless, elements of her brave if flawed analysis are prescient, such as the observation that both the natural and social sciences are thoroughly infused with patriarchal ideology. Like any good feminist killjoy, I both criticize and honor the work of my feminist elders simultaneously. On feminist practices of reflexivity and holding space for nuance, see Hammond, "Audre Lorde"; Halley, *Split Decisions*; Ahmed, "Feminist Killjoys."

25 Millett, *Sexual Politics*, 240.

26 For important feminist critiques of DEI, see Ahmed, *On Being Included*.

27 All lab members' names are pseudonyms.

28 Millett, *Sexual Politics*. See also my brief discussion of US "Tox Lab" founder E. M. K. Geiling in chapter 1. The fact that I so easily rolled into the lab's family fold is no doubt related to my social location and identity. Most lab members came from highly educated, white, middle-class backgrounds, and while there was some ethnic and racial diversity during the snapshot of time I spent with this lab, people of African, Indigenous, and Latin@ descent were underrepresented (across the lab's hosting academic institution as a whole), as were queer and trans folks and people living with disabilities. While I could not (and felt no desire to) join lab chit-chat about the best skiing destinations, for example—my own white, lower-middle-class upbringing did not afford me *that* level of luxury—it's worth noting that for me, such moments of socioeconomic discordance were few and far between.

29 I borrow the terms scientist feminist and feminist scientist from Roy, *Molecular Feminisms*.

30 Lab interview no. 1, 2021. Original emphasis.

31 Lab interview no. 1, 2021. Emphasis added.

32 Packer, "Finding the Man in the Glyphosate."

33 Roy, "Science Still Bears the Fingerprints of Colonialism."

34 Author field notes, lab meeting no. 11, 2021. Emphasis added. Lab meetings were not audio recorded so all quoted excerpts from field notes are approximate, not direct.

35 The lab maintained several channels on the web- and phone-based application Slack; one channel was strictly for science-related posts, whereas other channels were meant as spaces for other conversations, such as important dates on the school calendar, university and community events of interest, or random fun bits of information. The PI invited me at one point to share my list of "top ten" resources on critical feminist STS, asking that I post this list on one of the other(ed) Slack channels. In a small, hopefully harmless, act of rebellion, I posted my top ten list—which was nearly impossible to compile, as there are so much more than ten—on the core "science" Slack channel instead of the lab's peripheral channels.

From that point on, I must confess, I made a creatively incompetent habit of posting any content relating to environmental justice or critical theory on the main, "science only" channel.

36 Lab interview no. 6, 2021. Emphasis added.

37 Subramaniam, "Snow Brown and the Seven Detergents."

38 Author field notes, lab meeting no. 11, 2021.

39 Author field notes, lab meeting no. 18, 2021.

40 Gregory's comment also reminded me of conversations I have had with close colleagues, such as feminist biologist Ambika Kamath, about how many people are drawn to the *order* of dominant science because of trauma. Ambika and I have also discussed whether in their attempts to diversify science, the privileged are "inviting" marginalized peoples to share in that dominant mode of power—then how does it land to say "No you can't have that power anymore, we're changing it"? Do we want diversity within the existing scientific system or do we want to radically transform scientific practices? Bruno, a member of the lab profiled in this chapter, did express an interesting concern during one of our lab meeting discussions on the topic—that feminist and postcolonial critiques of science might in fact deter historically marginalized people from becoming scientists, out of anger and disgust.

41 Author field notes, lab meeting no. 19, 2021.

42 Herzig, *Suffering for Science*, 13.

43 Herzig, 101.

44 Ahmed, "Feminist Killjoys."

45 Author field notes, lab meeting no. 18, 2021.

46 For an excellent and more thorough discussion of the problematics of "invasive" species, see Kim, *Dangerous Crossings*.

47 Author field notes, lab meeting no. 18, 2021. Original emphasis.

48 Also see critiques in Perret, "Chemical Castration."

49 Author field notes, lab meeting no. 18, 2021. Original emphasis.

50 Ben later revealed to me, in a comment on this section of my draft chapter, that he "often says things that he doesn't actually believe, in order to provoke thought/discussion," implying that this was one of those instances. Personal communication, 2022.

51 Author field notes, lab meeting no. 18, 2021.

52 The last lab meeting I attended that academic year, as a participant-observer, was exceptionally heartwarming. The PI and his students were effusive with their praise and gratitude for my participation, and I remain equally thankful and buoyed by the experience.

53 Packer and Lambert, "What's Gender Got to Do with It?"

54 Max and I met through the Queer Ecologies | Feminist Biologies working group brilliantly assembled by scientist feminist Ashton Wesner, hosted at UC Berkeley 2018–2020.

55 Lambert and Packer, "How Gendered Language Leads Scientists Astray."

56 See the literature on environmental justice and activism, for example, United Church of Christ Commission for Racial Justice, "Toxic Wastes and Race in the United States"; Cushing et al., "The Haves, the Have-Nots, and the Health of Everyone"; Voyles, *Wastelanding*.

57 I took notes as best I could during the meeting, but all "quotes" are from my memory of the exchange, as unfortunately I did not think to ask whether I could record the session. I typed my immediate impressions and thoughts as soon as the meeting ended, but these are undoubtedly flawed and fragmented memories nonetheless.

58 Lab interviewee no. 8, personal communication, 2022.

59 Lab interviewee no. 2, personal communication, 2022. Emphasis added.

60 In general, I strive for an "epistemology of generosity," as I heard Charis Thompson describe it once (personal communication).

61 Lab interviewee no. 8, personal communication, 2022.

62 Haraway, "Situated Knowledges"; Harding, "Strong Objectivity."

63 As Lancaster writes: "I am convinced that sophisticated constructionist positions can be put into simple, accessible language—as with the exemplary antiracist ads that appeared on the sides of buses in 1998: 'Race is a fiction, racism is real.'" Lancaster, *Trouble with Nature*, 23.

64 Twombly, "Assault on the Male"; Di Chiro, "Polluted Politics?," 206–9.

65 For example, see Trasande, *Sicker, Fatter, Poorer*; Brockovich, "Plummeting Sperm Counts, Shrinking Penises"; Swan and Colino, *Count Down*.

66 For example, see Bederman, *Manliness & Civilization*; Herzig, *Suffering for Science*.

67 Frickel, *Chemical Consequences*, 98.

68 Frickel, 98.

69 Lab interviewee no. 2, personal communication, 2022. Emphasis added.

70 The negative blind peer reviews that Max and I received on earlier drafts of our paper, coincidentally, contained many of the same objections expressed by this reflexive PI and his thoughtful trainees. Our one queer feminist STS reviewer not only identified herself, but also offered exclusively and overwhelmingly positive reviews of the article.

71 Mortimer-Sandilands and Erickson, *Queer Ecologies*; Seymour, *Strange Natures*; Halberstam, *Wild Things*.

72 Lab interviewee no. 2, personal communication, 2022.

73 Lab interviewee no. 8, personal communication, 2022. Emphasis added.

74 For example, see Mitman, *State of Nature*; Gould, *Mismeasure of Man*; Panofsky, *Misbehaving Science*; Branch et al., "Discussions of the 'Not So Fit.'" See also Kamath and Packer, *Feminism in the Wild*.

75 For critical analyses of evolutionary fitness, sociobiology, and genetics from scientists and nonscientists alike, see Sahlins, *Use and Abuse of Biology*; Levins and Lewontin, *Dialectical Biologist*; Keller, *Century of the Gene*; Lancaster, *Trouble with Nature*; Reardon, *Race to the Finish*; Gould, *Mismeasure of Man*; TallBear, *Native*

American DNA; Nelson, *Social Life of DNA*; Ogbunugafor, "DNA, Basketball, and Birthday Luck." For a science studies critique of sociobiology and genetics in terms of animal behavior (or behavior-as-phenotype) see Crist, *Images of Animals*.

76 For a powerful indictment of famed sociobiologist E. O. Wilson's eugenicism, for example, see Farina and Gibbons, "Last Refuge of Scoundrels."

77 Crist, *Images of Animals*, 227n2.

78 Crist, 126, 128.

79 Frickel, *Chemical Consequences*, 106.

80 Packer and Lambert, "What's Gender Got to Do with It?," 115, 117.

81 Crist, *Images of Animals*, 136. Emphasis added.

82 For example, see Montford and Taylor, *Colonialism and Animality*.

83 Monk et al., "Alternative Hypothesis for the Evolution of Same-Sex Sexual Behaviour in Animals."

84 Lab interviewee no. 8, personal communication, 2022.

85 Lab interviewee no. 6., personal communication, 2022.

86 For example, see Shadaan and Murphy, "EDCs as Industrial Chemicals and Settler Colonial Structures"; Kojola and Pellow, "New Directions in Environmental Justice Studies."

87 SisterSong, "Reproductive Justice."

88 Ben wondered, while reading my chapter draft, whether it was in fact racist to question the reproductive effects of EDCs, given how exposures are racialized via their uneven distributions (personal communication, 2022).

89 Crist, *Images of Animals*, 142.

90 Thomas, "Toxic Responses of the Reproductive System"; Altman et al., "Pollution Comes Home and Gets Personal."

91 For more on the eugenicism of sex categories and evolutionary biology, respectively, see Velocci, *Binary Logic*; Kamath and Packer, *Feminism in the Wild*.

92 Lab interviewee no. 2, personal communication, 2022.

93 Lab interviewee no. 8, personal communication, 2022.

94 Taylor, *Beasts of Burden*, 189, as quoted in Packer and Lambert, "What's Gender Got to Do with It?"

95 One of these women clarified to me afterwards,

> I really wanted to say more during the conversation, I felt I had a lot more to say, but I am one to notice if I am speaking too much in a group and I want my other lab members to take their turn. I am also more generally quiet in larger groups (I think I find it difficult to speak up for myself, or rather it takes a lot of energy for me to do so, and I have realized about myself that it is kind of self-preserving, I do not find it worth my energy to argue with someone that will not listen . . .) I think I do also take a while to internalize things, I was still trying to acknowledge my own role in these issues—it is a hard thing to acknowledge in oneself and I want to take the time for self-reflection and working out how I can improve myself, and given these realizations did occur during the meeting, I did not always know how to

respond to them (i.e. the questions being asked) ESPECIALLY when there are speakers dominating the conversation to a topic I felt very unsure about whether was correct or not. The next day during lunch, when [there] were only all the ladies in the lab, including myself, we had another hour-long conversation about the article which was incredibly interesting. I don't remember a lot of what we talked about, but I feel we ended up siding with your article more towards the end. I think taking another day to reflect on it and our previous discussion was really helpful. Regardless, it was much more of a friendly discussion than the lab meeting." (Lab interviewee no. 2, personal communication, 2022; emphasis added.)

96 As feminist philosopher Kate Manne argues, misogyny is to sexism as law enforcement is to the law. As long as women play by the sexist rules, they escape misogynistic punishment. The absence of misogyny (hatred of women), of course, does not imply the absence of sexism. See Manne, *Down Girl*.

97 Personal communication with lab interviewees no. 2 and 6, 2022.

98 Lab interviewee no. 8, personal communication, 2022.

99 Toni Morrison, "Nobel Lecture." Nobel Prize, December 7, 1993, https://www.nobelprize.org.

100 Chandler, "Alabama Law Criminalizing Care for Transgender Youth Faces Federal Test"; Gibson, "Dreading the Knock at the Door."

101 Davis, "Florida Senate Passes a Controversial Schools Bill Labeled 'Don't Say Gay' by Critics."

102 Crenshaw, "Panic over Critical Race Theory"; Gerstein and Ward, "Supreme Court Has Voted to Overturn Abortion Rights, Draft Opinion Shows."

103 Lab interviewee no. 8, personal communication, 2022.

104 Author field notes, lab meeting no. 19, 2021.

105 Ruha Benjamin, "Catching Our Breath," 148. See also Anderson, "White Space"; Shabazz, "Black Women, White Campus."

106 Lab interviewee no. 8, personal communication, 2022.

107 During scene 2, act 1, in which Prince Ferdinand hears, but does not see, a song sung by the island spirit Ariel, suggesting that his father Alonso drowned in the shipwreck that left Ferdinand stranded on the island: "Full fathom five thy father lies / Of his bones are coral made / Those are pearls that were his eyes / Nothing of him that doth fade / But doth suffer a sea-change / into something rich and strange." Shakespeare, *The Tempest*, 35–36.

108 Including, for example, venture capital firms. "SeaChange," SeaChange, accessed May 22, 2024, https://seachangeventures.com.

109 Barad, *Meeting the Universe Halfway*.

110 Lab interviewee no. 8, personal communication, 2022.

111 Lab interview no. 8, 2021.

112 I thank lab interviewee no. 2 (personal communication, 2022) for pointing out the privilege inherent in her tenured PI's ability to say "fuck off" (in so many words) at an academic conference.

113 Author field notes, lab meeting no. 3, 2020.

114 Corbin et al., "(Re)Thinking the Tenure Process by Embracing Diversity in Scholars and Scholarship."

115 Tironi, "Hypo-Interventions."

116 Cohn, "Sex and Death in the Rational World of Defense Intellectuals," 708.

117 Never mind that we are each trying to deconstruct a thing from different positions that have both been constructed by and within that thing—a fundamental challenge noted by, among others, Fanon, *Black Skin, White Masks*; Lorde, "Master's Tools Will Never Dismantle the Master's House"; Spivak, "Can the Subaltern Speak?"; Butler, *Gender Trouble*; Scott, "Evidence of Experience"; Brown, "Wounded Attachments."

5. FISHY EXCEPTIONALISM

1 Gruen, *Entangled Empathy*, 36.

2 Michael E. Lynch (1988) comments on the use of the term "sacrifice" in this context, which denotes not only "that the animal serves the 'higher' interests of science" but also "a set of rituals [that transform] the animal from a living, holistic, 'naturalistic' animals into an 'analytic' one." Lynch, "Sacrifice and the Transformation of the Animal Body into a Scientific Object," as cited in Holmberg, "Feeling for the Animal," 326. See also Haraway, *When Species Meet*.

3 For a cheeky yet clever take on a rodent's experience of laboratory and field-based scientific research, see Nelson and Whitney, "Becoming a Research Rodent."

4 Holmberg, "Feeling for the Animal," 332. Emphasis added. For more on how both scientists and laboratory animals become transformed through the process of experimentation, see Daston and Mitman, "How and Why of Thinking with Animals."

5 Rader, *Making Mice*.

6 The US National Institutes of Health (NIH) places model organisms into two categories: "Non-human mammalian model organisms, such as: Mouse, Rat" and "Non-mammalian model organisms, such as: Budding yeast, Social amoebae, Roundworm, Arabidopsis, Fruit fly, Zebrafish, Frog." National Institute of Health, "Model Organism Sharing Policy," NIH Scientific Data Sharing, accessed May 31, 2022, https://sharing.nih.gov. Some intrepid STS scholar should research the historically and socially contingent process through which a particular more-than-human animal is made into a model organism, as Karen Rader (*Making Mice*) has done for mice, and, in different ways, Michelle Murphy and Robert E. Kohler have done for drosophila, or the fruit fly. Murphy, *Economization of Life*; Kohler, *Lords of the Fly*.

7 For example, see Brown, "She Experimented on Primates for Decades." For histories of antivivisectionist movements, often led by women and hence more readily dismissed, see Elston, "Women and Anti-Vivisection in Victorian England, 1870–1900"; Ritvo, *Animal Estate*; Beers, *For the Prevention of Cruelty*.

8 Nelson, *Model Behavior*. For more on the distinctly gendered dismissal of anti-vivisectionists in particular, see Ritvo, *Animal Estate*.

9 Albert, Luque, and Courchamp, "Twenty Most Charismatic Species."

10 Brown, "She Experimented on Primates for Decades."

11 Goodman, Chandna, and Roe, "Trends in Animal Use at US Research Facilities"; Tollefson, "Scientists Concerned over US Environment Agency's Plan to Limit Animal Research"; Grimm, "How Many Mice and Rats Are Used in U.S. Labs?"

12 On the politics and ethics of dominant science's use of more-than-human animals, see, for example: Haraway, *When Species Meet*; Chakrabarti, "Beasts of Burden"; Thompson, *Good Science*; Gluck, *Voracious Science & Vulnerable Animals*.

13 On the multispecies politics of defining fish as species themselves, see Miller, *Why Fish Don't Exist*.

14 At the ends of my feminist STS project, I am back to the beginnings of feminist STS, such as Birke, "Science, Feminism and Animal Natures II."

15 For example, see Hornblum, *Acres of Skin*; Ahuja, *Bioinsecurities*; Tu, *Experiments in Skin*. If nothing else, those of us who rely on toxicology today owe it to those *unwillingly* suffering for science to put that knowledge to greater use, namely toward more strict regulation, if not an end to production, of toxic chemicals, not to mention some form of financial or land-based reparations for those communities who have been historically, disproportionately more burdened, and will thus continue to remain so, due to EDCs' transgenerational health effects. On the transgenerational effects of EDC exposures, see Rothstein, Cai, and Marchant, "Ghost in Our Genes"; Thayer and Kuzawa, "Biological Memories of Past Environments"; Weasel, "Embodying Intersectionality."

16 On the interlockings of patriarchy, racism, and capitalism with environmental destruction and animal abuse, see Merchant, *Death of Nature*; Plumwood, *Feminism and the Mastery of Nature*; Kim, *Dangerous Crossings*; Boisseron, *Afro-Dog*; Ko, *Racism as Zoological Witchcraft*.

17 Hodge, foreword to *Toxicology*.

18 Rader, *Making Mice*; Nelson, *Model Behavior*; Fox and Bennett, "Laboratory Animal Medicine."

19 Lynch, "Sacrifice and the Transformation of the Animal Body into a Scientific Object."

20 Lab interview no. 5, 2021.

21 Lab interview no. 5, 2021. Emphasis added.

22 Russell and Burch, *Principles of Humane Experimental Technique*; Thompson, *Good Science*, 206.

23 Holmberg, "Feeling for the Animal," 329.

24 As cited in Brown, "She Experimented on Primates for Decades"; Gluck, *Voracious Science & Vulnerable Animals*.

25 Law professor and animal liberationist Gary L. Francione talks about such hierarchies as "selective speciesism." Francione, *Introduction to Animal Rights*. Notably,

Ben the PI did not offer this reasoning for himself, clarifying, "I don't study fish because I don't want to hurt mammals. I study fish because they are inherently important and useful as models for certain questions." Lab interviewee no. 8, personal communication 2022.

26 Balcombe, *What a Fish Knows*.

27 Balcombe, 232. I first came across this particular quote in Marris, *Wild Souls*, 27.

28 For fascinating discussion of how evolutionarily close the somewhat outdated category of "fish" indeed are to humans, see Yoon, *Naming Nature*; Balcombe, *What a Fish Knows*; Miller, *Why Fish Don't Exist*.

29 Thompson, *Good Science*, 192–93. Emphasis original.

30 Lab interview no. 3, 2021. Emphasis added.

31 Lab interview no. 3, 2021. Emphasis added.

32 Lab interview no. 3, 2021.

33 CRISPR, a novel genetic manipulation technology, stands for clustered regularly interspaced short palindromic repeats.

34 Lab interview no. 3, 2021. Emphasis added.

35 For example, see, Chakrabarti, "Beasts of Burden"; Ahuja, "Postcolonial Critique in a Multispecies World"; Schiebinger, "Feminist History of Colonial Science"; Anderson, *Race and the Crisis of Humanism*; Thompson, *Good Science*.

36 Plumwood, "Integrating Ethical Frameworks for Animals, Humans, and Nature"; Kim, *Dangerous Crossings*; Jackson, *Becoming Human*; Adams, *Sexual Politics of Meat*; Deckha, "Toward a Postcolonial, Posthumanist Feminist Theory"; Arvin, Tuck, and Morrill, "Decolonizing Feminism"; Federici, *Caliban and the Witch*.

37 Haraway, *When Species Meet*, 71. Emphasis original.

38 Haraway, 75.

39 I quote Haraway once more: "Unidirectional relations of use, ruled by practices of calculation and self-sure of hierarchy . . . [take] heart from the primary dualism that parses body one way and mind another. That dualism should have withered long ago in the light of feminist and many other criticisms, but the fantastic mind/body binary has proved remarkably resilient." Haraway, *When Species Meet*, 75.

40 Lab interview no. 7, 2021.

41 Holmberg, "Feeling for the Animal," 332.

42 Lab interview no. 7, 2021.

43 Lab interviewee no. 8, personal communication, 2022.

44 Gina M. Hilton, personal communication, 2022. See also Evisabel Craig et al., "Reducing the Need for Animal Testing."

45 Visvanathan, "From the Annals of the Laboratory State," 25, as cited in Thompson, *Good Science*, 220.

46 Barad, *Meeting the Universe Halfway*. By merging ethics (ways of relating), ontology (ways of being), and epistemology (ways of knowing), Barad encourages us to consider how we know what we think we know in terms of who and what we ought to care about.

47 Lab interview no. 7, 2021. Emphasis added.

48 Author field notes, lab meeting no. 20, 2021.

49 Visvanathan, "From the Annals of the Laboratory State," 43.

50 Holmberg, "Feeling for the Animal," 318. I believe Holmberg refers to "good science" here in the sense of methodological and intellectual rigor, whereas Thompson refers to "good science" in the sense of both scientific and ethical integrity.

51 On the darker side of care, see Glenn, *Forced to Care*; Hobart and Kneese, "Radical Care"; Seiler, "Origins of White Care."

52 For more on "the performance of [scientific] experiments . . . [as] itself a discipline of self-mastery" see White, "Experimental Animal in Victorian Britain," 67.

53 Lab interviewee no. 7, personal communication, 2022.

54 Lab interviewee no. 7, personal communication, 2022. Emphasis added.

55 Lab interviewee no. 7, personal communication, 2022.

56 Lab interviewee no. 7, personal communication, 2022. Emphasis added.

57 Haraway, *When Species Meet*, 75.

58 Lab interview no. 2, 2021. Emphasis added.

59 Expert interview no. 1, 2019.

60 White, "Experimental Animal in Victorian Britain," 74. Emphasis added.

61 Gruen, *Entangled Empathy*.

62 Author field notes, lab meeting no. 21, 2022.

63 Lab interview no. 6, 2021. Emphasis added.

64 Lab interview no. 5, 2021.

65 Lab interview no. 5, 2021.

66 Lab interview no. 5, 2021. Emphasis added.

67 Lab interview no. 4, 2021.

68 Lab interview no. 8, 2021. Emphasis added.

69 Lab interview no. 5, 2021.

70 For more on the inevitability of toxic disasters, see Fortun, "Learning Across Disaster"; Jill Lindsey Harrison, "'Accidents' and Invisibilities."

71 Thompson, *Good Science*, 221.

72 Thompson, 5, 27.

73 As Juno Parreñas asks, in the context of orangutan conservation efforts, "For people intervening, what forms of violence are permissible at the level of individuals for the good of a species' future?" Parreñas, *Decolonizing Extinction*, 85.

74 Tollefson, "Scientists Concerned over US Environment Agency's Plan to Limit Animal Research."

75 For numerous reasons to distrust chemical corporations, see Oreskes and Conway, *Merchants of Doubt*; Proctor, *Cancer Wars*; Markowitz and Rosner, *Deceit and Denial*; Ross and Amter, *Polluters*; Fortun, *Advocacy after Bhopal*.

76 For example, see Pellow, *Resisting Global Toxics*; Steingraber, *Living Downstream*; Wiebe, *Everyday Exposure*; Cordner, *Toxic Safety*.

77 Exxon Valdez Oil Spill Trustee Council, "Settlement," accessed July 25, 2022. https://evostc.state.ak.us; Stevens, "Exxon Mobil's First-Quarter Profit Rises, Even after $3.4 Billion Hit from Russia Charge."

78 Thompson, *Good Science*, 220. Original emphasis.

79 Respectfully challenging Frickel's claims regarding the "scientist social movement" that generated genetic toxicology, for example. Frickel, *Chemical Consequences*.

80 Nash, "Purity and Danger"; Sellers, *Hazards of the Job*; Davis, *Banned*; Murphy,
Sick Building Syndrome and the Problem of Uncertainty.

81 I saw this tagline in a Monsanto advertisement in a 1955 issue of *Scientific
American*; contemporary marketing researchers date this tagline back to the late
1930s, if not earlier. "Authors"; McDonald, Laverie, and Manis, "Interplay between
Advertising and Society."

82 Weheliye, *Habeas Viscus*.

83 Haraway, *When Species Meet*, 76.

84 Lab interview no. 9, 2021. Emphasis added.

85 There is a growing literature on animal cultures and animals' (own sense of) ethics. See Bekoff and Pierce, *Wild Justice*; Yarbrough, "Species, Race, and Culture in
the Space of Wildlife Management."

86 Luke, "Taming Ourselves or Going Feral?," 315.

87 Holmberg, "Feeling for the Animal," 333.

88 Lab interviewee no. 4, personal communication, 2022.

89 Prescod-Weinstein and McKittrick, "Public Thinker."

90 Historian of science Evan Hepler-Smith makes a similar "industry's game" argument, what he calls "molecular bureaucracy": "If the politics of environmental
chemicals is a game of chess, and chemicals are the pieces, environmental laws
the rules, and methods of toxicology and advocacy the strategies, then molecular
bureaucracy is the game board. The pieces exist apart from the board, but the
board structures how players make sense of the pieces." Hepler-Smith, "Molecular
Bureaucracy," 537.

91 On high-throughput screening, see Borrel et al., "High-Throughput Screening
to Predict Chemical-Assay Interference." On encouraging, innovative collaborations between natural scientists and scientist feminists (and feminist scientists),
for example, see CLEAR, "CLEAR Lab Book"; Wylie, Sara. "Public Lab." Sara
Wylie, January 15, 2018. https://sarawylie.com; Cynthia Foster, "Asking Different
Questions Archive Now on YouTube," Feminist Research Institute, November
19, 2020, https://fri.ucdavis.edu; Lasker and Simcox, "Using Feminist Theory
and Social Justice Pedagogy to Educate"; Cleo A. Woelfle-Erskine, "F.R.E.S.H.
Water Relations," F.R.E.S.H. Water Relations, accessed July 7, 2022, https://water
-relations.net; Ambika Kamath, "F.L.A.I.R. Lab," F.L.A.I.R. Lab, accessed July 7,
2022, https://kamathlab.com/.

92 For the full worksheet and additional resources, see Free Radicals, "Research
Justice Worksheet," n.d., https://freerads.org.

93 Lab interviewee no. 8, personal communication, 2022.

94 McCutcheon, "Toxicology and the Law."

95 Particularly in the wake of the Supreme Court's overturning of *Roe v. Wade*, I was doubly horrified to learn, from Olivia, that IACUC maintains no oversight over animal embryos; embryos don't count as organisms in this human-made, nonhuman world. This lack of institutional recognition of (and care for) animal embryos left Olivia in the deeply disturbing position of having to kill late-stage embryos without first euthanizing them, because the euthanizing chemical needed was not approved in her lab's budget, nor under her IACUC protocol, for that specific use. Lacking sodium barbital, and anyway prohibited from using it in such a manner, Olivia recalled in horror how she found herself decapitating late-stage embryos in order to kill and then dissect them: "Some of [the chick embryos] were already starting to get fuzzy and grow feathers, and some of them make noises—it was rough . . ." (lab interviewee no. 6, personal communication, 2022). And as I finalized this chapter, news broke of the US Supreme Court scuttling the Clean Water Act. Totenberg, "Supreme Court Has Narrowed the Scope of the Clean Water Act."

96 I borrow "otherwise" from Povinelli, "Routes/Worlds"; and "scientist feminist" from Roy, *Molecular Feminisms*.

OUTRO

1 Freeman, *Time Binds*, 173.
2 With this title I also purposefully reference Douglas, *Purity and Danger*; Kosek, "Purity and Pollution"; Nash, "Purity and Danger"; Zimring, *Clean and White*.
3 See similar and more specific critiques in Roberts, *Messengers of Sex*.
4 On the "drag of the race" in terms of dog breeding, for example, see Wehle, *Snakefoot*.
5 Bederman, *Manliness & Civilization*.
6 Butler, *Gender Trouble*; Pellegrini, *Performance Anxieties*.
7 See also Halberstam, *In a Queer Time and Place*; Halberstam, *Queer Art of Failure*.
8 Freeman, *Time Binds*, xxiii. Emphasis added.
9 Butler, "Merely Cultural."
10 Hayward, "Intoxifornicate"; Helmreich, "Left Hand of Nature and Culture," 378.
11 Freeman, *Time Binds*, xiii.
12 Freeman, xiii.
13 Freeman, xxi–xxii.
14 Shotwell, *Against Purity*.
15 Crews and McLachlan, "Epigenetics, Evolution, Endocrine Disruption, Health, and Disease," 16. For a more thorough critique of this review paper, see Packer, "Becoming with Toxicity."
16 Brockovich, "Plummeting Sperm Counts, Shrinking Penises"; Swan and Colino, *Count Down*.
17 Kevles, *In the Name of Eugenics*; Panofsky, *Misbehaving Science*; Schuller, *Biopolitics of Feeling*; Clare, *Brilliant Imperfection*; Benjamin, "Interrogating Equity."

18 Zimdahl, *History of Weed Science in the United States*, 137.
19 On potentially feminist crop breeding, for instance, see Tarjem, "Feminist Crops."
20 Aviv, "Valuable Reputation."
21 As argued in Perret, "Chemical Castration."
22 Packer and Lambert, "What's Gender Got to Do With It?"
23 As Kim (2015) writes: "Structured by the post-civil rights regime, the American left is thoroughly segmented. Each cause has its cluster of advocacy organizations and corresponding academic field(s). Each engages the enemy from a separate bunker. Each resists coercive universalisms and coalitional possibilities, except momentarily. In the meantime, the forces of neoliberal capitalism face few obstacles as they transform racialized others, animals, and the earth into 'resources' in the game of perpetual capital accumulation." Kim, *Dangerous Crossings*, 287. Perhaps there's a time and place in environmental toxicology for what Spivak called "strategic essentialism." Spivak, "Subaltern Studies."
24 Colborn, Dumanoski, and Myers, *Our Stolen Future*.
25 Howard, *Concentration and Power in the Food System*; Clapp, "Bigger Is Not Always Better."
26 Robbins and Moore, "Ecological Anxiety Disorder."
27 Here I quote, respectively: Murphy, "Alterlife and Decolonial Chemical Relations"; Combahee River Collective, "A Black Feminist Statement," April 1977, https://combaheerivercollective.weebly.com; Gilmore, *Golden Gulag*.
28 Glenn, *Forced to Care*; Parreñas, "Reproductive Labour of Migrant Workers."
29 I am not suggesting, *pace* psychologist Carol Gilligan, that women are somehow inherently more caring, nor that women's ethics magically flow from some essentialist tendency towards care. Gilligan, *In a Different Voice*.
30 See also anthropologist David Graeber's and archaeologist David Wengrow's sobering discussion of the enduring "particular nexus of violence and care": "Slavery finds its origins in war. But everywhere we encounter it slavery is also, at first, a domestic institution. Hierarchy and property may derive from notions of the sacred, but the most brutal forms of exploitation have their origins in the most intimate of social relations: as perversions of nurture, love and caring." Graeber and Wengrow, *Dawn of Everything*, 510, 208.
31 Lab interview no. 8, 2021.
32 Lab interview no. 8, 2021. Emphasis added.
33 O'Brien, "Being a Scientist Means Taking Sides."
34 For inspiring examples of critical feminism deeply integrated into scientific training, see CLEAR, "CLEAR Lab Book"; Foster, "Asking Different Questions Archive Now on YouTube"; Kamath, "F.L.A.I.R. Lab"; Cleo A. Woelfle-Erskine, "F.R.E.S.H. Water Relations," F.R.E.S.H. Water Relations, accessed July 7, 2022, https://water-relations.net; GeoContext, "Welcome to GeoContext!," accessed January 15, 2021, https://geo-context.github.io.
35 Lab interview no. 8, 2021.

36 Benotti et al., "Pharmaceuticals and Endocrine Disrupting Compounds in U.S. Drinking Water"; Boxall et al., "Pharmaceuticals and Personal Care Products in the Environment."

37 For a beautiful reflection on a STS critic's necessary embrace of plastic, to cite another example, see Roberts, "Reflections of an Unrepentant Plastiphobe."

APPENDIX

1 Ward, "Dyke Methods," 71.

2 On queer time, see Halberstam, *In a Queer Time and Place*; Freeman, *Time Binds*. Also discussed in this book's outro, "Purity and Drag."

3 Nader, "Up the Anthropologist"; Tuck, "Suspending Damage"; Tuck and Yang, "R-Words."

4 This research was approved by my sponsoring institutions' respective Committees for the Protection of Human Subjects, protocol numbers 2018-10-11488 (University of California, Berkeley) and HS-20–276 (University of California, Riverside).

BIBLIOGRAPHY

Adams, Carol J. *Sexual Politics of Meat: A Feminist-Vegetarian Critical Theory*. 20th ed. New York: Bloomsbury Publishing, 2010.

Adams, Vincanne. *Glyphosate and the Swirl: An Agroindustrial Chemical on the Move*. Critical Global Health: Evidence, Efficacy, Ethnography. Durham, NC: Duke University Press, 2023.

Agard-Jones, Vanessa. "Bodies in the System." *Small Axe: A Caribbean Journal of Criticism* 17, no. 3 (42) (November 1, 2013): 182–92. https://doi.org/10.1215/07990537-2378991.

Ah-King, Malin, and Eva Hayward. "Toxic Sexes: Perverting Pollution and Queering Hormone Disruption." *O-Zone: A Journal of Object Oriented Studies*, no. 1 (Spring 2013): 1–12.

Ahmed, Sara. "Feminist Killjoys (and Other Willful Subjects)." *Scholar & Feminist Online* 8, no. 3 (2010). http://sfonline.barnard.edu.

———. *On Being Included: Racism and Diversity in Institutional Life*. Durham, NC: Duke University Press, 2012.

Ahuja, Neel. *Bioinsecurities: Disease Interventions, Empire, and the Government of Species*. ANIMA: Critical Race Studies Otherwise. Durham, NC: Duke University Press, 2016.

———. "Postcolonial Critique in a Multispecies World." *PMLA* 124, no. 2 (2009): 556–63.

Akaba, Azibuike. "Science as a Double-Edged Sword: Research Has Often Rewarded Polluters, but EJ Activists Are Taking It Back." *Race, Poverty & the Environment* 11, no. 2 (2004): 9–11.

Albert, Céline, Gloria M. Luque, and Franck Courchamp. "The Twenty Most Charismatic Species." *PLOS ONE* 13, no. 7 (July 9, 2018): e0199149. https://doi.org/10.1371/journal.pone.0199149.

Aleksunes, Lauren M., and David L. Eaton. "Principles of Toxicology." In *Casarett & Doull's Toxicology: The Basic Science of Poisons*, 9th ed. New York: McGraw Hill Medical, 2019.

Allen, Garland E. "Science Misapplied: The Eugenics Age Revisited." *Technology Review* 99, no. 6 (1996): 23–31.

Altman, Rebecca Gasior, Rachel Morello-Frosch, Julia Green Brody, Ruthann Rudel, Phil Brown, and Mara Averick. "Pollution Comes Home and Gets Personal: Women's Experience of Household Chemical Exposure." *Journal of Health and Social Behavior* 49, no. 4 (December 2008): 417–35.

Anderson, Elijah. "The White Space." *Sociology of Race and Ethnicity* 1, no. 1 (January 2015): 10–21. https://doi.org/10.1177/2332649214561306.

Anderson, Kay. *Race and the Crisis of Humanism*. London: Routledge, 2006.

Anderson, Warwick. *The Cultivation of Whiteness: Science, Health, and Racial Destiny in Australia*. Durham, NC: Duke University Press, 2006.

Anker, Peder. *Imperial Ecology: Environmental Order in the British Empire, 1895–1945*. Cambridge, MA: Harvard University Press, 2001.

Antonini, Francesca. "Pessimism of the Intellect, Optimism of the Will: Gramsci's Political Thought in the Last Miscellaneous Notebooks." *Rethinking Marxism* 31, no. 1 (January 2, 2019): 42–57. https://doi.org/10.1080/08935696.2019.1577616.

Arvin, Maile, Eve Tuck, and Angie Morrill. "Decolonizing Feminism: Challenging Connections between Settler Colonialism and Heteropatriarchy." *Feminist Formations* 25, no. 1 (2013): 8–34. https://doi.org/10.1353/ff.2013.0006.

Austin, Daniel F. "Bindweed (Convolvulus Arvensis, Convolvulaceae) in North America, from Medicine to Menace." *Journal of the Torrey Botanical Society* 127, no. 2 (2000): 172–77. https://doi.org/10.2307/3088694.

"The Authors." *Scientific American* 192, no. 5 (1955): 18–30.

Aviv, Rachel. "A Valuable Reputation." *New Yorker*, February 3, 2014. https://www.newyorker.com.

Bagemihl, Bruce. *Biological Exuberance: Animal Homosexuality and Natural Diversity*. Stonewall Inn Editions. New York: St. Martin's Press, 2000.

Balcombe, Jonathan P. *What a Fish Knows: The Inner Lives of Our Underwater Cousins*. New York: Scientific American; Farrar, Straus and Giroux, 2016.

Baltzell, E. Digby. *The Protestant Establishment: Aristocracy & Caste in America*. New Haven, CT: Yale University Press, 1987.

Barad, Karen Michelle. *Meeting the Universe Halfway: Quantum Physics and the Entanglement of Matter and Meaning*. Durham, NC: Duke University Press, 2007.

Barba, Mayra G. Sánchez. "'Keeping Them Down': Neurotoxic Pesticides, Race, and Disabling Biopolitics." *Catalyst: Feminism, Theory, Technoscience* 6, no. 1 (2020): 1–31. https://doi.org/10.28968/cftt.v6i1.32253.

Bederman, Gail. *Manliness & Civilization: A Cultural History of Gender and Race in the United States, 1880–1917*. Women in Culture and Society. Chicago: University of Chicago Press, 1995.

Beers, Diane L. *For the Prevention of Cruelty: The History and Legacy of Animal Rights Activism in the United States*. Athens: Swallow Press, an imprint of Ohio University Press, 2006.

Bekoff, Marc, and Jessica Pierce. *Wild Justice: The Moral Lives of Animals*. Chicago: University of Chicago Press, 2010.

Benbrook, Charles M. "How Did the US EPA and IARC Reach Diametrically Opposed Conclusions on the Genotoxicity of Glyphosate-Based Herbicides?" *Environmental Sciences Europe* 31, no. 1 (2019): 1–16. https://doi.org/10.1186/s12302-018-0184-7.

———. "Trends in Glyphosate Herbicide Use in the United States and Globally." *Environmental Sciences Europe* 28, no. 1 (2016): 1–15. https://doi.org/10.1186/s12302-016 -0070-0.

———. "Why Regulators Lost Track and Control of Pesticide Risks: Lessons from the Case of Glyphosate-Based Herbicides and Genetically Engineered-Crop Technology." *Current Environmental Health Reports* 5, no. 3 (2018): 387–95. https://doi.org /10.1007/s40572-018-0207-y.

Benbrook, Charles, Melissa J. Perry, Fiorella Belpoggi, Philip J. Landrigan, Michelle Perro, Daniele Mandrioli, Michael N. Antoniou, Paul Winchester, and Robin Mesnage. "Commentary: Novel Strategies and New Tools to Curtail the Health Effects of Pesticides." *Environmental Health* 20, no. 1 (August 3, 2021): 87. https://doi .org/10.1186/s12940-021-00773-4.

Benjamin, Ruha. "Catching Our Breath: Critical Race STS and the Carceral Imagination." *Engaging Science, Technology, and Society* 2 (July 1, 2016): 145–56. https://doi .org/10.17351/ests2016.70.

———. "Interrogating Equity: A Disability Justice Approach to Genetic Engineering." In *Issues in Science & Technology* 32, no. 3 (2016): 50–54.

Benotti, Mark J., Rebecca A. Trenholm, Brett J. Vanderford, Janie C. Holady, Benjamin D. Stanford, and Shane A. Snyder. "Pharmaceuticals and Endocrine Disrupting Compounds in U.S. Drinking Water." *Environmental Science & Technology* 43, no. 3 (2009): 597–603. https://doi.org/10.1021/es801845a.

Bergman, Åke, Jerrold J Heindel, Susan Jobling, Karen Ann Kidd, R. Thomas Zoeller, World Health Organization, and United Nations Environment Programme. *State of the Science of Endocrine Disrupting Chemicals—2012: An Assessment of the State of the Science of Endocrine Disruptors Prepared by a Group of Experts for the United Nations Environment Programme (UNEP) and WHO.* Geneva, Switzerland: United Nations Environment Programme and the World Health Organization, 2013. http://www.who.int.

Bernal, Martin. *Black Athena: The Afroasiatic Roots of Classical Civilization.* New Brunswick, NJ: Rutgers University Press, 1987.

———. "Race, Class and Gender in the Formation of the Aryan Model of Greek Origins." *South Atlantic Quarterly* 94, no. 4 (1995): 987–1008.

Bhattacharya, Tithi, ed. *Social Reproduction Theory: Remapping Class, Recentering Oppression.* London: Pluto Press, 2017.

Birke, Lynda I. A. "Science, Feminism and Animal Natures II: Feminist Critiques and the Place of Animals in Science." *Women's Studies International Forum* 14, no. 5 (1991): 451–58. https://doi.org/10.1016/0277-5395(91)90047-L.

Birnbaum, Linda S. "When Environmental Chemicals Act like Uncontrolled Medicine." *Trends in Endocrinology & Metabolism* 24, no. 7 (July 2013): 321–23. https://doi .org/10.1016/j.tem.2012.12.005.

Blum, Joel D., Jeffrey C. Drazen, Marcus W. Johnson, Brian N. Popp, Laura C. Motta, and Alan J. Jamieson. "Mercury Isotopes Identify Near-Surface Marine Mercury in

Deep-Sea Trench Biota." *Proceedings of the National Academy of Sciences* 117, no. 47 (November 24, 2020): 29292–98. https://doi.org/10.1073/pnas.2012773117.

Boast, Hannah. "Theorizing the Gay Frog." *Environmental Humanities* 14, no. 3 (November 1, 2022): 661–79. https://doi.org/10.1215/22011919-9962959.

Boisseron, Bénédicte. *Afro-Dog: Blackness and the Animal Question*. New York: Columbia University Press, 2018.

Bomgardner, Melody M. "Palmer Amaranth, the King of Weeds, Cripples New Herbicides." *Chemical & Engineering News*, August 3, 2019. https://cen.acs.org.

Bordo, Susan. "The Cartesian Masculinization of Thought." *Signs* 11, no. 3 (1986): 439–56.

Borrel, Alexandre, Ruili Huang, Srilatha Sakamuru, Menghang Xia, Anton Simeonov, Kamel Mansouri, Keith A. Houck, Richard S. Judson, and Nicole C. Kleinstreuer. "High-Throughput Screening to Predict Chemical-Assay Interference." *Scientific Reports* 10, no. 1 (2020): 3986. https://doi.org/10.1038/s41598-020-60747-3.

Borzelleca, Joseph F. "Paracelsus: Herald of Modern Toxicology." *Toxicological Sciences* 53, no. 1 (January 2000): 2–4. https://doi.org/10.1093/toxsci/53.1.2.

Boudia, Soraya. "Managing Scientific and Political Uncertainty. Environmental Risk Assessment in an Historical Perspective." In *Powerless Science? Science and Politics in a Toxic World*, edited by Soraya Boudia and Nathalie Jas, 95–114. The Environment in History, vol. 2. New York: Berghahn Books, 2014.

Boudia, Soraya, Angela N. H. Creager, Scott Frickel, Emmanuel Henry, Nathalie Jas, Carsten Reinhardt, and Jody A. Roberts. "Residues: Rethinking Chemical Environments." *Engaging Science, Technology, and Society* 4, no. 0 (June 28, 2018): 165–78. https://doi.org/10.17351/ests2018.245.

Boudia, Soraya, and Nathalie Jas, eds. *Powerless Science? Science and Politics in a Toxic World*. The Environment in History, vol. 2. New York: Berghahn Books, 2014.

Boxall, Alistair B. A., Murray A. Rudd, Bryan W. Brooks, Daniel J. Caldwell, Kyungho Choi, Silke Hickmann, Elizabeth Innes, et al. "Pharmaceuticals and Personal Care Products in the Environment: What Are the Big Questions?" *Environmental Health Perspectives* 120, no. 9 (September 2012): 1221–29. https://doi.org/10.1289/ehp.1104477.

Branch, Haley A., Amanda N. Klingler, Kelsey J. R. P. Byers, Aaron Panofsky, and Danielle Peers. "Discussions of the 'Not So Fit': How Ableism Limits Diverse Thought and Investigative Potential in Evolutionary Biology." *American Naturalist* 200, no. 1 (2022): 101–13. https://doi.org/10.1086/720003.

Brockovich, Erin. "Plummeting Sperm Counts, Shrinking Penises: Toxic Chemicals Threaten Humanity." *The Guardian*, March 18, 2021, sec. Opinion. http://www.theguardian.com.

Brookshire, Bethany. *Pests. How Humans Create Animal Villains*. New York: Harper-Collins, 2022.

brown, adrienne maree, and Walidah Imarisha, eds. *Octavia's Brood: Science Fiction Stories from Social Justice Movements*. Oakland, CA: AK Press, 2015.

Brown, Harriet. "She Experimented on Primates for Decades. Now She Wants to Shut down the Labs." *The Guardian*, May 31, 2022, sec. World. https://www.theguardian.com.

Brown, John R., and John L. Thornton. "Percivall Pott (1714–1788) and Chimney Sweepers' Cancer of the Scrotum." *British Journal of Industrial Medicine* 14, no. 1 (January 1957): 68–70.

Brown, Phil. *Toxic Exposures: Contested Illnesses and the Environmental Health Movement*. New York: Columbia University Press, 2007.

Brown, Phil, Stephen Zavestoski, Sabrina McCormick, Meadow Linder, Joshua Mandelbaum, and Theo Luebke. "A Gulf of Difference: Disputes over Gulf War-Related Illnesses." *Journal of Health and Social Behavior* 42, no. 3 (2001): 235–57. https://doi.org/10.2307/3090213.

Brown, Wendy. "Finding the Man in the State." *Feminist Studies* 18, no. 1 (1992): 7–34. https://doi.org/10.2307/3178212.

———. "Wounded Attachments." *Political Theory* 21, no. 3 (August 1, 1993): 390–410.

Bullard, Robert D. *Dumping in Dixie: Race, Class, and Environmental Quality*. 3rd ed. Boulder, CO: Westview Press, 2000.

Bullard, Robert D., Paul Mohai, Robin Saha, and Beverly Wright. "Toxic Wastes and Race at Twenty: Why Race Still Matters After All These Years." *Environmental Law* 38, no. 2 (2008): 371–411.

Butler, Judith. *Gender Trouble: Feminism and the Subversion of Identity*. Thinking Gender. New York: Routledge, 1990.

———. "Merely Cultural." *New Left Review*, no. 227 (January/February 1998): 33–44.

Cajete, Gregory. *Native Science: Natural Laws of Interdependence*. 1st ed. Santa Fe: Clear Light Publishers, 2000.

Canavan, Gerry. "'There's Nothing New / Under the Sun, / But There Are New Suns': Recovering Octavia E. Butler's Lost Parables." *Los Angeles Review of Books*, June 9, 2014. https://lareviewofbooks.org.

Carson, Rachel. *Silent Spring*. New York: Fawcett Crest, 1962.

Casarett, Louis J. "Origin and Scope of Toxicology." In *Toxicology: The Basic Science of Poisons*, edited by Louis J. Casarett and John Doull, 3–10. New York: Macmillan, 1975.

———. "Toxicologic Evaluation." In *Toxicology: The Basic Science of Poisons*, edited by Louis J. Casarett and John Doull, 11–25. New York: Macmillan, 1975.

Casarett, Louis J., and John Doull. Preface to *Toxicology: The Basic Science of Poisons*, edited by Louis J. Casarett and John Doull, vii. New York: Macmillan, 1975.

———, eds. *Toxicology: The Basic Science of Poisons*. New York: Macmillan, 1975.

Chakrabarti, Pratik. "Beasts of Burden: Animals and Laboratory Research in Colonial India." *History of Science* 48, no. 2 (2010): 125–51. https://doi.org/10.1177/007327531004800201.

Chandler, Kimberly. "Alabama Law Criminalizing Care for Transgender Youth Faces Federal Test." *PBS NewsHour*, May 5, 2022. https://www.pbs.org.

ChemicalSafetyFacts.org. "Debunking the Myths: Are There Really 84,000 Chemicals?" *ChemicalSafetyFacts.Org* (blog), 2022. https://www.chemicalsafetyfacts.org.

Chen, Eli. "Monsanto and Growers Groups Sue California over Adding Warning Labels to Glyphosate Herbicides." *St. Louis Public Radio*, November 15, 2017. http://news.stlpublicradio.org.

Chen, Mel Y. "Toxic Animacies, Inanimate Affections." *GLQ: A Journal of Lesbian and Gay Studies* 17, no. 2 (2011): 265–86.

Cho, Sumi, Kimberlé Williams Crenshaw, and Leslie McCall. "Toward a Field of Intersectionality Studies: Theory, Applications, and Praxis." *Signs* 38, no. 4 (2013): 785–810. https://doi.org/10.1086/669608.

Clapp, Jennifer. *Bigger Is Not Always Better: The Drivers and Implications of the Recent Agribusiness Megamergers*. Waterloo, ON: Global Food Politics Group, University of Waterloo, 2017. https://www.researchgate.net.

Clare, Eli. *Brilliant Imperfection: Grappling with Cure*. Durham, NC: Duke University Press, 2017.

Civic Laboratory for Environmental Action Research (CLEAR). "CLEAR Lab Book." *CLEAR* (blog), December 30, 2017. https://civiclaboratory.nl.

Cohn, Carol. "Sex and Death in the Rational World of Defense Intellectuals." *Signs* 12, no. 4 (1987): 687–718.

Colborn, Theo, and Coralie Clement, eds. *Chemically-Induced Alterations in Sexual and Functional Development: The Wildlife/Human Connection*. Princeton, NJ: Princeton Scientific Publishing, 1992.

Colborn, Theo, Dianne Dumanoski, and John Peterson Myers. *Our Stolen Future: Are We Threatening Our Fertility, Intelligence, and Survival?: A Scientific Detective Story*. New York: Dutton, 1996.

Cone, Marla. *Silent Snow: The Slow Poisoning of the Arctic*. New York: Grove Press, 2005.

Conis, Elena. "DDT Disbelievers: Health and the New Economic Poisons in Georgia after World War II." *Southern Spaces*, October 28, 2016. https://southernspaces.org.

Connell, R. W. *Masculinities*. 2nd ed. Berkeley: University of California Press, 2005.

Corbin, C. N. E., Guillermo Douglass-Jaimes, Jesse Williamson, Ashton Wesner, Margot Higgins, and Jenny L. Palomino. "(Re)Thinking the Tenure Process by Embracing Diversity in Scholars and Scholarship." *University of California Student Association Graduate and Professional Student Policy Journal* 1, no. 1 (2015): 4–9.

Cordner, Alissa. *Toxic Safety: Flame Retardants, Chemical Controversies, and Environmental Health*. New York: Columbia University Press, 2016.

Craig, Evisabel, Kelly Lowe, Gregory Akerman, Jeffrey Dawson, Brenda May, Elissa Reaves, and Anna Lowit. "Reducing the Need for Animal Testing While Increasing Efficiency in a Pesticide Regulatory Setting: Lessons from the EPA Office of Pesticide Programs' Hazard and Science Policy Council." *Regulatory Toxicology and Pharmacology* 108 (November 1, 2019): 104481. https://doi.org/10.1016/j.yrtph.2019.104481.

Cram, Shannon. "Living in Dose: Nuclear Work and the Politics of Permissible Exposure." *Public Culture* 28, no. 3 (80) (2016): 519–39. https://doi.org/10.1215/08992363-3511526.

Crenshaw, Kimberlé. "Demarginalizing the Intersection of Race and Sex: A Black Feminist Critique of Antidiscrimination Doctrine, Feminist Theory and Antiracist Politics." *University of Chicago Legal Forum* 1989, no. 1 (1989): 139–67.

——. "Mapping the Margins: Intersectionality, Identity Politics, and Violence against Women of Color." *Stanford Law Review* 43, no. 6 (1991): 1241–99.

——. "The Panic over Critical Race Theory Is an Attempt to Whitewash U.S. History." *Washington Post*, July 2, 2021, sec. Perspective. https://www.washingtonpost.com.

Crenshaw, Kimberlé, Neil Gotanda, Garry Peller, and Kendall Thomas. *Critical Race Theory: The Key Writings That Formed the Movement*. New York: New Press, 1995.

Crews, David, and John A. McLachlan. "Epigenetics, Evolution, Endocrine Disruption, Health, and Disease." Supplement, *Endocrinology* 147, no. S6 (June 2006): S4–10. https://doi.org/10.1210/en.2005-1122.

Crist, Eileen. *Images of Animals: Anthropomorphism and Animal Mind*. Animals, Culture, and Society. Philadelphia: Temple University Press, 1999.

Cronon, William. "The Uses of Environmental History." *Environmental History Review* 17, no. 3 (1993): 1. https://doi.org/10.2307/3984602.

Cummings, Brian. "Michael Gallo Receives 2021 SOT Founders Award (for Outstanding Leadership in Toxicology)." *Toxchange* (blog), January 21, 2021. https://toxchange.toxicology.org.

Cushing, Lara, Rachel Morello-Frosch, Madeline Wander, and Manuel Pastor. "The Haves, the Have-Nots, and the Health of Everyone: The Relationship Between Social Inequality and Environmental Quality." *Annual Review of Public Health* 36, no. 1 (2015): 193–209. https://doi.org/10.1146/annurev-publhealth-031914-122646.

Dally, Ann. "Thalidomide: Was the Tragedy Preventable?" *The Lancet* 351, no. 9110 (1998): 1197–99. https://doi.org/10.1016/S0140-6736(97)09038-7.

Daston, Lorraine, and Peter Galison. *Objectivity*. Paperback ed. New York: Zone Books, 2010.

Daston, Lorraine, and Gregg Mitman. "The How and Why of Thinking with Animals." In *Thinking with Animals: New Perspectives on Anthropomorphism*, edited by Lorraine Daston and Gregg Mitman, 1–14. New York: Columbia University Press, 2005.

Davis, Angela Y. *Women, Race & Class*. New York: Vintage Books, 1983.

Davis, Frederick Rowe. *Banned: A History of Pesticides and the Science of Toxicology*. New Haven, CT: Yale University Press, 2014.

——. "Pesticides and the Paradox of the Anthropocene: From Natural to Synthetic to Synthesised Nature." *Global Environment* 10, no. 1 (2017): 114–36.

Davis, Georgiann. *Contesting Intersex: The Dubious Diagnosis*. New York: New York University Press, 2015.

Davis, Wynne. "Florida Senate Passes a Controversial Schools Bill Labeled 'Don't Say Gay' by Critics." *NPR*, March 8, 2022, sec. Politics. https://www.npr.org.

De Chadarevian, Soraya. *Heredity under the Microscope*. Chicago: University of Chicago Press, 2020.

Deckha, Maneesha. "Toward a Postcolonial, Posthumanist Feminist Theory: Centralizing Race and Culture in Feminist Work on Nonhuman Animals." *Hypatia* 27, no. 3 (2012): 527–45. https://doi.org/10.1111/j.1527-2001.2012.01290.x.

Descartes, René. *Descartes: Philosophical Letters*. Translated by Anthony Kenny. Oxford: Clarendon Press, 1970.

DeVault, Marjorie L. *Feeding the Family: The Social Organization of Caring as Gendered Work*. Women in Culture and Society. Chicago: University of Chicago Press, 1991.

Di Chiro, Giovanna. "Polluted Politics? Confronting Toxic Discourse, Sex Panic, and Eco-Normativity." In *Queer Ecologies: Sex, Nature, Politics, Desire*, edited by Catriona Mortimer-Sandilands and Bruce Erickson, 199–230. Bloomington: Indiana University Press, 2010.

Diamanti-Kandarakis, Evanthia, Jean-Pierre Bourguignon, Linda C. Giudice, Russ Hauser, Gail S. Prins, Ana M. Soto, R. Thomas Zoeller, and Andrea C. Gore. "Endocrine-Disrupting Chemicals: An Endocrine Society Scientific Statement." *Endocrine Reviews* 30, no. 4 (June 2009): 293–342. https://doi.org/10.1210/er.2009-0002.

Dominiczak, Marek H. "International Year of Chemistry 2011: Paracelsus: In Praise of Mavericks." *Clinical Chemistry* 57, no. 6 (June 1, 2011): 932–34. https://doi.org/10.1373/clinchem.2011.165894.

Douglas, Mary. *Purity and Danger: An Analysis of Concepts of Pollution and Taboo*. New York: Routledge and Kegan Paul, 1966.

Drugs.com. "Thalidomide (Monograph)." Last updated April 7, 2023. https://www.drugs.com.

Duong, Natalia. "Homing Toxicity: The Domestication of Herbidical Warfare." *Catalyst: Feminism, Theory, Technoscience* 9, no. 1 (2023): 1–24.

"DuPont Song: "Better Things for Better Living . . . through Chemistry" (1964 New York World's Fair)." DuPont's Wonderful World of Chemistry show at the 1964 New York World's Fair. YouTube video, 00:00:36, November 18, 2012. https://www.youtube.com/watch?v=tJtKkBYlHFw.

Egede, Leonard E., and Rebekah J. Walker. "Structural Racism, Social Risk Factors, and Covid-19—A Dangerous Convergence for Black Americans." *New England Journal of Medicine* 383, no. 12 (September 17, 2020): e77. https://doi.org/10.1056/NEJMp2023616.

Elston, Mary Ann. "Women and Anti-Vivisection in Victorian England, 1870–1900." In *Vivisection in Historical Perspective*, edited by Nicolaas A. Rupke, 259–94. London: Croom Helm, 1987.

Engels, Friedrich. *The Origin of the Family, Private Property and the State*. Chicago: C. H. Kerr, 1902.

Enloe, Cynthia H. *Bananas, Beaches and Bases: Making Feminist Sense of International Politics*. 2nd ed. Berkeley, CA: University of California Press, 2014.

Erickson, Britt E. "US EPA to Impose Atrazine Restrictions." *Chemical & Engineering News*, July 1, 2022. https://cen.acs.org.

Fanon, Frantz. *Black Skin, White Masks*. Translated by Charles Lam Markmann. London, UK: Pluto Press, 2008.

———. "Colonial Violence and Mental Disorders." In *The Wretched of the Earth*, translated by Richard Philcox. New York: Grove Press, 1961.

Farina, Stacy, and Matthew Gibbons. "The Last Refuge of Scoundrels." *Science for the People Magazine*, February 1, 2022. https://magazine.scienceforthepeople.org.

Faustman, Elaine M. "Risk Assessment." In *Casarett & Doull's Toxicology: The Basic Science of Poisons*, edited by Curtis D. Klaassen, 9th ed. New York: McGraw Hill Education, 2019.

Faustman, Elaine M., and Gilbert S. Omenn. "Risk Assessment." In *Casarett & Doull's Toxicology: The Basic Science of Poisons*, edited by Louis J. Casarett, Curtis D. Klaassen, Mary O. Amdur, and John Doull, 5th ed., 75–88. New York: McGraw Hill, Health Professions Division, 1996.

Fausto-Sterling, Anne. *Sexing the Body: Gender Politics and the Construction of Sexuality*. New York: Basic Books, 2000.

Federici, Silvia. *Caliban and the Witch: Women, the Body and Primitive Accumulation*. New York: Autonomedia, 2004.

———. *Wages Against Housework*. Bristol, UK: Power of Women Collective and Falling Wall Press, 1975. https://caringlabor.files.wordpress.com.

Ferguson, Roderick A. "Of Our Normative Strivings: African American Studies and the Histories of Sexuality." *Social Text* 23, nos. 3–4 (84–85) (Fall–Winter 2005): 85–100. https://doi.org/10.1215/01642472-23-3-4_84-85-85.

Flynn, James, Paul Slovic, and C. K. Mertz. "Gender, Race, and Perception of Environmental Health Risks." *Risk Analysis: An Official Publication of the Society for Risk Analysis* 14, no. 6 (December 1994): 1101–8. https://doi.org/10.1111/j.1539-6924.1994.tb00082.x.

Food and Agriculture Organization of the United Nations. *Pesticides Use: Global, Regional and Country Trends 1990–2018*. FAOSTAT Analytical Brief. Geneva, Switzerland: United Nations, 2020. https://www.fao.org.

Fortun, Kim. *Advocacy after Bhopal: Environmentalism, Disaster, New Global Orders*. Chicago: University of Chicago Press, 2001.

———. "Learning Across Disaster." In *Health in Disasters: A Science and Technology Studies Practicum for Medical Students and Healthcare Professionals*, edited by Rethy Kieth Chhem and Gregory Clancey. N.p.: International Atomic Energy Agency, National University of Singapore, 2015.

Foster, John Bellamy. *Marx's Ecology: Materialism and Nature*. New York: Monthly Review Press, 2000.

Foster, Steven, and Christopher Hobbs. *A Field Guide to Western Medicinal Plants and Herbs*. Peterson Field Guide Series. Boston: Houghton Mifflin, 2002.

Fox, James G., and B. Taylor Bennett. "Laboratory Animal Medicine: Historical Perspectives." In *Laboratory Animal Medicine*, edited by James G. Fox, Lynn C. Anderson, Glen M. Otto, Kathleen R. Pritchett-Corning, Mark T. Whary, and American College of Laboratory Animal Medicine, 3rd ed., 1–22. American College of Laboratory Animal Medicine Series. Amsterdam: Elsevier; Academic Press, 2015.

Francione, Gary L. *Introduction to Animal Rights: Your Child or the Dog?* Philadelphia: Temple University Press, 2000.

Franco, N. H., and I. A. S. Olsson. "Scientists and the 3Rs: Attitudes to Animal Use in Biomedical Research and the Effect of Mandatory Training in Laboratory Animal

Science." *Laboratory Animals* 48, no. 1 (January 1, 2014): 50–60. https://doi.org/10
.1177/0023677213498717.

Frederick, Peter, and Nilmini Jayasena. "Altered Pairing Behaviour and Reproductive
Success in White Ibises Exposed to Environmentally Relevant Concentrations of
Methylmercury." *Proceedings of the Royal Society B: Biological Sciences* 278, no. 1713
(December 1, 2010): 1851–57. https://doi.org/10.1098/rspb.2010.2189.

Freeman, Elizabeth. *Time Binds: Queer Temporalities, Queer Histories.* Durham, NC:
Duke University Press, 2010.

Frickel, Scott. *Chemical Consequences: Environmental Mutagens, Scientist Activism, and
the Rise of Genetic Toxicology.* New Brunswick, NJ: Rutgers University Press, 2004.

Gallo, Michael A. "History and Scope of Toxicology." In *Casarett & Doull's Toxicology:
The Basic Science of Poisons,* edited by Mary O. Amdur, John Doull, and Curtis D.
Klaassen, 4th ed., 3–11. New York: McGraw Hill Education, 1991.

———. "History and Scope of Toxicology." In *Casarett & Doull's: Toxicology the Basic
Science of Poisons,* edited by Curtis D. Klaassen, Louis J. Casarett, and John Doull,
8th ed., 3–11. New York: McGraw Hill Education, Medical, 2013.

Garcia, Angela. *The Pastoral Clinic: Addiction and Dispossession along the Rio Grande.*
Berkeley: University of California Press, 2010.

Guerre, Marc de. *The Disappearing Male.* Documentary. Eggplant Picture & Sound,
Optix Digital Pictures, Red Apple Entertainment, November 6, 2008.

Goldstein, Daniel. *LinkedIn* profile. Accessed August 6, 2020. https://www.linkedin
.com/in/daniel-goldstein-76b06b9.

Spivak, Gayatri Chakravorty. "Subaltern Studies: Deconstructing Historiography." In
Selected Subaltern Studies, edited by Ranajit Guha and Gayatri Chakravorty Spivak,
3–32. New Delhi, India: Oxford University Press, 1988.

Gerstein, Josh, and Alexander Ward. "Supreme Court Has Voted to Overturn Abortion
Rights, Draft Opinion Shows." *POLITICO,* May 2, 2022. https://www.politico.com.

Gibson, Caitlin. "Dreading the Knock at the Door: Parents of Trans Kids in Texas
Are Terrified for Their Families." *Washington Post,* March 17, 2022. https://www
.washingtonpost.com.

Gillam, Carey. *The Monsanto Papers: Deadly Secrets, Corporate Corruption, and One
Man's Search for Justice.* Washington, DC: Island Press, 2021.

———. *Whitewash: The Story of a Weed Killer, Cancer, and the Corruption of Science.*
Washington, DC: Island Press, 2017.

Gilligan, Carol. *In a Different Voice: Psychological Theory and Women's Development.*
Cambridge, MA: Harvard University Press, 2003.

Gilmore, Ruth Wilson. *Golden Gulag. Prisons, Surplus, Crisis, and Opposition in
Globalizing California.* American Crossroads 21. Berkeley: University of California
Press, 2007.

Glenn, Evelyn Nakano. *Forced to Care: Coercion and Caregiving in America.* Cambridge, MA: Harvard University Press, 2012.

———. "From Servitude to Service Work: Historical Continuities in the Racial Division
of Paid Reproductive Labor." *Signs* 18, no. 1 (1992): 1–43.

———. "Settler Colonialism as Structure: A Framework for Comparative Studies of U.S. Race and Gender Formation." *Sociology of Race and Ethnicity* 1, no. 1 (January 1, 2015): 52–72. https://doi.org/10.1177/2332649214560440.

Gluck, John P. *Voracious Science & Vulnerable Animals: A Primate Scientist's Ethical Journey.* Animal Lives. Chicago: University of Chicago Press, 2016.

Goodman, Justin, Alka Chandna, and Katherine Roe. "Trends in Animal Use at US Research Facilities." *Journal of Medical Ethics* 41, no. 7 (July 1, 2015): 567–69. https://doi.org/10.1136/medethics-2014-102404.

Goodrich, Jennie, and Claudia Lawson. *Kashaya Pomo Plants.* Los Angeles: American Indian Studies Center, University of California, Los Angeles, 2000.

Gottlieb, Robert. "Where We Live, Work, Play . . . and Eat: Expanding the Environmental Justice Agenda." *Environmental Justice* 2, no. 1 (March 2009): 7–8. https://doi.org/10.1089/env.2009.0001.

Gould, Stephen Jay. *The Mismeasure of Man.* Revised and expanded with a new introduction. New York: W. W. Norton, 2008.

Graeber, David, and David Wengrow. *The Dawn of Everything: A New History of Humanity.* First American edition. New York: Farrar, Straus and Giroux, 2021.

Grier, James W. "Ban of DDT and Subsequent Recovery of Reproduction in Bald Eagles." *Science* 218 (December 17, 1982): 1232–35.

Grimm, David. "How Many Mice and Rats Are Used in U.S. Labs? Controversial Study Says More than 100 Million." *Science News*, January 12, 2021. https://www.science.org.

Gross, Liza, and Linda S. Birnbaum. "Regulating Toxic Chemicals for Public and Environmental Health." *PLOS Biology* 15, no. 12 (December 18, 2017): e2004814. https://doi.org/10.1371/journal.pbio.2004814.

Gruen, Lori. *Entangled Empathy: An Alternative Ethic for Our Relationships with Animals.* Brooklyn: Lantern Books, 2015.

Guthman, Julie. *Agrarian Dreams: The Paradox of Organic Farming in California.* California Studies in Critical Human Geography. Berkeley: University of California Press, 2004.

———. *Weighing In: Obesity, Food Justice, and the Limits of Capitalism.* Berkeley: University of California Press, 2011.

Guthman, Julie, and Sandy Brown. "Whose Life Counts: Biopolitics and the 'Bright Line' of Chloropicrin Mitigation in California's Strawberry Industry." *Science, Technology, & Human Values* 41, no. 3 (May 2016): 461–82. https://doi.org/10.1177/0162243915606804.

Guyton, Kathryn Z., Linda Rieswijk, Amy Wang, Weihsueh A. Chiu, and Martyn T. Smith. "Key Characteristics Approach to Carcinogenic Hazard Identification." *Chemical Research in Toxicology* 31, no. 12 (December 17, 2018): 1290–92. https://doi.org/10.1021/acs.chemrestox.8b00321.

Hacking, Ian. "Language, Truth, and Reason." In *Rationality and Relativism*, edited by Martin Hollis and Steven Lukes, 48–66. Cambridge, MA: MIT Press, 1982.

Halberstam, J. Jack. *In a Queer Time and Place: Transgender Bodies, Subcultural Lives.* Sexual Cultures. New York: New York University Press, 2005.

————. *The Queer Art of Failure*. Durham, NC: Duke University Press, 2011.

————. *Wild Things: The Disorder of Desire*. Perverse Modernities. Durham, NC: Duke University Press, 2020.

Hall, Stuart. "The West and the Rest: Discourse and Power." In *Formations of Modernity*, edited by Bram Gieben and Stuart Hall, 184–227. Understanding Modern Societies 1. Cambridge: Polity Press, 1993.

Halley, Janet E. *Split Decisions: How and Why to Take a Break from Feminism*. Princeton, NJ: Princeton University Press, 2006.

Hammond, Carla M. "Audre Lorde: Interview." *Denver Quarterly* 16, no. 1 (1981): 10–27.

Haraway, Donna. "Situated Knowledges: The Science Question in Feminism and the Privilege of Partial Perspective." *Feminist Studies* 14, no. 3 (1988): 575–99. https://doi .org/10.2307/3178066.

————. "Teddy Bear Patriarchy: Taxidermy in the Garden of Eden, New York City, 1908–1936." *Social Text*, no. 11 (Winter 1984–1985): 20–64. https://doi.org/10.2307 /466593.

————. *When Species Meet*. Posthumanities 3. Minneapolis: University of Minnesota Press, 2008.

Harding, Sandra. "'Strong Objectivity': A Response to the New Objectivity Question." *Synthese* 104, no. 3 (September 1, 1995): 331–49. https://doi.org/10.1007 /BF01064504.

Harding, Sandra G., ed. *The Postcolonial Science and Technology Studies Reader*. Durham, NC: Duke University Press, 2011.

Harrison, Jill Lindsey. "'Accidents' and Invisibilities: Scaled Discourse and the Naturalization of Regulatory Neglect in California's Pesticide Drift Conflict." *Political Geography* 25, no. 5 (June 1, 2006): 506–29. https://doi.org/10.1016/j.polgeo.2006.02.003.

————. *From the Inside Out: The Fight for Environmental Justice within Government Agencies*. Urban and Industrial Environments. Cambridge, MA: MIT Press, 2019.

————. *Pesticide Drift and the Pursuit of Environmental Justice*. Food, Health, and the Environment. Cambridge, MA: MIT Press, 2011.

Hayden, Cori. *When Nature Goes Public: The Making and Unmaking of Bioprospecting in Mexico*. In-Formation Series. Princeton, NJ: Princeton University Press, 2003.

Hayward, Eva. "Intoxifornicate." Presented at the Society for Social Studies of Science, San Diego, CA, October 6, 2013. https://prezi.com/ydv706bionad/intoxifornicate/.

Helmreich, Stefan. "The Left Hand of Nature and Culture." *HAU: Journal of Ethnographic Theory* 4, no. 3 (December 2014): 373–81. https://doi.org/10.14318/hau4.3.024.

Hendlin, Yogi Hale. "Surveying the Chemical Anthropocene: Chemical Imaginaries and the Politics of Defining Toxicity." *Environment and Society* 12, no. 1 (September 1, 2021): 181–202. https://doi.org/10.3167/ares.2021.120111.

Henke, Christopher. *Cultivating Science, Harvesting Power: Science and Industrial Agriculture in California*. Inside Technology. Cambridge, MA: MIT Press, 2008.

Hepler-Smith, Evan. "Molecular Bureaucracy: Toxicological Information and Environmental Protection." *Environmental History* 24, no. 3 (July 2019): 534–60. https://doi .org/10.1093/envhis/emy134.

Herzig, Rebecca M. *Suffering for Science: Reason and Sacrifice in Modern America.* New Brunswick, NJ: Rutgers University Press, 2006.

Hine, Darlene C. "Female Slave Resistance: The Economics of Sex." *Western Journal of Black Studies* 3, no. 2 (1979): 123–27.

Hird, Myra J. "Naturally Queer." *Feminist Theory* 5, no. 1 (April 2004): 85–89. https://doi.org/10.1177/1464700104040817.

Hobart, Hiʻilei Julia Kawehipuaakahaopulani, and Tamara Kneese. "Radical Care: Survival Strategies for Uncertain Times." *Social Text* 38, no. 1 (142) (March 1, 2020): 1–16. https://doi.org/10.1215/01642472-7971067.

Hochschild, Arlie Russell. "Inside the Clockwork of Male Careers." In *At the Heart of Work and Family: Engaging the Ideas of Arlie Hochschild*, edited by Anita Ilta Garey and Karen V. Hansen, 17–60. New Brunswick, NJ: Rutgers University Press, 2011.

———. *The Second Shift: Working Parents and the Revolution at Home.* New York: Viking, 1989.

———. *The Time Bind: When Work Becomes Home and Home Becomes Work.* New York: Metropolitan Books, 1997.

Hodge, Harold. Foreword to *Toxicology: The Basic Science of Poisons*, edited by Louis J. Casarett and John Doull, v–vi. New York: Macmillan, 1975.

Holmberg, Tora. "A Feeling for the Animal: On Becoming an Experimentalist." *Society & Animals* 16, no. 4 (October 2008): 316–35. https://doi.org/10.1163/156853008X357658.

hooks, bell. *Feminist Theory from Margin to Center.* Boston, MA: South End Press, 1984.

Horkeimer, Max, and Theodor Adorno. "The Concept of Enlightenment." In *Dialectic of Enlightenment*, translated by John Cumming. New York: Herder & Herder, 1944.

Hornblum, Allen M. *Acres of Skin: Human Experiments at Holmesburg Prison; A Story of Abuse and Exploitation in the Name of Medical Science.* New York: Routledge, 1998.

Howard, Philip H. *Concentration and Power in the Food System: Who Controls What We Eat?* London: Bloomsbury Academic, 2020.

———. "The Myth of 'Feeding the World': Subsidizing Agricultural Overproduction and Industrial Technologies, and Marginalizing Alternatives." *Journal of Agriculture, Food Systems, and Community Development* 12, no. 3 (Spring 2023): 1–2. https://doi.org/10.5304/jafscd.2023.123.008.

Irigaray, Luce. *This Sex Which Is Not One.* Translated by Catherine Porter and Carolyn Burke. Ithaca, NY: Cornell University Press, 1985.

Jackson, Zakiyyah Iman. *Becoming Human: Matter and Meaning in an Antiblack World.* Sexual Cultures. New York: New York University Press, 2020.

Jensen, Derrick. "Amid Plenty: Anuradha Mittal on the True Cause of World Hunger." *Sun Magazine*, February 2002. https://www.thesunmagazine.org.

Johnson, Valerie Ann. "Bringing Together Feminist Disability Studies and Environmental Justice." In *Disability Studies and the Environmental Humanities: Toward an Eco-Crip Theory*, edited by Sarah Jaquette Ray and Jay Sibara, 73–93. Lincoln: University of Nebraska Press, 2017.

Justice Pesticides. "Dewayne Johnson v. Monsanto (Bayer)." *Justice Pesticides* (blog), 2023. https://justicepesticides.org.

Kaba, Mariame. "Free Us All." *New Inquiry* (blog), May 8, 2017. https://thenewinquiry .com.

Kamath, Ambika, and Melina Packer. *Feminism in the Wild: How Human Biases Shape Our Understanding of Animal Behavior*. Cambridge, MA: MIT Press, forthcoming 2025.

Karkazis, Katrina. "The Misuses of 'Biological Sex.'" *The Lancet* 394, no. 10212 (November 23, 2019): 1898–99. https://doi.org/10.1016/S0140-6736(19)32764-3.

Kasymova, Salima, Jean Marie S. Place, Deborah L. Billings, and Jesus D. Aldape. "Impacts of the COVID-19 Pandemic on the Productivity of Academics Who Mother." Supplement, *Gender, Work & Organization* 28, no. S2 (2021): S419–33. https://doi .org/10.1111/gwao.12699.

Keel, Terence. *Divine Variations: How Christian Thought Became Racial Science*. Stanford, CA: Stanford University Press, 2018.

Keller, Evelyn Fox. *Refiguring Life: Metaphors of Twentieth-Century Biology*. The Wellek Library Lecture Series at the University of California, Irvine. New York: Columbia University Press, 1995.

———. *The Century of the Gene*. Cambridge, MA: Harvard University Press, 2002.

Kevles, Daniel J. *In the Name of Eugenics: Genetics and the Uses of Human Heredity*. Cambridge, MA: Harvard University Press, 1995.

Kim, Claire Jean. *Dangerous Crossings: Race, Species, and Nature in a Multicultural Age*. Cambridge: Cambridge University Press, 2015.

Kimbrell, Andrew, ed. *Fatal Harvest: The Tragedy of Industrial Agriculture*. Washington, DC: Island Press, 2002.

Kimmerer, Robin Wall. "The Covenant of Reciprocity." In *The Wiley Blackwell Companion to Religion and Ecology*, edited by John Hart, 368–81. Hoboken, NJ: John Wiley & Sons, 2017.

Klaassen, Curtis D., ed. *Casarett & Doull's Toxicology: The Basic Science of Poisons*. 9th ed. New York: McGraw Hill Education, 2019.

Klaassen, Curtis D. Dedication in *Casarett & Doull's Toxicology: The Basic Science of Poisons*, edited by Louis J Casarett and John Doull, 8th ed. New York: McGraw Hill, 2013.

Kloppenburg, Jack Ralph. *First the Seed: The Political Economy of Plant Biotechnology, 1492–2000*. 2nd ed. Science and Technology in Society. Madison: University of Wisconsin Press, 2004.

Ko, Aph. *Racism as Zoological Witchcraft: A Guide for Getting Out*. Brooklyn: Lantern Books, 2019.

Kohler, Robert E. *Lords of the Fly: Drosophila Genetics and the Experimental Life*. Chicago: University of Chicago Press, 1994.

Kojola, Erik, and David N. Pellow. "New Directions in Environmental Justice Studies: Examining the State and Violence." *Environmental Politics* 30, no. 1–2 (October 25, 2020): 100–118. https://doi.org/10.1080/09644016.2020.1836898.

Kosek, Jake. "Purity and Pollution: Racial Degradation and Environmental Anxieties." In *Liberation Ecologies*, edited by Richard Peet and Michael Watts, 2nd ed., 125–65. New York: Routledge, 2004.

Kreeger, Pamela K., Amy Brock, Holly C. Gibbs, K. Jane Grande-Allen, Alice H. Huang, Kristyn S. Masters, Padmini Rangamani, Michaela R. Reagan, and Shannon L. Servoss. "Ten Simple Rules for Women Principal Investigators during a Pandemic." *PLOS Computational Biology* 16, no. 10 (October 29, 2020): e1008370. https://doi.org/10.1371/journal.pcbi.1008370.

Krimsky, Sheldon. "Essay: Monsanto's Ghostwriting and Strong-Arming Threaten Sound Science—and Society." Environmental Health News, June 26, 2018. http://www.ehn.org.

———. "An Epistemological Inquiry into the Endocrine Disruptor Thesis." *Annals of the New York Academy of Sciences* 948, no. 1 (December 2001): 130–42.

Krimsky, Sheldon, and Carey Gillam. "Roundup Litigation Discovery Documents: Implications for Public Health and Journal Ethics." *Journal of Public Health Policy* 39 (June 8, 2018): 318–26. https://doi.org/10.1057/s41271-018-0134-z.

La Merrill, Michele A., Laura N. Vandenberg, Martyn T. Smith, William Goodson, Patience Browne, Heather B. Patisaul, Kathryn Z. Guyton, et al. "Consensus on the Key Characteristics of Endocrine-Disrupting Chemicals as a Basis for Hazard Identification." *Nature Reviews: Endocrinology* 16, no. 1 (January 2020): 45–57. https://doi.org/10.1038/s41574-019-0273-8.

Lambert, Max, and Melina Packer. "How Gendered Language Leads Scientists Astray." *Washington Post*, June 10, 2019, sec. Perspective. https://www.washingtonpost.com.

Lambert, Max R., Tien Tran, Andrzej Kilian, Tariq Ezaz, and David K. Skelly. "Molecular Evidence for Sex Reversal in Wild Populations of Green Frogs (Rana Clamitans)." *PeerJ* 7 (February 8, 2019): e6449. https://doi.org/10.7717/peerj.6449.

Lancaster, Roger N. *The Trouble with Nature*. Berkeley: University of California Press, 2003.

Landecker, Hannah. "Antibiotic Resistance and the Biology of History." *Body & Society* 22, no. 4 (2016): 19–52. https://doi.org/10.1177/1357034X14561341.

Landecker, Hannah, and Aaron Panofsky. "From Social Structure to Gene Regulation, and Back: A Critical Introduction to Environmental Epigenetics for Sociology." *Annual Review of Sociology* 39, no. 1 (2013): 333–57. https://doi.org/10.1146/annurev-soc-071312-145707.

Langston, Nancy. *Toxic Bodies: Hormone Disruptors and the Legacy of DES*. New Haven, CT: Yale University Press, 2010.

Lanphear, Bruce P. "Low-Level Toxicity of Chemicals: No Acceptable Levels?" *PLOS Biology* 15, no. 12 (December 19, 2017): e2003066. https://doi.org/10.1371/journal.pbio.2003066.

Lasker, Grace A., and Nancy J. Simcox. "Using Feminist Theory and Social Justice Pedagogy to Educate a New Generation of Precautionary Principle Chemists." *Catalyst: Feminism, Theory, Technoscience* 6, no. 1 (May 15, 2020). https://doi.org/10.28968/cftt.v6i1.32084.

Laskow, Sarah. "The Sad Sex Lives of Suburban Frogs." *Atlas Obscura*, September 9, 2015. http://www.atlasobscura.com.

Latham, Jonathan. "Unsafe at Any Dose? Diagnosing Chemical Safety Failures, from DDT to BPA." *Independent Science News*, May 16, 2016. https://www .independentsciencenews.org.

Latour, Bruno. *Science in Action: How to Follow Scientists and Engineers through Society*. Cambridge, MA: Harvard University Press, 1988.

Lerner, Steve. *Sacrifice Zones: The Front Lines of Toxic Chemical Exposure in the United States*. Cambridge, MA: MIT Press, 2010.

Levin, Sam. "Monsanto Trial: Cancer Patient Says He Used Herbicide for Three Decades." *The Guardian*, March 5, 2019, sec. Business. https://www.theguardian.com.

Levins, Richard, and Richard Charles Lewontin. *The Dialectical Biologist*. Cambridge, MA: Harvard University Press, 1987.

Liboiron, Max. *Pollution Is Colonialism*. Durham, NC: Duke University Press, 2021.

———. "There's No Such Thing as 'We.'" *Discard Studies*, October 12, 2020. https://discardstudies.com.

———. "Toxins or Toxicants? Why the Difference Matters." *Discard Studies*, September 11, 2017. https://discardstudies.com.

Liboiron, Max, Manuel Tironi, and Nerea Calvillo. "Toxic Politics: Acting in a Permanently Polluted World:" *Social Studies of Science* 48, no. 3 (2018): 331–49. https://doi .org/10.1177/0306312718783087.

Lorde, Audre. "The Master's Tools Will Never Dismantle the Master's House." In her *Sister Outsider: Essays and Speeches*, 110–13. Berkeley, CA: Crossing Press, 1984.

Lugones, Maria. "The Coloniality of Gender." In *The Palgrave Handbook of Gender and Development: Critical Engagements in Feminist Theory and Practice*, edited by Wendy Harcourt, 13–33. London: Palgrave Macmillan UK, 2016. https://doi.org/10 .1007/978-1-137-38273-3_2.

Luke, Brian. "Taming Ourselves or Going Feral? Toward a Nonpatriarchal Metaethic of Animal Liberation." In *Animals and Women: Feminist Theoretical Explorations*, edited by Carol J. Adams and Josephine Donovan, 290–319. Durham, NC: Duke University Press, 1995.

Lynch, Michael E. "Sacrifice and the Transformation of the Animal Body into a Scientific Object: Laboratory Culture and Ritual Practice in the Neurosciences." *Social Studies of Science* 18, no. 2 (May 1, 1988): 265–89. https://doi.org/10.1177 /030631288018002004.

Lyons, Kristina. "Chemical Warfare in Colombia, Evidentiary Ecologies and Senti-Actuando Practices of Justice." *Social Studies of Science* 48, no. 3 (June 1, 2018): 414–37. https://doi.org/10.1177/0306312718765375.

MacKendrick, Norah. *Better Safe than Sorry: How Consumers Navigate Exposure to Everyday Toxics*. Oakland: University of California Press, 2018.

Manne, Kate. *Down Girl: The Logic of Misogyny*. Oxford, New York: Oxford University Press, 2017.

———. *Entitled: How Male Privilege Hurts Women*. First edition. New York: Crown, an imprint of Random House, 2020.

Mansfield, Becky. "Environmental Health as Biosecurity: 'Seafood Choices,' Risk, and the Pregnant Woman as Threshold." *Annals of the Association of American Geographers* 102, no. 5 (September 2012): 969–76. https://doi.org/10.1080/00045608.2012.657496.

Markowitz, Gerald E., and David Rosner. *Deceit and Denial: The Deadly Politics of Industrial Pollution*. California/Milbank Books on Health and the Public 6. Berkeley: University of California Press; New York: Milbank Memorial Fund, 2002.

Markowitz, Sally. "Pelvic Politics: Sexual Dimorphism and Racial Difference." *Signs* 26, no. 2 (2001): 389–414.

Marris, Emma. *Wild Souls: Freedom and Flourishing in the Non-Human World*. New York: Bloomsbury Publishing, 2021.

Martin, Emily. "The Egg and the Sperm: How Science Has Constructed a Romance Based on Stereotypical Male-Female Roles." *Signs* 16, no. 3 (1991): 485–501.

Masco, Joseph. "Mutant Ecologies: Radioactive Life in Post–Cold War New Mexico." *Cultural Anthropology* 19, no. 4 (November 1, 2004): 517–50. https://doi.org/10.1525/can.2004.19.4.517.

Masri, Shahir, Claudia S. Miller, Raymond F. Palmer, and Nicholas Ashford. "Toxicant-Induced Loss of Tolerance for Chemicals, Foods, and Drugs: Assessing Patterns of Exposure behind a Global Phenomenon." *Environmental Sciences Europe* 33, no. 1 (May 27, 2021): 65. https://doi.org/10.1186/s12302-021-00504-z.

Matchar, Emily. *Homeward Bound: Why Women Are Embracing the New Domesticity*. 1st hardcover edition. New York: Simon & Schuster, 2013.

McClintock, Anne. *Imperial Leather: Race, Gender, and Sexuality in the Colonial Contest*. New York: Routledge, 1995.

McCutcheon, Rob S. "Toxicology and the Law." In *Toxicology: The Basic Science of Poisons*, edited by Louis J. Casarett and John Doull, 728–41. New York: Macmillan, 1975.

McDonald, Robert E., Debra A. Laverie, and Kerry T. Manis. "The Interplay between Advertising and Society: An Historical Analysis." *Journal of Macromarketing* 41, no. 4 (December 1, 2021): 585–609. https://doi.org/10.1177/0276146720964324.

McWilliams, Carey. *Factories in the Field: The Story of Migratory Farm Labor in California*. Berkeley: University of California Press, 2000.

Merchant, Carolyn. *The Death of Nature: Women, Ecology, and the Scientific Revolution*. New York: Harper & Row, 1989.

Merton, Robert K. *The Sociology of Science: Theoretical and Empirical Investigations*. Chicago: University of Chicago Press, 1974.

Messing, Karen, and Donna Mergler. "'The Rat Couldn't Speak, But We Can': Inhumanity in Occupational Health Research." In *Reinventing Biology: Respect for Life and the Creation of Knowledge*, edited by Lynda Birke and Ruth Hubbard, 21–49. Race, Gender, and Science. Bloomington: Indiana University Press, 1995.

Michaels, David. *Doubt Is Their Product: How Industry's Assault on Science Threatens Your Health*. Oxford: Oxford University Press, 2008.

Miller, Lulu. *Why Fish Don't Exist: A Story of Loss, Love, and the Hidden Order of Life*. New York: Simon & Schuster Paperbacks, 2021.

Millett, Kate. *Sexual Politics*. New York: Avon Books, 1970.

Mills, Charles W. "White Supremacy." In *The Routledge Companion to Philosophy of Race*, edited by Paul C. Taylor, Linda Martín Alcoff, and Luvell Anderson, 475–88. New York: Routledge, 2017.

Mitich, Larry W. "Intriguing World of Weeds: Weed Science Society of America." *Field Bindweed* (blog), accessed July 18, 2019. http://wssa.net.

Mitman, Gregg. *The State of Nature: Ecology, Community, and American Social Thought, 1900–1950*. Science and Its Conceptual Foundations. Chicago: University of Chicago Press, 1992.

Monk, Julia D., Erin Giglio, Ambika Kamath, Max R. Lambert, and Caitlin E. McDonough. "An Alternative Hypothesis for the Evolution of Same-Sex Sexual Behaviour in Animals." *Nature Ecology & Evolution* 3, no. 12 (December 2019): 1622–31. https://doi.org/10.1038/s41559-019-1019-7.

Montford, Kelly Struthers, and Chloë Taylor, eds. *Colonialism and Animality: Anti-Colonial Perspectives in Critical Animal Studies*. Routledge Advances in Critical Diversities. Abingdon, UK: Routledge, 2020.

Moore, Martha Gilchrist, Heather R. Rose-Glowacki, Keith Belton, Emily Sanchez, David Lan, and Zahra Saifi. *2023 Guide to the Business of Chemistry*. Washington, DC: American Chemistry Council, 2023. https://www.americanchemistry.com.

Morales, Helda, and Ivette Perfecto. "Traditional Knowledge and Pest Management in the Guatemalan Highlands." *Agriculture and Human Values* 17, no. 1 (March 2000): 49–63. https://doi.org/10.1023/A:1007680726231.

Morrison, Toni. "Academic Whispers [2004]." In *The Source of Self-Regard: Selected Essays, Speeches, and Meditations*, 198–204. New York: Vintage International, 2020.

Morrow, Paul E., Margaret C. Bruce, and John Doull. "Louis James Casarett (1927–1972)." *Toxicological Sciences* 63, no. 2 (October 2001): 151–52. https://doi.org/10.1093/toxsci/63.2.151.

Mortimer-Sandilands, Catriona, and Bruce Erickson, eds. *Queer Ecologies: Sex, Nature, Politics, Desire*. Bloomington: Indiana University Press, 2010.

Murphy, Michelle. "Alterlife and Decolonial Chemical Relations." *Cultural Anthropology* 32, no. 4 (2017): 494–503. https://doi.org/10.14506/ca32.4.02.

———. *Sick Building Syndrome and the Problem of Uncertainty: Environmental Politics, Technoscience, and Women Workers*. Durham, NC: Duke University Press, 2006.

———. *The Economization of Life*. Durham, NC: Duke University Press, 2017.

Nader, Laura. "Up the Anthropologist: Perspectives Gained from Studying Up." In *Reinventing Anthropology*, edited by Dell Hymes, 284–311. New York: Pantheon, 1972.

Nagel, Thomas. *The View from Nowhere*. Oxford: Oxford University Press, 1989.

Nash, Jennifer C. *Black Feminism Reimagined: After Intersectionality*. Next Wave New Directions in Women's Studies. Durham, NC: Duke University Press, 2019.

Nash, Linda. "Purity and Danger: Historical Reflections on the Regulation of Environmental Pollutants." *Environmental History* 13, no. 4 (2008): 651–58.

Nash, Margaret A. "Entangled Pasts: Land-Grant Colleges and American Indian Dispossession." *History of Education Quarterly* 59, no. 4 (November 2019): 437–67. https://doi.org/10.1017/heq.2019.31.

Neil, Nancy, Torbjörn Malmfors, and Paul Slovic. "Intuitive Toxicology: Expert and Lay Judgments of Chemical Risks." *Toxicologic Pathology* 22, no. 2 (March/April 1994): 198–201. https://doi.org/10.1177/019262339402200214.

Nelson, Alondra. *The Social Life of DNA.* Boston: Beacon Press, 2016.

Nelson, Nicole. *Model Behavior: Animal Experiments, Complexity, and the Genetics of Psychiatric Disorders.* Chicago: University of Chicago Press, 2018.

Nelson, Nicole C., and Kaitlin Stack Whitney. "Becoming a Research Rodent." In *Living with Animals: Bonds across Species,* edited by Natalie Porter and Ilana Gershon, 199–208. Ithaca, NY: Cornell University Press, 2018.

Nixon, Rob. *Slow Violence and the Environmentalism of the Poor.* Cambridge, MA: Harvard University Press, 2013.

O'Brien, Mary H. "Being a Scientist Means Taking Sides." *BioScience* 43, no. 10 (1993): 706–8. https://doi.org/10.2307/1312342.

Ogbunugafor, C. Brandon. "DNA, Basketball, and Birthday Luck. A Review of *The Genetic Lottery: Why DNA Matters for Social Equality.*" *American Journal of Biological Anthropology* 179, no. 3 (August 6, 2022): 501–4. https://doi.org/10.1002/ajpa.24599.

Olson, Mary. "Females Exposed to Nuclear Radiation Are Far Likelier Than Males to Suffer Harm." *PassBlue: Independent Coverage of the UN* (blog), July 5, 2017. https://www.passblue.com.

Omenn, Gilbert S. *Report on the Accomplishments of the Commission on Risk Assessment and Risk Management.* Washington, DC: Presidential/Congressional Commission on Risk Assessment and Risk Management, September 26, 1997. https://cfpub.epa.gov.

Oreskes, Naomi, and Erik M. Conway. *Merchants of Doubt: How a Handful of Scientists Obscured the Truth on Issues from Tobacco Smoke to Global Warming.* New York: Bloomsbury Press, 2010.

Oyěwùmí, Oyèrónkẹ́. *The Invention of Women: Making an African Sense of Western Gender Discourses.* Minneapolis: University of Minnesota Press, 1997.

Pachá, Paulo. "Why the Brazilian Far Right Loves the European Middle Ages." *Pacific Standard,* February 18, 2019. https://psmag.com.

Packer, Melina. "Becoming with Toxicity: Chemical Epigenetics as 'Racializing and Sexualizing Assemblage.'" *Hypatia* 37, no. 1 (Winter 2022): 2–26. https://www.doi.org/10.1017/hyp.2021.68.

———. "Chemical Agents: The Biopolitical Science of Toxicity." *Environment and Society* 12, no. 1 (September 1, 2021): 25–43. https://doi.org/10.3167/ares.2021.120103.

———. "Finding the Man in the Glyphosate." PhD Dissertation, University of California, Berkeley, 2020.

Packer, Melina, and Max R. Lambert. "What's Gender Got to Do with It? Dismantling the Human Hierarchies in Evolutionary Biology and Environmental Toxicology for

Scientific and Social Progress." *American Naturalist* 200, no. 1 (July 2022): 114–28. https://doi.org/10.1086/720131.

Pagel, Walter. *Paracelsus: An Introduction to Philosophical Medicine in the Era of the Renaissance*. 2nd, rev. ed. Basel; New York: Karger, 1982.

Panofsky, Aaron. *Misbehaving Science: Controversy and the Development of Behavior Genetics*. Chicago: University of Chicago Press, 2014.

Parreñas, Juno Salazar. *Decolonizing Extinction: The Work of Care in Orangutan Rehabilitation*. Experimental Futures: Technological Lives, Scientific Arts, Anthropological Voices. Durham, NC: Duke University Press, 2018.

———. "Hunting." In *Gender: Animals*, edited by Juno Salazar Parreñas, 165–80. Macmillan Interdisciplinary Handbooks. Farmington Hills, MI: Macmillan Reference USA, 2017.

Parreñas, Rhacel Salazar. "The Reproductive Labour of Migrant Workers." *Global Networks* 12, no. 2 (April 2012): 269–75. https://doi.org/10.1111/j.1471-0374.2012 .00351.x.

Patel, Raj. "The Long Green Revolution." *Journal of Peasant Studies* 40, no. 1 (2013): 1–63. https://doi.org/10.1080/03066150.2012.719224.

Patil, Vrushali. "The Heterosexual Matrix as Imperial Effect." *Sociological Theory* 36, no. 1 (March 2018): 1–26. https://doi.org/10.1177/0735275118759382.

Pellegrini, Ann. *Performance Anxieties: Staging Psychoanalysis, Staging Race*. New York: Routledge, 2014.

Pellow, David N. *Resisting Global Toxics: Transnational Movements for Environmental Justice*. Urban and Industrial Environments. Cambridge, MA: MIT Press, 2007.

Peña, Devon G. "Structural Violence, Historical Trauma, and Public Health: The Environmental Justice Critique of Contemporary Risk Science and Practice." In *Communities, Neighborhoods, and Health*, edited by Linda Burton, Susan Kemp, ManChui Leung, Stephen Matthews, and D. T. Takeuchi, 203–18. New York: Springer, 2011.

Perret, Meg. "'Chemical Castration': White Genocide and Male Extinction in Rhetoric of Endocrine Disruption." *NiCHE* (blog), June 9, 2020. https://niche-canada.org.

Petryna, Adriana. *Life Exposed: Biological Citizens after Chernobyl*. Princeton, NJ: Princeton University Press, 2013.

Pico, Tamara. "The Darker Side of John Wesley Powell." *Scientific American Blog Network* (blog), September 9, 2019. https://blogs.scientificamerican.com.

Piepzna-Samarasinha, Leah Lakshmi. *Care Work: Dreaming Disability Justice*. Vancouver, Canada: Arsenal Pulp Press, 2018.

Plumwood, Val. *Feminism and the Mastery of Nature*. New York: Routledge, 1994.

———. "Integrating Ethical Frameworks for Animals, Humans, and Nature: A Critical Feminist Eco-Socialist Analysis." *Ethics and the Environment* 5, no. 2 (2000): 285–322.

Polcha, Elizabeth. "Breeding Insects and Reproducing White Supremacy in Maria Sibylla Merian's Ecology of Dispossession." *Lady Science* (blog), 2019. www.ladyscience .com.

Pollock, Anne. "Queering Endocrine Disruption." In *Object-Oriented Feminism*, edited by Katherine Behar, 183–99. Minneapolis: University of Minnesota Press, 2016.

Popper, Nicholas. Review of *Paracelsus: Medicine, Magic and Mission at the End of Time*, by Charles Webster. *American Historical Review* 115, no. 3 (2010): 904–5.

Porter, Theodore M. *Trust in Numbers: The Pursuit of Objectivity in Science and Public Life*. Princeton, NJ: Princeton University Press, 2020.

Povinelli, Elizabeth A. *Geontologies: A Requiem to Late Liberalism*. Durham, NC: Duke University Press, 2016.

——. "Routes/Worlds." *E-Flux Journal*, no. 27 (September 2011). https://www.e-flux .com.

——. "Windjarrameru, the Stealing C*nts." *E-Flux Journal 56th Venice Biennale— SUPERCOMMUNITY*, May 21, 2015. http://supercommunity.e-flux.com.

Pratt, Mary Louise. *Imperial Eyes: Travel Writing and Transculturation*. 2nd ed. London: Routledge, 2008.

Prescod-Weinstein, Chanda. "Making Black Women Scientists under White Empiricism: The Racialization of Epistemology in Physics." *Signs: Journal of Women in Culture and Society* 45, no. 2 (Winter 2020): 421–47. https://doi.org/10.1086/704991.

Prescod-Weinstein, Chanda, and Katherine McKittrick. "Public Thinker: Katherine McKittrick on Black Methodologies and Other Ways of Being." *Public Books* (blog), February 1, 2021. https://www.publicbooks.org.

Proctor, Robert. *Cancer Wars: How Politics Shapes What We Know and Don't Know about Cancer*. New York: Basic Books, 1995.

Proctor, Robert N. "'Everyone Knew but No One Had Proof': Tobacco Industry Use of Medical History Expertise in US Courts, 1990–2002." Supplement, *Tobacco Control* 15, no. S4 (December 2006): iv117–25. https://doi.org/10.1136/tc.2004.009928.

Pulido, Laura. *Environmentalism and Economic Justice: Two Chicano Struggles in the Southwest*. Society, Environment, and Place. Tucson: University of Arizona Press, 1996.

Rader, Karen. *Making Mice: Standardizing Animals for American Biomedical Research, 1900–1955*. Princeton, NJ: Princeton University Press, 2004.

Ray, Sarah Jaquette. *The Ecological Other: Environmental Exclusion in American Culture*. Tucson: University of Arizona Press, 2013.

Ray, Sarah Jaquette, and Jay Sibara. Introduction to *Disability Studies and the Environmental Humanities: Toward an Eco-Crip Theory*, edited by Sarah Jaquette Ray and Jay Sibara, 1–25. Lincoln: University of Nebraska Press, 2017.

Reardon, Jenny. *Race to the Finish: Identity and Governance in an Age of Genomics*. In-Formation Series. Princeton, NJ: Princeton University Press, 2005.

Richardson, Sarah S., Cynthia R. Daniels, Matthew W. Gillman, Janet Golden, Rebecca Kukla, Christopher Kuzawa, and Janet Rich-Edwards. "Society: Don't Blame the Mothers." *Nature News* 512, no. 7513 (August 14, 2014): 131–32. https://doi.org/10 .1038/512131a.

Richardson, Sarah S., Meredith Reiches, Heather Shattuck-Heidorn, Michelle Lynne LaBonte, and Theresa Consoli. "Focus on Preclinical Sex Differences Will Not

Address Women's and Men's Health Disparities." *Proceedings of the National Academy of Sciences* 112, no. 44 (November 3, 2015): 13419–20. https://doi.org/10.1073/pnas.1516958112.

Riskin, Jessica. *The Restless Clock: A History of the Centuries-Long Argument over What Makes Living Things Tick*. Chicago: University of Chicago Press, 2018.

Ritvo, Harriet. *The Animal Estate: The English and Other Creatures in the Victorian Age*. Cambridge, MA: Harvard University Press, 1987.

———. *The Platypus and the Mermaid, and Other Figments of the Classifying Imagination*. Cambridge, MA: Harvard University Press, 1998.

Robbins, Paul, and Sarah A. Moore. "Ecological Anxiety Disorder: Diagnosing the Politics of the Anthropocene." *Cultural Geographies* 20, no. 1 (January 2013): 3–19. https://doi.org/10.1177/1474474012469887.

Roberts, Celia. *Messengers of Sex: Hormones, Biomedicine, and Feminism*. Cambridge Studies in Society and the Life Sciences. Cambridge: Cambridge University Press, 2007.

Roberts, Elizabeth F. S. "What Gets Inside: Violent Entanglements and Toxic Boundaries in Mexico City." *Cultural Anthropology* 32, no. 4 (November 18, 2017): 592–619. https://doi.org/10.14506/ca32.4.07.

Roberts, Jody A. "Reflections of an Unrepentant Plastiphobe: Plasticity and the STS Life." *Science as Culture* 19, no. 1 (March 2010): 101–20. https://doi.org/10.1080/09505430903557916.

Rosenblatt, Joel. "Bayer Loses Second Roundup Appeal, A Blow to Curbing Suits." *Bloomberg*, May 14, 2021. https://www.bloomberg.com.

Ross, Benjamin, and Steven Amter. *The Polluters: The Making of Our Chemically Altered Environment*. New York: Oxford University Press, 2010.

Rossiter, Margaret W. "The Matthew Matilda Effect in Science." *Social Studies of Science* 23, no. 2 (1993): 325–41.

Rothfels Lab. "The Rothfels Lab Stands against Racism Everywhere." *Rothfels Lab* (blog), June 5, 2020. https://rothfelslab.berkeley.edu.

Rothstein, Mark, Yu Cai, and Gary Marchant. "The Ghost in Our Genes: Legal and Ethical Implications of Epigenetics." *Health Matrix: The Journal of Law-Medicine* 19, no. 1 (Winter 2009): 1–62.

Roy, Deboleena. "Asking Different Questions: Feminist Practices for the Natural Sciences." *Hypatia* 23, no. 4 (2008): 134–56. https://doi.org/10.1111/j.1527-2001.2008.tb01437.x.

———. *Molecular Feminisms: Biology, Becomings, and Life in the Lab*. Feminist Technosciences. Seattle: University of Washington Press, 2018.

Roy, Rohan Deb. "Science Still Bears the Fingerprints of Colonialism." *Smithsonian Magazine*, April 9, 2018. https://www.smithsonianmag.com.

Rusert, Britt. *Fugitive Science: Empiricism and Freedom in Early African American Culture*. New York: New York University Press, 2017.

Russell, William M. S., and Rex L. Burch. *The Principles of Humane Experimental Technique*. 1959. Accessed June 5, 2022. http://caat.jhsph.edu.

Russett, Cynthia E. *Sexual Science: The Victorian Construction of Womanhood*. Cambridge, MA: Harvard University Press, 1995.

Ryerson, Kelly. "A Blended Bifurcation." *Glyphosate Girl* (blog), January 29, 2019. https://glyphosategirl.com.

Sahlins, Marshall. *The Use and Abuse of Biology: An Anthropological Critique of Sociobiology*. Ann Arbor, MI: University of Michigan Press, 1977.

Schiebinger, Londa, ed. *Colonial Botany: Science, Commerce, and Politics in the Early Modern World*. Philadelphia: University of Pennsylvania Press, 2007.

———. "Feminist History of Colonial Science." *Hypatia* 19, no. 1 (2004): 233–54.

———. *Nature's Body: Gender in the Making of Modern Science*. New Brunswick, NJ: Rutgers University Press, 2004.

Schor, Juliet. *The Overworked American: The Unexpected Decline of Leisure*. New York: Basic Books, 1991.

Schroer, Sara Asu, Thom van Dooren, Ursula Münster, and Hugo Reinert. "Introduction: Multispecies Care in the Sixth Extinction." *Society for Cultural Anthropology*, January 26, 2021. https://culanth.org.

Schubert, Charlotte. "US Pushes Limits on Ozone Destroyer." *Nature*, December 2, 2005. https://doi.org/10.1038/news051128-13.

Schuller, Kyla. *The Biopolitics of Feeling: Race, Sex, and Science in the Nineteenth Century*. Anima. Durham, NC: Duke University Press, 2017.

Scott, Dayna Nadine, ed. *Our Chemical Selves: Gender, Toxics, and Environmental Health*. Vancouver, Canada: University of British Columbia Press, 2015.

Scott, Dayna Nadine, Jennie Haw, and Robyn Lee. "'Wannabe Toxic-Free?' From Precautionary Consumption to Corporeal Citizenship." *Environmental Politics* 26, no. 2 (2017): 322–42. https://doi.org/10.1080/09644016.2016.1232523.

Scott, Joan W. "Gender: A Useful Category of Historical Analysis." *American Historical Review* 91, no. 5 (December 1986): 1053–75. https://doi.org/10.2307/1864376.

———. "The Evidence of Experience." *Critical Inquiry* 17, no. 4 (1991): 773–97.

SeaChange. "SeaChange." Accessed May 22, 2024. https://seachangeventures.com.

Seiler, Cotten. "The Origins of White Care." *Social Text* 38, no. 1 (142) (March 1, 2020): 17–38. https://doi.org/10.1215/01642472-7971079.

Sellers, Christopher C. *Hazards of the Job: From Industrial Disease to Environmental Health Science*. Chapel Hill: University of North Carolina Press, 1997.

Seymour, Nicole. *Strange Natures: Futurity, Empathy, and the Queer Ecological Imagination*. Urbana: University of Illinois Press, 2013.

Shabazz, Khalilah Annette. "Black Women, White Campus: Students Living through Invisibility." PhD diss., Indiana University, 2015.

Shadaan, Reena, and Michelle Murphy. "EDCs as Industrial Chemicals and Settler Colonial Structures: Towards a Decolonial Feminist Approach." *Catalyst: Feminism, Theory, Technoscience* 6, no. 1 (2020). https://doi.org/10.28968/cftt.v6i1.32089.

Shakespeare, William. *The Tempest*. Edited by Burton Raffel. With contributions from Harold Bloom. New Haven, CT: Yale University Press, 2006.

Shapiro, Nicholas. "Attuning to the Chemosphere: Domestic Formaldehyde, Bodily Reasoning, and the Chemical Sublime." *Cultural Anthropology* 30, no. 3 (2015): 368–93. https://doi.org/10.14506/ca30.3.02.

Shapiro, Nicholas, Nasser Zakariya, and Jody Roberts. "A Wary Alliance: From Enumerating the Environment to Inviting Apprehension." *Engaging Science, Technology, and Society* 3, no. 0 (2017): 575–602. https://doi.org/10.17351/ests2017.133.

Shattuck, Annie. "Risky Subjects: Embodiment and Partial Knowledges in the Safe Use of Pesticide." *Geoforum*, May 7, 2019. https://doi.org/10.1016/j.geoforum.2019.04.029.

Shostak, Sara. "Environmental Justice and Genomics: Acting on the Futures of Environmental Health." *Science as Culture* 13, no. 4 (2004): 539–62. https://doi.org/10.1080/0950543042000311850.

———. *Exposed Science: Genes, the Environment, and the Politics of Population Health.* Berkeley: University of California Press, 2013.

Shotwell, Alexis. *Against Purity: Living Ethically in Compromised Times.* Minneapolis: University of Minnesota Press, 2016.

Siegel, Seth M. "Troubled Water: Estrogen and Its Doppelgängers." *Environmental Health News*, October 28, 2019. https://www.ehn.org.

Sigerist, Henry E., ed. *Four Treatises of Theophrastus von Hohenheim, Called Paracelsus.* Translated by Clarice Lilian Temkin, George Rosen, and Gregory Zilboory. Baltimore: Johns Hopkins University Press, 1996.

SisterSong. "Reproductive Justice." Women of Color Reproductive Justice Collective, accessed July 16, 2019. https://www.sistersong.net.

Smith, Linda Tuhiwai. *Decolonizing Methodologies: Research and Indigenous Peoples.* Dunedin, New Zealand: University of Otago Press, 1999.

Solnit, Rebecca. *Men Explain Things to Me.* Chicago: Haymarket Books, 2014.

Somerville, Siobhan. "Scientific Racism and the Emergence of the Homosexual Body." *Journal of the History of Sexuality* 5, no. 2 (1994): 243–66.

Sosnoskie, Lynn M. "The Biology of Field Bindweed." *Notes In the Margins: Agronomy and Weed Science Musings* (blog), August 29, 2018. https://ucanr.edu.

Spade, Dean. "Solidarity Not Charity: Mutual Aid for Mobilization and Survival." *Social Text* 38, no. 1 (142) (March 1, 2020): 131–51. https://doi.org/10.1215/01642472-7971139.

Spanier, Bonnie. *Im/Partial Science: Gender Ideology in Molecular Biology.* Race, Gender, and Science. Bloomington: Indiana University Press, 1995.

Spivak, Gayatri. "Can the Subaltern Speak?" In *Marxism and the Interpretation of Culture,* edited by Cary Nelson and Larry Grossberg, 271–313. Urbana: University of Illinois Press, 1988.

Stein, Rachel, ed. *New Perspectives on Environmental Justice: Gender, Sexuality, and Activism.* New Brunswick: Rutgers University Press, 2004.

Steingraber, Sandra. *Living Downstream: An Ecologist's Personal Investigation of Cancer and the Environment.* 2nd ed. Cambridge, MA: Da Capo Press, 2010.

Stern, Alexandra Minna. *Eugenic Nation: Faults and Frontiers of Better Breeding in Modern America*. 2nd ed. Berkeley: University of California Press, 2015.

Stevens, Pippa. "Exxon Mobil's First-Quarter Profit Rises, Even after $3.4 Billion Hit from Russia Charge." *CNBC*, April 29, 2022. https://www.cnbc.com.

Stoler, Ann Laura. *Carnal Knowledge and Imperial Power: Race and the Intimate in Colonial Rule*. Berkeley: University of California Press, 2002.

Subramaniam, Banu. *Ghost Stories for Darwin: The Science of Variation and the Politics of Diversity*. Urbana: University of Illinois Press, 2014.

———. "Snow Brown and the Seven Detergents: A Metanarrative on Science and the Scientific Method." *Women's Studies Quarterly* 28, no. 1/2 (2000): 296–304.

———. "The Aliens Have Landed! Reflections on the Rhetoric of Biological Invasions." *Meridians* 2, no. 1 (2001): 26–40.

Swan, Shanna H., and Stacey Colino. *Count Down: How Our Modern World Is Threatening Sperm Counts, Altering Male and Female Reproductive Development, and Imperiling the Future of the Human Race*. New York: Simon & Schuster, 2021.

Sweet, Paige L. "The Sociology of Gaslighting." *American Sociological Review* 84, no. 5 (October 2019): 851–75. https://doi.org/10.1177/0003122419874843.

Sze, Julie. "Boundaries and Border Wars: DES, Technology, and Environmental Justice." *American Quarterly* 58, no. 3 (September 2006): 791–814. https://doi.org/10.1353/aq.2006.0070.

Székács, András, and Béla Darvas. "Forty Years with Glyphosate." In *Herbicides—Properties, Synthesis and Control of Weeds*, edited by Mohammed Naguib Abd El-Ghany Hasaneen, 247–84. Croatia: InTech, 2012. https://www.intechopen.com/chapters/25624.

TallBear, Kimberly. *Native American DNA: Tribal Belonging and the False Promise of Genetic Science*. Minneapolis: University of Minnesota Press, 2013.

Tarjem, Ida. "Feminist Crops: A More-than-Human Concept for Advancing Feminist Crop Breeding for Development." *Catalyst: Feminism, Theory, Technoscience* 8, no. 2 (Fall 2022). https://doi.org/10.28968/cftt.v8i2.37243.

Taylor, Charles. *Sources of the Self: The Making of the Modern Identity*. Cambridge, MA: Harvard University Press, 1989.

Taylor, Dorceta E. *The Rise of the American Conservation Movement: Power, Privilege, and Environmental Protection*. Durham, NC: Duke University Press, 2016.

———. "The Rise of the Environmental Justice Paradigm: Injustice Framing and the Social Construction of Environmental Discourses." *American Behavioral Scientist* 43, no. 4 (January 2000): 508–80. https://doi.org/10.1177/0002764200043004003.

———. *Toxic Communities: Environmental Racism, Industrial Pollution, and Residential Mobility*. New York: New York University Press, 2014.

Taylor, Sunaura. *Beasts of Burden: Animal and Disability Liberation*. New York: New Press, 2017.

Temkin, Clarice Lilian. "Seven Defensiones, the Reply to Certain Calumniations of His Enemies." In *Four Treatises of Theophrastus von Hohenheim, Called Paracelsus*, 1–42. Baltimore, MD: The Classics of Medicine Library, 1988.

Terry, Jennifer. "'Unnatural Acts' in Nature: The Scientific Fascination with Queer Animals." *GLQ: A Journal of Lesbian and Gay Studies* 6, no. 2 (April 2000): 151–93.

Thayer, Zaneta M., and Christopher W. Kuzawa. "Biological Memories of Past Environments: Epigenetic Pathways to Health Disparities." *Epigenetics* 6, no. 7 (July 2011): 798–803. https://doi.org/10.4161/epi.6.7.16222.

Thomas, John A. "Toxic Responses of the Reproductive System." In *Casarett & Doull's Toxicology: The Basic Science of Poisons*, edited by Curtis D. Klaassen, 5th ed., 547–82. New York: McGraw Hill, Health Professions Division, 1996.

Thompson, Charis. "Critique in the Era of Trump." *Center for Race and Gender: News* (blog), August 1, 2017. http://crg.berkeley.edu.

———. *Good Science: The Ethical Choreography of Stem Cell Research*. Inside Technology. Cambridge, MA: MIT Press, 2013.

Tilley, Helen. *Africa as a Living Laboratory: Empire, Development, and the Problem of Scientific Knowledge, 1870–1950*. Chicago: University of Chicago Press, 2011.

Tironi, Manuel. "Hypo-Interventions: Intimate Activism in Toxic Environments." *Social Studies of Science* 48, no. 3 (June 2018): 438–55. https://doi.org/10.1177/0306312718784779.

Tollefson, Jeff. "Scientists Concerned over US Environment Agency's Plan to Limit Animal Research." *Nature*, September 10, 2019. https://doi.org/10.1038/d41586-019-02715-0.

Tonn, Jenna. "The Evolutionary Brotherhood: Manliness and Experimental Zoology in Nineteenth-Century America." YouTube video from the Science History Institute, 00:48:58, February 24, 2021. https://www.youtube.com/watch?v=LNRbsAHhBBY.

Totenberg, Nina. "The Supreme Court Has Narrowed the Scope of the Clean Water Act." *NPR*, May 25, 2023, sec. Law. https://www.npr.org.

Trasande, Leonardo. *Sicker, Fatter, Poorer: The Urgent Threat of Hormone-Disrupting Chemicals on Our Health and Future . . . and What We Can Do about It*. Boston: Houghton Mifflin Harcourt, 2019.

Tu, Thuy Linh N. *Experiments in Skin: Race and Beauty in the Shadows of Vietnam*. Durham, NC: Duke University Press, 2021.

Tuck, Eve. "Suspending Damage: A Letter to Communities." *Harvard Educational Review* 79, no. 3 (2009): 409–27.

Tuck, Eve, and K. Wayne Yang. "R-Words: Refusing Research." In *Humanizing Research: Decolonizing Qualitative Inquiry with Youth and Communities*, edited by Django Paris and Maisha T. Winn, 223–47. Thousand Oaks, CA: SAGE, 2014.

Tullo, Alexander H. "DowDuPont Names Its Three Planned Spin-Offs." *Chemical & Engineering News*, February 26, 2018. https://cen.acs.org.

Twombly, R. "Assault on the Male." *Environmental Health Perspectives* 103, no. 9 (September 1995): 802–5. https://doi.org/10.1289/ehp.95103802.

United Church of Christ and Commission for Racial Justice. *Toxic Wastes and Race in the United States: A National Report on the Racial and Socio-Economic*

Characteristics of Communities with Hazardous Waste Sites. New York: United Church of Christ, 1987.

United States Environmental Protection Agency. "Chemical Production Data." Chemical Data Reporting, September 20, 2022. https://www.epa.gov.

University of California Academic Senate. *University of California: In Memoriam, 1990*. University of California History Digital Archives. Berkely: University of California Regents, 1990. http://texts.cdlib.org.

Vandenberg, Laura N., Theo Colborn, Tyrone B. Hayes, Jerrold J. Heindel, David R. Jacobs, Duk-Hee Lee, Toshi Shioda, et al. "Hormones and Endocrine-Disrupting Chemicals: Low-Dose Effects and Nonmonotonic Dose Responses." *Endocrine Reviews* 33, no. 3 (June 1, 2012): 378–455. https://doi.org/10.1210/er.2011-1050.

Velocci, Beans. "The Battle Over Trans Rights Is About Power, Not Science." *Washington Post*, October 29, 2018, sec. Perspective. https://www.washingtonpost.com.

———. *Binary Logic: The Power of Incoherence in American Sex Science*. Durham, NC: Duke University Press, forthcoming.

Viloria, Hida, and Maria Nieto. *The Spectrum of Sex: The Science of Male, Female, and Intersex*. Vancouver: University of British Columbia Press, 2020.

Visvanathan, Shiv. "From the Annals of the Laboratory State." *Alternatives* 12, no. 1 (January 1987): 37–59. https://doi.org/10.1177/030437548701200102.

Vogel, Sarah A. "From 'The Dose Makes the Poison' to 'The Timing Makes the Poison': Conceptualizing Risk in the Synthetic Age." *Environmental History* 13, no. 4 (2008): 667–73.

Voyles, Traci Brynne. "Toxic Masculinity: California's Salton Sea and the Environmental Consequences of Manliness." *Environmental History* 26, no. 1 (January 2021): 127–41. https://doi.org/10.1093/envhis/emaa076.

———. *Wastelanding: Legacies of Uranium Mining in Navajo Country*. Minneapolis: University of Minnesota Press, 2015.

Walker, Richard. *The Conquest of Bread: 150 Years of Agribusiness in California*. New York: New Press, 2004.

Ward, Jane. "Dyke Methods: A Meditation on Queer Studies and the Gay Men Who Hate It." *WSQ: Women's Studies Quarterly* 44, no. 3/4 (Fall/Winter 2016): 68–85. https://doi.org/10.1353/wsq.2016.0036.

———. *The Tragedy of Heterosexuality*. Sexual Cultures. New York: New York University Press, 2020.

Washington, Harriet A. *Medical Apartheid: The Dark History of Medical Experimentation on Black Americans from Colonial Times to the Present*. New York: Doubleday, 2006.

Weasel, Lisa H. "Embodying Intersectionality: The Promise (and Peril) of Epigenetics for Feminist Science Studies." In *Mattering: Feminism, Science, and Materialism*, edited by Victoria Pitts-Taylor, 104–21. New York: New York University Press, 2016.

Webster, Charles. *Paracelsus: Medicine, Magic and Mission at the End of Time*. New Haven, CT: Yale University Press, 2008.

Weheliye, Alexander G. *Habeas Viscus: Racializing Assemblages, Biopolitics, and Black Feminist Theories of the Human*. Durham, NC: Duke University Press, 2014.

Wehle, Robert G. *Snakefoot: The Making of a Champion*. Henderson, NY: Country Press, 1996.

Weir, Lorna. *Pregnancy, Risk, and Biopolitics: On the Threshold of the Living Subject*. Abingdon, UK: Routledge, 2006.

Welsome, Eileen. *The Plutonium Files: America's Secret Medical Experiments in the Cold War*. New York: Dial Press, 1999.

Wexler, Philip, and Antoinette N. Hayes. "The Evolving Journey of Toxicology: An Historical Glimpse." In *Casarett & Doull's Toxicology: The Basic Science of Poisons*, edited by Curtis D. Klaassen, 9th ed., 3–23. New York: McGraw Hill Education, 2019.

White, Paul S. "The Experimental Animal in Victorian Britain." In *Thinking with Animals: New Perspectives on Anthropomorphism*, edited by Lorraine Daston and Gregg Mitman, 59–82. New York: Columbia University Press, 2005.

Wiebe, Sarah Marie. *Everyday Exposure: Indigenous Mobilization and Environmental Justice in Canada's Chemical Valley*. Vancouver, Canada: University of British Columbia Press, 2016.

Wiesinger, Helene, Zhanyun Wang, and Stefanie Hellweg. "Deep Dive into Plastic Monomers, Additives, and Processing Aids." *Environmental Science & Technology* 55, no. 13 (2021): 9339–51. https://doi.org/10.1021/acs.est.1c00976.

Williams, Brian. "'That We May Live': Pesticides, Plantations, and Environmental Racism in the United States South." *Environment and Planning E: Nature and Space* 1, no. 1–2 (March–June 2018): 243–67. https://doi.org/10.1177/2514848618778085.

Winerip, Michael. "The Death and Afterlife of Thalidomide." *New York Times*, September 23, 2013. https://www.nytimes.com.

Wohlforth, Charles. "Conservation and Eugenics." *Orion Magazine* (July/August) 2010. https://orionmagazine.org.

Wynter, Sylvia. "Unsettling the Coloniality of Being/Power/Truth/Freedom: Towards the Human, after Man, Its Overrepresentation—An Argument." *CR: The New Centennial Review* 3, no. 3 (2003): 257–337.

Wynter, Sylvia, and Katherine McKittrick. "Unparalleled Catastrophe for Our Species? Or, to Give Humanness a Different Future: Conversations." In *Sylvia Wynter: On Being Human as Praxis*, edited by Katherine McKittrick, 9–89. Durham, NC: Duke University Press, 2015.

Yarbrough, Anastasia. "Species, Race, and Culture in the Space of Wildlife Management." In *Critical Animal Geographies*, edited by Kathryn Gillespie and Rosemary-Claire Collard, 108–26. London: Routledge, 2015. https://doi.org/10.4324/9781315762760-9.

Yoon, Carol Kaesuk. *Naming Nature: The Clash between Instinct and Science*. New York: W. W. Norton, 2009.

Zimdahl, Robert L. *A History of Weed Science in the United States*. Elsevier Insights. London: Elsevier, 2010.

Zimring, Carl A. *Clean and White: A History of Environmental Racism in the United States*. New York: New York University Press, 2015.

Zota, Ami R., and Bhavna Shamasunder. "The Environmental Injustice of Beauty: Framing Chemical Exposures from Beauty Products as a Health Disparities Concern." *American Journal of Obstetrics and Gynecology* 217, no. 4 (October 2017): 418–22. https://doi.org/10.1016/j.ajog.2017.07.020.

INDEX

Page numbers in italics indicate Figures and Tables

Weed Science Societies (WSS), 117; presidential addresses, 111–12; weed contests of, 122, 129–32

weed scientists, 108; on dose-response, 70; hypermasculinity of, 16, 95–97, 127; on pesticides, 133; visual assessments of, 100, *101*; on weed science masculinism and militarism, 97–98; women, 120, 121; Zimdahl on, 122, 132–33

Weheliye, Alexander, 209

Welsome, Eileen, 34–35

Wengrow, David, 268n30

Western Liberal Man Master Subject, 209

Wexler, Philip, 48–49, 90–91

What a Fish Knows (Balcombe), 187

When Species Meet (Haraway), 191–92

White, Paul S., 199

white empiricism, 55, 66

white epistemic entitlement, 115

white man's burden, 133

white supremacism: of EDC toxicology, 10, 13; of primitive masculinity, 127; of toxicology, 106; wilderness intertwined with, 15

WHO. *See* World Health Organization

Wiebe, Sarah, 12

wilderness, white supremacism and masculinism intertwined with, 15

William S. Merrell Company, 42

women, 111, 251n18; care work of, 138, 268n29; Casarett, Louis J., on, 14, 84, 107–8, 109; distaff set, 14, 84, 108, 109, 239n72; in ecotoxicology lab, 260n95; nonwhite, 67; poisoners, 61, 105, 107, 110; toxicant masculinity of, 115–16; toxic exposure impacting, 105, 138, 256n16; weed scientists, 120, 121; in workforce, 11

women, Black: identity intersectionality of, 11; physicists, 66

women of color, 104, 247n41

workday, women and men impacted by, 11

World Health Organization (WHO), 79, 82, 104

World War II, toxicants from, 22

WSS. *See* Weed Science Societies

xenophobia, of US agriculture, 254n70

Yang, K. Wayne, 232

Zimdahl, Robert L.: on weed science, 98, 102, 103, 108–9, 111–12, 253n59; on weed scientists, 122, 132–33

ABOUT THE AUTHOR

MELINA PACKER is Assistant Professor of Race, Gender, and Sexuality Studies at the University of Wisconsin–La Crosse, on Ho-Chunk Nation land, where she teaches courses on queer feminist science studies and antiracist animal studies. She is co-author, with Ambika Kamath, of *Feminism in the Wild: How Human Biases Shape Our Understanding of Animal Behavior.*

Printed in the United States
by Baker & Taylor Publisher Services